AF446848

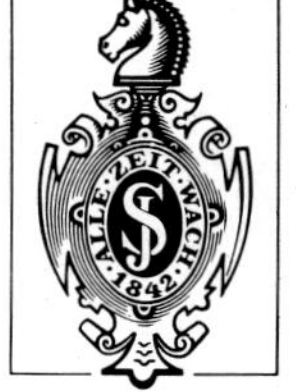

J.S. Smolen   J.R. Kalden
R.N. Maini   (Eds.)

Rheumatoid Arthritis

Recent Research Advances

With 53 Figures and 58 Tables

Springer-Verlag
Berlin Heidelberg New York
London Paris Tokyo
Hong Kong Barcelona
Budapest

Professor Dr. Josef S. Smolen
2. Medizinische Abteilung
Zentrum für Diagnostik und Therapie
rheumatischer Erkrankungen
Krankenhaus der Stadt Wien-Lainz
und Ludwig Boltzmann Institut
für Rheumatologie und Balneologie
Wolkersbergenstraße 1, A-1130 Wien, Austria

Professor Dr. Joachim R. Kalden
Medizinische Klinik III mit Poliklinik
und Institut für Klinische Immunologie
und Rheumatologie
Friedrich-Alexander-Universität Erlangen-Nürnberg
Krankenhausstraße 12, W-8520 Erlangen
Federal Republic of Germany

Professor Dr. Ravinder N. Maini
Mathilda and Terence Kennedy Institute
of Rheumatology
6 Bute Gardens, Hammersmith
London W6 7DW, United Kingdom

ISBN 3-540-53315-X Springer-Verlag Berlin Heidelberg New York
ISBN 0-387-53315-X Springer-Verlag New York Berlin Heidelberg

Library of Congress Cataloging-in-Publication Data
Rheumatoid arthritis : recent research advances / J. S. Smolen, J. R. Kalden, R. N. Maini (eds.).
p.   cm.   Includes bibliographical references and index.
ISBN 3-540-53315-X (alk. paper). --
ISBN 0-387-53315-X (alk. paper)
1. Rheumatoid arthritis. I. Smolen, Josef S., 1950–   . II. Kalden, J. R. (Joachim Robert)
III. Maini, R. N. [DNLM: 1. Arthritis, Rheumatoid.   WE 346 R47307]   RC933.R4288   1992
616.7'227--dc20   DLC for Library of Congress   91-5068   CIP

Typesetting: Elsner & Behrens GmbH, D-6836 Oftersheim
27/3145-5 4 3 2 1 0 – Printed on acid-free paper

To our families

Preface

Clinical medicine first recognized rheumatoid arthritis (RA) as a disease entity in the nineteenth century. In the early days the major development in understanding this disease came at the bedside, in distinguishing it from rheumatic fever and gout. Later, with the advances in medicine and the powerful ideas emanating from the fast-growing fields of pathology and microbiology, interest turned to the description of its morbid anatomy and the quest for an infectious etiology. The development of immunology and biochemistry made an impact too, and hypotheses tracing RA to infection, fibrinoid degeneration of collagen, and eventually autoimmunity had their proponents by the middle of this century.

RA was meanwhile being split up into further nosological entities as a result of developments emerging on at least two fronts: first, with the discovery of IgM rheumatoid factor, seropositive and seronegative disease were differentiated; second, on clinicopathological grounds, adherents of rheumatoid spondylitis were conceded the existence of ankylosing spondylitis, a movement which eventually led to the concept of spondyloarthropathies. The heterogeneity of RA was further emphasized more recently with the description of "marker" autoantibodies and associated with the chronic polyarthritis of conditions such as systemic lupus erythematosus (SLE), primary Sjögren's syndrome, overlap, and mixed connective tissue disease, usefully distinguished from RA.

These introductory comments provide a background to our interest in promoting this book. Having recognized the influence of scientific thought and technology on clinical research in arthritis and the central importance of clinical observation in posing questions and guiding enquiry, it seemed appropriate to ask whether the time was ripe to attempt to take stock of progress in the field. Recent information presented by leading researchers at meetings and in journals convinced us that this was indeed the case and that there were exciting new prospects for progress. The generosity of the individuals we approached, in agreeing to write for this book, will, we hope, bear testimony to there being grounds for our optimism.

The book begins with a challenging chapter by an epidemiologist on the incidence and prevalence of RA. Considerable interest surrounds the question whether RA is a new disease and whether, as has been claimed, it is already beginning to disappear. To a large extent such issues depend on definitions and ascertainment. However, there is little doubt now that there are geographic variations in disease expression. The part that genes play in this process can now be addressed to a degree, and the two succeeding chapters examine this by reviewing molecular research and taking a fresh look at RA in the southeastern region of Europe.

The next section deals with aspects of progress in cellular and immunological fields which have contributed to our understanding of the pathogenesis of RA. The role that cytokines and surface molecules play in regulating cellular function and interactions has been in the forefront of progress recently and is covered here. This inevitably leads to contributions on T and B cells, endothelial cells and dendritic cells, polymorphs, and finally regulation and expression of MHC class II antigens and the V genes involved in rheumatoid factors.

In the next section, we have selected contributions that highlight the possible role of environmental factors – principally infectious agents – and of autoimmunity in initiating and perpetuating RA. This includes most current candidates, namely, heat shock proteins, mycobacterial antigens, collagen, streptococcal antigens, retroviruses, and Epstein-Barr virus. Autoantibodies observed in RA, including antiperinuclear factor and antikeratin antibodies, are reevaluated, and new findings on anti-RA 33 are presented. Discussion of the acute phase response, amyloid, and markers of cartilage destruction provides necessary vignettes to mark progress in the field.

In the final section, therapeutic initiatives are dealt with in two chapters. Although modern drugs, monoclonal antibodies, and T cell vaccination are covered, the information is most likely to prove to be outdated in the near future as a result of intense activity in this area.

Progress in research is not an orderly affair, and our initial approach in getting the contents of this book together was to make a list of areas that we felt were witnessing advances. It is a sign of the times that even though we did this relatively recently, it is likely that other fields will have opened up which are not covered. However, by inviting some of the key figures in research we expected to gain from their perceptions and knowledge and thereby secure maximum coverage of the cutting edge in research. We trust that the result will justify our hopes and that the contents, individually or as a whole, will coalesce into a worthwhile statement of the state of the art. If it inspires new ideas or a debate, so much the better. It is quite likely that we have failed to be comprehensive, but for this we do not apologize, since our wish was not to publish a reference volume but to put together an enjoyable and readable book.

Wien, Erlangen, and London, May 1992

J. S. Smolen
J. R. Kalden
R. N. Maini

Contents

Etiologic Factors –
Bacterial Antigens, Autoantigens, Viruses

Autoantibodies and Markers of Disease Activity

Therapy

List of Contributors

Aicher, W. K.
Division of Clinical Immunology and Rheumatology,
Department of Medicine, University of Alabama at Birmingham,
Birmingham, AL 35294, USA

Alsalameh, S.
Institute of Clinical Immunology and Rheumatology,
Department of Medicine III, University of Erlangen-Nürnberg,
Krankenhausstrasse 12, W-8520 Erlangen, FRG

Barnum, S. R.
Division of Clinical Immunology and Rheumatology,
Department of Medicine, University of Alabama at Birmingham,
Birmingham, AL 35294, USA

Boog, C. J. P.
Department of Infectious Diseases and Immunology,
Veterinary Faculty, University of Utrecht, P.O. Box 80.165,
3508 TD Utrecht, The Netherlands

Breedveld, F. C.
Department of Rheumatology, University Hospital Leiden,
P.O. Box, 9600 RC Leiden, The Netherlands

Brennan, F. M.
Charing Cross Sunley Research Centre, Lurgan Avenue,
Hammersmith, London W6 8LW, UK

Burmester, G. R.
Institute of Clinical Immunology and Rheumatology,
Department of Medicine III, University of Erlangen-Nürnberg,
Krankenhausstrasse 12, W-8520 Erlangen, FRG

Crofford, L. J.
Arthritis and Rheumatism Branch, National Institute of Arthritis
and Musculoskeletal and Skin Diseases, National Institutes of
Health, Building 10, Room 9N240, Bethesda, MD 20892, USA

Dumay, A.
Laboratory of Immunology and Clinic of Rheumatology,
Brest University Medical School Hospital, BP 824,
29285 Brest Cédex, France

van Eden, W.
Department of Infectious Diseases and Immunology,
Veterinary Faculty, University of Utrecht, P.O. Box 80.165,
3508 TD Utrecht, The Netherlands

van Embden, J. D. A.
Department of Bacteriology, National Institute of Public Health
and Environmental Hygiene, P.O. Box 1, 3720 BA Bilthoven,
The Netherlands

Feldmann, M.
Charing Cross Sunley Research Centre, Lurgan Avenue,
Hammersmith, London W6 8LW, UK

Field, M.
Kennedy Institute of Rheumatology, 6 Bute Gardens,
Hammersmith, London W6 7DM, UK

Førre, Ø.
Oslo Sanitetsforenings Rheumatism Hospital, Akersbakken 27,
0172 Oslo 1, Norway

Gay, R. E.
Division of Clinical Immunology and Rheumatology,
Department of Medicine, University of Alabama at Birmingham,
Birmingham, AL 35294, USA

Gay, S.
Division of Clinical Immunology and Rheumatology,
Department of Medicine, University of Alabama at Birmingham,
Birmingham, AL 35294, USA

Graninger, W.
Second Department of Medicine, University of Vienna,
Garnisongasse 13, 1090 Vienna, Austria

Hassfeld, W.
Second Department of Medicine, Center for Rheumatic Diseases,
Lainz Hospital, Wolkersbergenstrasse 1, 1130 Vienna, Austria

Hoet, R. M.
Department of Biochemistry, University of Nijmegen,
P.O. Box 9101, 6500 HB Nijmegen, The Netherlands

Hogervorst, E. J. M.
Department of Infectious Diseases and Immunology,
Veterinary Faculty, University of Utrecht, P.O. Box 80.165,
3508 TD Utrecht, The Netherlands

Holmdahl, R.
Department of Medical and Physiological Chemistry, Box 575,
Uppsala University, 75123 Uppsala, Sweden

Husby, G.
Department of Rheumatology, The University Hospital of Tromsø,
9000 Tromsø, Norway

Kalden, J. R.
Institute of Clinical Immunology and Rheumatology,
Department of Internal Medicine III,
Friedrich Alexander University Erlangen-Nürnberg,
Krankenhausstrasse 12, W-8530 Erlangen, FRG

Klareskog, L.
Department of Clinical Immunology, Uppsala University Hospital,
75185 Uppsala, Sweden

Krapf, E. F.
Institute of Clinical Immunology and Rheumatology,
Department of Internal Medicine III,
Friedrich Alexander University Erlangen-Nürnberg,
Krankenhausstrasse 12, W-8530 Erlangen, FRG

Lamour, A.
Laboratory of Immunology and Clinic of Rheumatology,
Brest University Medical School Hospital, BP 824,
29285 Brest Cédex, France

Lanchbury, J. S. S.
Molecular Immunogenetics and Rheumatology Units,
Division of Medicine, United Medical and Dental Schools,
Guy's Hospital, London SE1 9RT, UK

Lazary, S.
Institute of Animal Husbandry, University of Berne,
Länggass-Strasse 122, 3012 Berne, Switzerland

Le Goff, P.
Laboratory of Immunology and Clinic of Rheumatology,
Brest University Medical School Hospital, BP 824,
29285 Brest Cédex, France

Lotz, M.
Department of Medicine, University of California, San Diego,
La Jolla, CA 92093, USA

Maini, R. N.
Kennedy Institute of Rheumatology, 6 Bute Gardens,
Hammersmith, London W6 7DW, UK

Mollenhauer, J.
Institute of Pharmacology and Toxicology,
University of Erlangen-Nürnberg, Krankenhausstrasse 12,
W-8520 Erlangen, FRG

Moutsoupoulos, H. M.
Department of Internal Medicine, School of Medicine,
University of Ioannina, Greece

Natvig, J. B.
Institute of Immunology and Rheumatology,
The National Hospital, Oslo, Norway

Panayi, G.
Molecular Immunogenetics and Rheumatology Units, UMDS,
Guy's Hospital, London SE1 9RT, UK

Peterhans, E.
Institute of Veterinary Virology, University of Berne,
Länggass-Strasse 122, 3012 Berne, Switzerland

Plater-Zyberk, C.
Kennedy Institute of Rheumatology, 6 Bute Gardens,
Hammersmith, London W6 7DW, UK

Pohl, B.
Institute of Veterinary Virology, University of Berne,
Länggass-Strasse 122, 3012 Berne, Switzerland

Randen, I.
MRC Centre, Molecular Immunopathology Unit, Cambridge, UK

Roudier, J.
Université d'Aix Marseille, 13385 Marseille Cedex 5, France

Sakkas, L. I.
Molecular Immunogenetics and Rheumatology Units, UMDS,
Guy's Hospital, London SE1 9RT, UK

Saxne, T.
Department of Rheumatology and Department of Physiological
Chemistry, University of Lund, Lund, Sweden

Silman, A. J.
Arthritis and Rheumatism Council Epidemiology Research Unit,
Manchester University Medical School, Manchester, UK

Smolen, J. S.
2nd Department of Medicine and Ludwig Boltzmann Institute
for Rheumatology, Krankenhaus der Stadt Wien-Lainz,
Wolkersbergenstrasse 1, 1130 Wien, Austria

Steiner, G.
Ludwig Boltzmann Institute for Rheumatology and Balneology,
c/o 2nd Dept. of Medicine, Lainz Hospital,
Wolkersbergenstrasse 1, 1130 Vienna, Austria

Stransky, G.
Division of Clinical Immunology and Rheumatology,
Department of Medicine, University of Alabama at Birmingham,
Birmingham, AL 35294, USA

Thompson, K.
Department of Immunology, Institute of Animal Physiology and
Genetics Research, Cambridge, UK

Trabandt, A.
Division of Clinical Immunology and Rheumatology,
Department of Medicine, University of Alabama at Birmingham,
Birmingham, AL 35294, USA

Venables, P. J. W.
Division of Clinical Immunology, Kennedy Institute,
London W6 7DW, UK

van Venrooij, W. J.
Department of Biochemistry, University of Nijmegen, P.O. Box 9101,
6500 HB Nijmegen, The Netherlands

Vlachoyiannopoulos, P. G.
Department of Internal Medicine, School of Medicine,
University of Ioannina, Greece

de Vries, R. R. P.
Department of Immunohematology, University Hospital,
2300 RC Leiden, The Netherlands

Waalen, K.
Department of Animal Genetics, Norwegian College of Veterinary
Medicine, Oslo, Norway

Wauben, M. H. M.
Department of Infectious Diseases and Immunology,
Veterinary Faculty, University of Utrecht, P.O. Box 80.165,
3508 TD Utrecht, The Netherlands

Wilder, T. L.
Arthritis and Rheumatism Branch, National Institute of Arthritis
and Musculoskeletal and Skin Diseases, National Institutes of
Health, Building 10, Room 9N240, Bethesda, MD 20892, USA

Wollheim, F. A.
Department of Rheumatology, Lund University Hospital,
Lund, Sweden

Youinou, P.
Laboratory of Immunology and Clinic of Rheumatology,
Brest University Medical School Hospital, BP 824,
29285 Brest Cédex, France

Zanoni, R.
Institute of Veterinary Virology, University of Berne,
Länggass-Strasse 122, 3012 Berne, Switzerland

van der Zee, R.
Department of Bacteriology, National Institute of Public Health
and Environmental Hygiene, P.O. Box 1, 3720 BA Bilthoven,
The Netherlands

Ziff, M.
The University of Texas Southwestern Medical Center, Dallas,
Texas, USA

Introduction

Is Rheumatoid Arthritis a Disappearing Disease?

A. J. Silman

Arthritis and Rheumatism Council Epidemiology Research Unit, Manchester University Medical School, Manchester, UK

Introduction

Rheumatoid arthritis (RA) is not a new disease and has been described in historical writings and portrayed in paintings probably for at least 1000 years. Compared to osteoarthritis, however, paleopathological evidence from skeletal remains of its early existence is difficult to obtain. It was hypothesized over 10 years ago [1] that RA, commonly agreed to be triggered by a virus, could behave like other major chronic infectious diseases, many of which showed large temporal swings in epidemicity. Further, following the example of other diseases, it was suggested that there was an epidemic of RA in the middle of this century and that it will ultimately disappear perhaps by the end of the next century. Such ideas have subsequently been fuelled by anecdotal reports, and it is of interest to evaluate the available data to support or refute the hypothesis that RA is either declining in incidence or severity and to consider possible explanations. If the hypothesis of a recent decline is true, then, in addition to its relevance to those planning health services, such a reduction might suggest new avenues of etiologic inquiry or provide insight into the effectiveness of current approaches to disease management.

Measuring Trends

The main method for examining trends in a disease is a comparison of incidence rates, i. e., the rate of new cases arising in a population over the time period of interest. There are two approaches to achieving this: The first is to survey the same population at many different points in time and to estimate the number of new cases occurring between those surveys. The problem with such an approach is that to ascertain change with any statistical precision, in a disease as relatively rare as RA, requires surveying a very large population (at least 20000), which is both expensive and difficult logistically. Further, individuals that develop RA and either die or fully recover between surveys will be missed by subsequent

Smolen, Kalden, Maini (Eds.)
Rheumatoid Arthritis
© Springer-Verlag Berlin Heidelberg 1992

surveys. The alternative and much cheaper approach is to constantly monitor prospectively the clinical facilities where patients with RA are likely to attend with a view to "capturing" all new cases. The major problem with this approach is that standardization of diagnosis is more difficult to achieve and completeness of notification by the attending physician wanes. One commonly adopted strategy is to retrospectively identify patients, who attended the target unit, by using (preferably) computerized diagnostic indices. There are two further difficulties with relying on physician attendance. First, patients with either mild RA and/or not who were referred will be missed. Second, particularly in urban areas, it may be difficult to enroll all possible physicians seeing patients from the target denominator population selected. Under-ascertainment is likely to occur as a result.

Period of Onset or Period of Birth

RA is a disease whose onset is difficult to define in time and indeed serological change, which might be etiologically more important, can antedate clinical presentation by many years [2]. Thus, trends in calendar year of presentation or diagnosis may not reflect true temporal patterns of disease. Further, if the presumed environmental exposure which triggers RA occurs early in life, it might be more appropriate to examine trends in disease in successive generations defined by their cohort of birth. An illustrative example of this is that most studies of the incidence of RA carried out over a short period of time demonstrate a marked increase in risk with increasing age [3]. Although this might represent a true age effect on incidence, an alternative explanation is that the oldest groups in that population were at highest risk based on their year of birth and that follow-up over a longer period would confirm that the succeeding generation to reach the oldest age-group would experience a fall in their age specific incidence rate.

Incidence of Severity

Trends in RA can be considered either in terms of disease incidence or of severity in those who develop the disease, although there is an inherent circularity in the distinction. Currently accepted diagnostic criteria include recognized indices of severity: positive rheumatoid factor and radiological erosions [4, 5]. Failure to satisfy the criteria might reflect absence of disease or a less severe form. Changes in severity could also reflect both the underlying aggressiveness of the disorder or changes in therapy, despite evidence from formal clinical trials that current therapeutic options offer little prognostically [6]. One problem in examining trends of severity is that such studies are frequently based on samples of patients attending specialized hospital units and could therefore reflect changes in patterns of referral or attendance.

Disease Definition

There is considerable difficulty in defining RA for epidemiological studies. Current criteria [5] were derived from those with long-standing disease and do not reflect many short-lived cases of inflammatory polyarthritis arising in the population. Over the recent decades many different criteria have been in use [4, 5, 7, 8]. Thus, comparison of different studies conducted at different times may not yield anything of use about change in incidence but rather might reflect differences in diagnostic assignment. As an example, the revised American Rheumatism Association (ARA) criteria are probably less sensitive at detecting what was previously described as "definite RA" at the gain of improved specificity [9].

Trends in Incidence

The earliest reliable data on the incidence of RA come from population samples studied in Leigh and Wensleydale, in the north of England, in the 1950s and 1960s [10]. In the first survey, in 1954–1959, those in the population surveyed found to have RA were asked to recall age at first symptoms. From these data an average annual incidence of approximately 2 per 1000 in adults over age 35 was found. Such data are, as the author of that survey pointed out, subject to error as they exclude those individuals who had either died or fully recovered from RA prior to the survey date. A follow-up survey was undertaken after 5 years in the 620 individuals who had participated in the initial survey. A total of 36 people, or 6% of the original population, who were initially free of arthritis, developed it in follow-up period. This is equivalent to an annual incidence of 12 per 1000, which probably seriously overestimates the true occurrence of the disease and reflects a case definition of low specificity. It is unlikely that the incidence increased sixfold between these surveys. These surveys were also too small (total populations around 2800) to obtain estimates with reasonable precision.

The examination of trends probably requires the continual monitoring of a population and access to contemporary medical records; the latter permitting retrospective correct diagnostic assignment. Such a system can only work if the monitoring system can detect all the affected individuals in a defined population. Such a system exists in the Rochester Epidemiology Program based at the Mayo Clinic. This institution, together with the Olmsted Medical Practice, provides the only source of medical care for the population of Olmsted County in Minnesota. Although retrospective examination of medical records will omit those who never seek medical attention for their symptoms and standardization of diagnosis is difficult, the utility of such a system in documenting trends in new cases is clear. Figure 1 shows the published results from 1950–1975 [3]; there was an increase in incidence in the first part of this

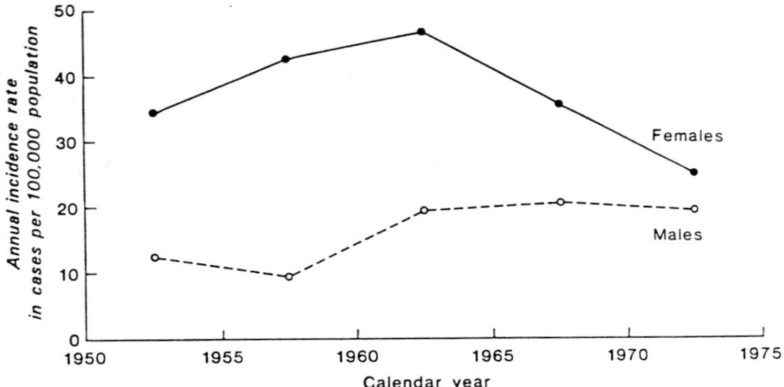

Fig. 1. Incidence rate of definite in Rochester Minnesota, 1950–74, age adjusted to 1960 US white population. (From [3])

25 year period and a marked subsequent decline in females but not in males. Although there have been considerable changes in diagnostic practice over the period, with increasing recognition of the need to separate out the HLA B27 related seronegative arthritis group of disorders, this is unlikely to explain the patterns observed. Specifically, such a diagnostic reassignment would have been expected to alter the trends in both sexes in the opposite manner, i. e., a greater decline in males. Possible reasons for the difference between the sexes will be considered further in this review. A recent study from Seattle [11], aiming to "capture" all incident cases in women in 1987 in a fixed population, yielded an annual incidence rate of 0.23 per 1000 women age 18–64, compared to a rate of 0.46 per 1000 in the same age group in the Rochester population; that is, the rate had halved. Whether such a comparison is valid given the different study approaches is difficult to assess, but the Seatlle study, being prospective, is perhaps more likely to have complete ascertainment. Thus, this source of bias is unlikely to explain the reduction.

Trends in the United Kingdom are difficult to obtain. There is a widespread opinion that the number of new RA patients referred to rheumatology specialists is declining. For example, at a major London teaching hospital, the number of new patient referrals showed a steady decline of around 50% over the period 1970–1980, although it could reflect changing referral patterns rather than a change in local incidence [12]. Probably the only direct source of date is from the Royal College of General Practitioners (RCGP) morbidity surveys. The first source of data is an ongoing survey of all patients attending 1 of 30 participating general practitioners. The latter send back to the central unit a "weekly return" of the number of attending patients with a new episode, as defined by a list of specific diagnoses which include RA [13]. Data from this source were recently analyzed (Fig. 2) [14]. A statistically significant decline of approximately 7.5 per 100000 per year in new consultations for RA between 1976 and 1987, equivalent to a halving in the incidence rate was found. Although most of the participating doctors had remained the same during the

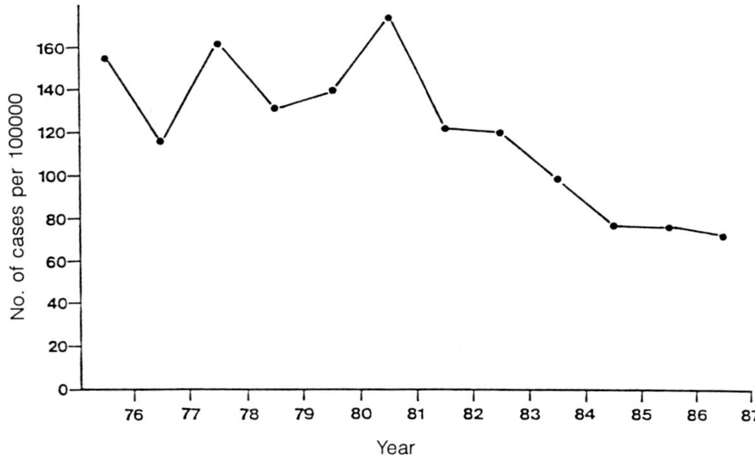

Fig. 2. Estimated annual incidence of RA in United Kingdom 1976–1987, based on first consultations to general practitioners. (Not adjusted for age or sex) (From [14])

Table 1. Incidence of first episodes of rheumatoid arthritis presenting to general practitioners

Age	Males		Females	
	1971	1981	1971	1981
15–24	0.5	0.4	0.6	0.6
25–44	1.1	0.9	2.3	1.8
45–64	2.2	2.4	6.4	5.6
65–74	3.0	2.4	8.2	5.7
>75	2.1	3.3	5.4	5.2

Source: Royal College of General Practitioners, national morbidity surveys

period of observation the possibility cannot be excluded that there was a decline in completeness of recording during this period. The other source of data from the RCGP come from ad hoc national morbidity surveys conducted by a much larger group of general practitioners who were required during the survey year to make a diagnosis based on every patient consultation. These surveys, in 1971–1972 [15] and 1981–82 [16], all relied on the recorded diagnosis from the general practitioner and diagnoses were not standardized. The results show (Table 1) that in the 10 years between the two surveys there was no significant decline in incidence in males; however in females there were declines in all but the youngest age-group with an overall incidence decline in adult females of around 20%.

Whole population data are also available from those countries which have population morbidity register for specific disorders. Interpretation of trends from such sources is difficult as in addition to the persistent problem of changes in registration completeness, there may be selective changes in the severity of cases recorded. Such registers are extensively available in Scandinavia and data from Finland [17] have recently been published. This source demonstrated an annual incidence of registered seropositive RA of 0.46 per 1000 in 1980 which was unchanged from that recorded in the early 1970s.

Birth Cohort Trends

Lawrence [10] was the first to point out the possibility that the risk of RA could be related to the period in which an individual was born. In a population study in Oberhorlen in the Federal Republic of Germany [18] in the 1960s there was a steep rise in the prevalence of existing cases in the sixth decade which was not reflected in the age curve of new developing cases. Lawrence postulated that this meant that those born in the last decade of the nineteenth century were at greater risk than those born in subsequent decades.

More interesting perhaps are the data from the Leigh and Wensleydale population surveys on the prevalence of rheumatoid factor positivity (using the SCAT test) in relation to period of birth [10]. In brief, the observations that: (a) in urban populations rheumatoid factor positivity increases with age in cross-sectional studies [19, 20], (b) in a 10 year follow-up period in an urban population there was a tendency for individuals to have a fall in titre and (c) in an analysis by year of birth the rate of positivity fell in successive cohorts from those born in 1885–1894, indicating perhaps that the latter group had a peculiarly high risk. One hypothesis [10] was that the reduction in titre in the older age-groups was consistent with an effect of improvement in atmospheric pollution resulting from the Clean Air Acts (1956).

Trends in Severity

There is a commonly accepted view that RA is declining in severity [21] and indeed a recent survey of Australian rheumatologists confirmed this view in a large group of observers [22]. Such a conclusion may, however, result from changes in referral patterns of primary care physicians and thus may not reflect the true status of RA in the community.

Mortality data can be used as a proxy for the combined effects of both incidence and patient survival. Thus a declining population mortality for RA would be consistent either with a decrease in incidence or a reduction in severity of diagnosed patients. The inherent problem is the frequent failure to mention RA on death certificates (the source of population mortality rates) and there are a number of studies confirming the high rate of under-recording of this disease as a contributor to death [23]. The largest long-term population study of trends in mortality comes from Australia and covers the period 1950–1981 [24],

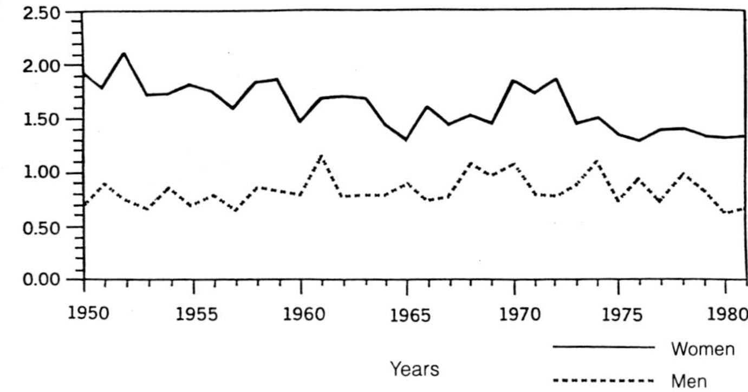

Fig. 3. Age standardised mortality rate from RA by sex, Australia 1950–1981. (From [23])

although it is not clearly stated in that report whether it covers all mentions of RA on death certificates or only those with RA as underlying cause of death. In brief, there was no significant trend apparent overall in age adjusted death rates during this period, althoug there was evidence of a recent decline in mortality in women, particularly those in the older age-group (Fig. 3). What was interesting from that data set was the observation that there was no improvement in survival of men with RA as judged by age at death, particularly against a background of decreasing mortality generally in the population.

Data on disease severity were analyzed directly on a birth cohort basis using three indicators of disease severity: ever seropositive, ever erosive and ever having subcutaneous nodules. If there was no birth cohort effect on severity, then the proportion of those with disease onset, for example, at age 35–44, who were ever seropositive should be the same for all periods of birth. This was not the situation and the results from all three indicators were similar (Fig. 4). The figures show that successively more recent generations were less likely to be positive for any of the above features. Further examination showed that the trends were not linear and that there was a "severity peak" in patients presenting in around 1960 with the majority of the birth cohorts displaying their maximum severity around that year [12].

Support for the hypothesis that RA is becoming less severe comes from Finland with the observation of a decline in the proportion of those registered disabled with musculoskeletal conditions having RA [17]. Furthermore, there was a marked decline in the number receiving disability pensions due to RA.

There have obviously been a number of prospective studies of RA looking at outcome, but few have been repeated with more recently diagnosed cohorts from the same population to examine trends in prognosis. In one such "paired" survey, a 9 year follow-up study of seropositive RA ending in 1958 showed that 38% progressed to severe handicap [25] compared to less than 3% for a similarly derived cohort followed for 8 years up to 1982 [21].

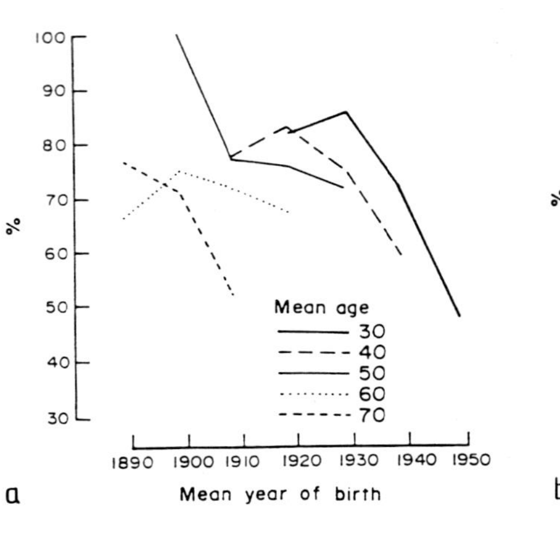

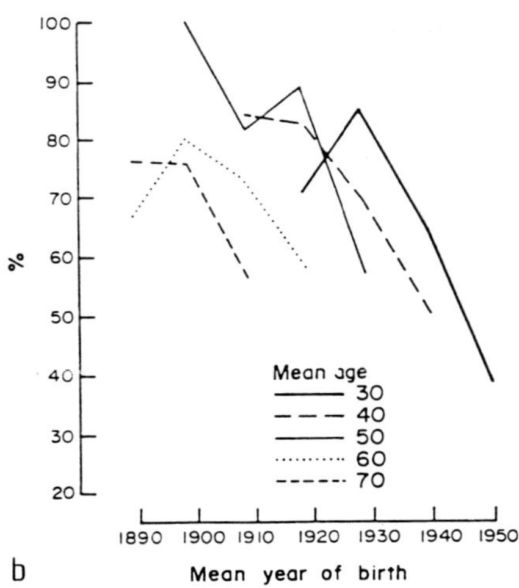

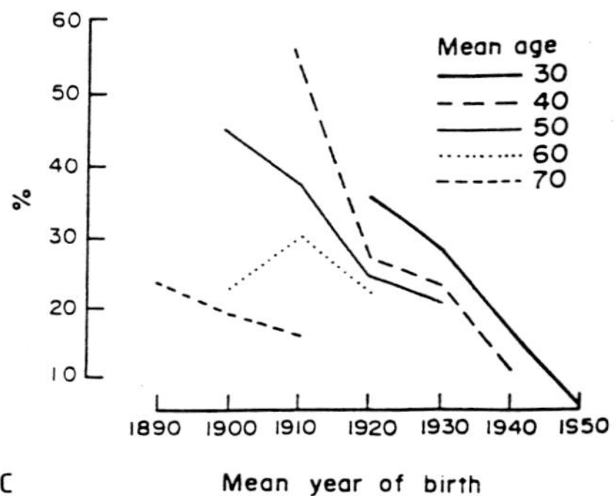

Fig. 4a–c. Proportion of patients, by decade of birth, by age at presentation who were **a** ever seropositive; **b** ever erosive; and **c** ever had nodules. If there was no effect of decade of birth then the age curves should approximate to horizontal lines. (From [12])

Possible Explanations

A reasonable summary from the data presented above is that there is a marked consistency with a decline both in the incidence and the severity of RA in the past 20 years or so, although conclusive proof is not available. Further, if there is a pointer to a possible cause it is that the decline is more marked in females than in males. It is this observation that led some to consider the role of increasing use of the oral contraceptive pill (OCP) [3, 26], based on an earlier prospective study suggesting that such use was associated with a reduction in RA risk [27]. There have been a large number of subsequent studies testing this hypothesis, including one surveying the same Mayo clinic population in whom the sex difference trend was first noted. Interestingly, in that population there was no evidence that OCP use could explain the trends [28, 29], but other studies have suggested that the opposite is the case, with most reports now finding a

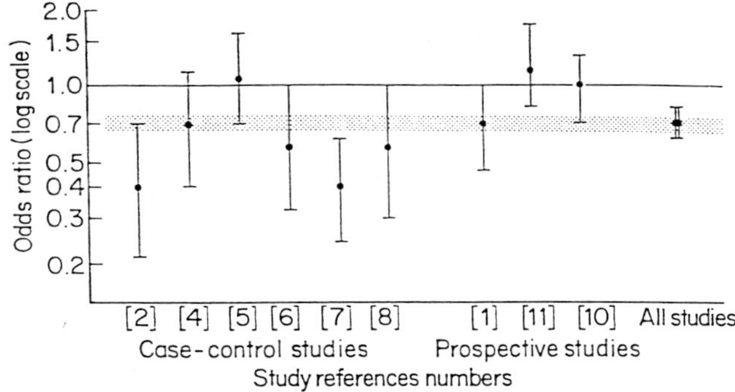

Fig. 5. Summary of results from studies examining the protective effect of oral contraceptive use on susceptibility to RA. (From [36])

protective effect of OCP use [26, 30–33] (Fig. 5). A recent consensus conference attempted to resolve the conflicting results and concluded that OCP use was likely both to postpone the development and reduce the severity of RA rather than affect the incidence per se [34]. Such a conclusion is consistent with the epidemiological data on trends summarized above.

Data concerning other possible explanations for the decline is speculative given the lack of etiologic clues concerning the onset of RA. Whether the trends in RA reflect changing patterns of viral or other infection, as postulated by Buchanan and Murdock [1], remain unclear but the problems associated with this were recently summarized [35]. Similarly, the possibility that changes in therapy have influenced severity remains untested in a population setting, although the evidence from clinical trials of the effectiveness of specific agents would argue against this being a major part of the story.

In summary, the available data point towards the interesting possibility that RA has or is declining in occurrence (particularly in females) and severity which perhaps, in part, is related to the pattern of hormonal consumption in Western countries.

References

1. Buchanan WW, Murdoch RM (1979) Hypothesis: that rheumatoid arthritis will disappear. J Rheumatol 6:324–329
2. Aho K, Palosuo T, Raunio V, Puska P, Aromaa A, Salonen T (1985) When does rheumatoid disease start? Arthritis Rheum 28(5):485–489
3. Linos A, Worthington JW, O'Fallon WM, Kurland LT (1980) The epidemiology of rheumatoid in Rochester, Minnesota: a study of incidence, prevalence and mortality. Am J Epidemiol 111:87–98
4. Ropes MW, Bennett GA, Cobb S et al (1957) Proposed diagnostic criteria for rheumatoid arthritis. Ann Rheum Dis 16:118–123

5. Arnett FC, Edworthy SM, Bloch DA et al (1988) The American Rheumatism Association 1987 revised criteria for the classification of rheumatoid arthritis. Arthritis Rheum 31(3):315–323
6. Goddard DH, Butler R (1989) Rheumatoid arthiritis: the treatment controversy. MacMillan, London
7. Bennett PH, Wood PHN (1968) Population studies of the rheumatic diseases. Excerpta Medica, Amsterdam, pp 477–478
8. Kellgren JH, Jeffrey MR, Ball J (1963) The epidemiology of chronic rheumatism, vol I. Blackwell, Oxford pp 324–327
9. Dugowson CE, Nelson JL, Koepsell TD, Daling JR (1989) Evaluation of the 1988 criteria for rheumatoid arthritis: application to a newly diagnosed cohort. Arthritis Rheum 22 (suppl):B79
10. Lawrence JS (1977) Rheumatism in Populations. Heinemann, London
11. Dugowson CE, Bley L, Koepsell TD, Nelson JL, Daling JR (1989) Incidence of rheumatoid arthritis in women. Arthritis Rheum 22 (suppl):A83
12. Silman AJ, Davies P, Currey HLF, Evans SJW (1983) Is rheumatoid arthritis becoming less severe? J Chronic Dis 36:891–897
13. Royal College of General Practitioners. Weekly returns of selected diagnoses 1976–1987. RCGP Research Unit, Birmingham, UK
14. Silman AJ (1988) Has the incidence of rheumatoid arthritis declined in the United Kingdom? Br J Rheumatol 27:77–79
15. Royal College of General Practitioners, Office of Population, Census and Surveys. Department of Health and Social Security (1979) Morbidity statistics from general practice: the 2nd national morbidity survey 1971/72. HMSO London
16. Royal College of General Practitioners, Office of Population, Census and Surveys. Department of Health and Social Security (1987) Morbidity statistics from general practice: the 3rd national morbidity survey 1981/82. HMSO London
17. Isomaki HA (1989) Rheumatoid arthritis as seen from official data registers. Experience in Finland. Scand J Rheumatol 79 (suppl):21–24
18. Behrend T, Lawrence JS, Behrend, H, Koch R (1972) Eine longitudinale Studie in Hinblick auf rheumatische Erkrankungen in der ländlichen Bevölkerung von Oberhörlen in Hessen. Z Rheumaforsch 31:153
19. Ball J, Lawrence JS (1961) Epidemiology of the sheep cell agglutination test. Ann Rheum Dis 20:235
20. Valkenburg HA, Hijmans W, Klein F (1968) Rheumatoid factor in patients suffering from chronic infectious diseases living in various temperate and non-temperate areas. In: Bennett PH, Wood PHN (eds) Population studies of rheumatic diseases. Exerpta Medica, Amsterdam p 181
21. Aho K, Tuomi T, Palosuo T, Kaarela K, Von Essen R, Isomaki H (1989) Is seropositive rheumatoid arthritis becoming less severe? Clin Exp Rheumatol 7:287–290
22. Laurent R, Robinson RG, Beller EM, Buchanan WW (1989) Incidence and severity of rheumatoid arthritis – the view from Australia. Brit J Rheum 28:360–361
23. Lindahl BIB (1985) In what sense is rheumatoid arthritis the principal cause of death? J Chronic Dis 38:963–72
24. Wicks IP, Moore J, Fleming A (1988) Australian mortality statistics for rheumatoid arthritis 1950–81: analysis of death certificate data. Ann Rheum Dis 47:563–569
25. Aho K, Kirpila J, Wager O (1959) The persistance of the agglutination activating factor (AAF) in the circulation. A nine year study of twenty seven patients. Ann Med Exp Fenn 37:377–381
26. Vandenbroucke JP, Valkenburg HA, Boersma HA et al (1982) Oral contraceptives and rheumatoid arthritis: further evidence for a preventive effect. Lancet 2:839–842
27. Wingrave SJ, Kay CR (1978) Reduction in incidence of rheumatoid arthritis associated with oral contraceptives. Lancet 1:569–571
28. Linos A, Worthington JW, O'Fallon WM, Kurland LT (1983) Case-control study of rheumatoid arthritis and prior use of oral contraceptives. Lancet 1:1299–1300

29. Del Junco DJ, Annegers JF, Luthtra HS, Coulam CB, Kurland LT (1985) Do oral contraceptives prevent rheumatoid arthritis? JAMA 254:1938–1941
30. Vandenbroucke JP, Witteman JCM, Valkenburg HA et al. (1986) Non-contraceptive hormones and rheumatoid arthritis in perimenopausal and postmenopausal women. JAMA 255:1299–1303
31. Hazes JMW, Dijkmans BAC, Vandenbroucke JP, De Vries RRP, Cats A (1990) Reduction of the risk of rheumatoid arthritis among women who take oral contraceptives. Arthritis Rheum 33:173–179
32. Spector TD, Roman E, Silman AJ (1990) The pill, parity and rheumatoid arthritis. Arthritis Rheum 33:782–789
33. Hazes JMW, Silman AJ, Brand R, Spector TD, Walker DJ, Vandenbroucke JP (1990) Influence of oral contraception on the occurrence of rheumatoid arthritis in female sibs. Scand J Rheumatol 19:306–310
34. Silman AJ, Vandenbroucke JP (1989) Female sex hormones and rheumatoid arthritis. Brit J Rheumatol 28 (suppl 1):1–73
35. Silman AJ (1989) Rheumatoid arthritis and infection: a population approach. Ann Rheum Dis 48:707–710

Genetics

Genetic Factors in Rheumatoid Arthritis

J. S. S. Lanchbury, L. I. Sakkas, and G. S. Panayi

Molecular Immunogenetics & Rheumatology Units, UMDS, Guy's Hospital,
London SE1 9RT, UK

Introduction

For many years the paradigm for genetic studies in rheumatoid arthritis (RA)
has been based around multifactorial determination of susceptibility including
an oligo- or polygenic component. Given the massive investment of resources in
this field of rheumatology research it is saluatory to consider data which suggest
the genetic component may account for as little as 12% of the total variability
[1]. Genetic studies, however, should not be dismissed on this basis since the
aetiology of RA is unknown. As will be discussed later, fine structural analysis
of the HLA-DR4 molecule, the best characterised genetic association, implicates specific immune regulation as a key area in the pathogenesis of RA. The
immediate potential of this type of approach is to facilitate the step towards
rational experimental design and eventually therapeutic intervention.

What Should We Study?

Problems arise when one sets out to study a spectrum disease for which there is
no single diagnostic test. Comparison of early with more recent data sets should
therefore be approached with caution. However, the lesson of recent molecular
studies of HLA-DR4 determinants among racially disparate definite or classical
RA patients is one of relative genetic homogeneity. This is particularily true for
some rigorously defined subsets of patients such as those with Felty's syndrome
[36]. What is the likely scope of these findings? Most genetic studies are carried
out on hospital ascertained patients, who by definition express more serious
disease than those who are treated at the community level. RA patients
ascertained in one random population survey showed no HLA-DR4 association in contrast to those treated in hospital [7]. In addition to HLA, the overall
genetic component is likely to be sensitive to the method of patient ascertain-

Smolen, Kalden, Maini (Eds.)
Rheumatoid Arthritis
© Springer-Verlag Berlin Heidelberg 1992

ment. One preliminary survey has shown that MZ (monozygotic) and DZ (dizygotic) twin concordance rates are doubled when RA patients are ascertained at the hospital rather than at the population level [37]. These data suggest that earlier work may have overestimated the MZ:DZ concordance ratio and may have provided an urealistically high MZ concordance rate. A ratio of 2.5 rather than 3.5 and 12% MZ concordance in contrast to 32% may be more realistic.

Family Approaches

Genetic studies in RA have utilised family material (pedigree, MZ and DZ twins, linkage and sibling pair analyses) and single gene marker surveys in populations. HLA markers identified in populations have subsequently been examined in multicase RA families to assess their correlation with disease. Several earlier reviews have dealt with family studies and classical marker associations, and we will concentrate here on recent data, especially those provided by molecular genetic approaches. Linkage analysis using the log odds (LOD) score method among multicase RA families has failed to find evidence of genetic linkage to the HLA region [30, 12, 42]. Studies of HLA haplotype sharing among affected sibling pairs suggest non-random distribution of one or two haplotypes [17], although this is not a universal finding [42]. This rather confusing picture may be reconciled if one considers HLA-DR to be one of several genetic not to mention environmental factors which are necessary for the development of RA. At the population level, if the correct HLA alleles are necessary but not sufficient for disease expression, most individuals with RA will carry the population associated alleles. Similarly, affected siblings will tend to share disease associated HLA haplotypes. However, classical linkage analysis will be confounded by the independent segregation of several susceptibility loci on different chromosomes.

HLA and RA

Prior to the explosion of novel restriction fragment length polymorphism (RFLP) allelic markers, which occurred during the 1980s, most known, polymorphic, single locus markers had been examined for association with RA [29]. By far the most consistent associations were found with alleles encoded in the human MHC (Fig. 1) and in particular the HLA-DR4 antigen. The fact that several alleles at distinct MHC loci are associated with RA reflects a phenomenon known as linkage disequilibrium. That is, particular combination of alleles exist more frequently than expected and are inherited as single units

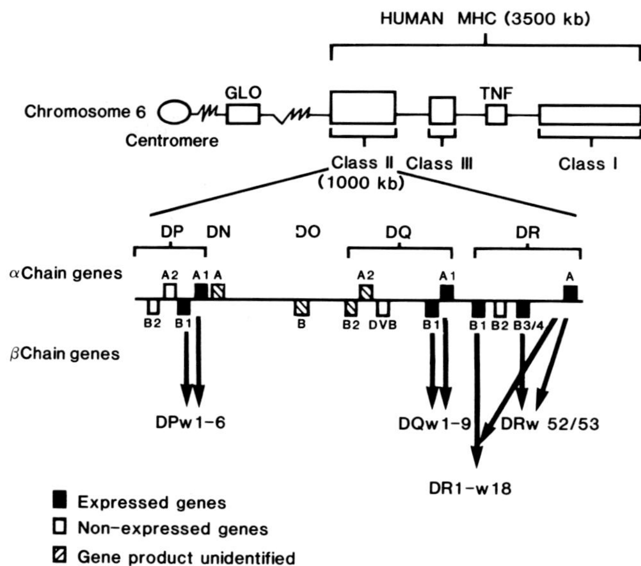

Fig. 1. The genomic organization of the human major histocompatibility complex (MHC) with the class II region shown in detail. The human MHC is located on the short arm of chromosome 6 and divided into class I, class II and class III regions. The class I region encodes the classical transplantation HLA-A, -B and -Cw antigens whose biological function is to present fragments of cellularly synthesized proteins to cytotoxic T lymphocytes. The class III region contains genes for C2, factor B, C4A and C4B components of the complement pathways together with 21 hydroxylase A and B genes. The class II region is divided into DR, DQ and DP subregions which each contain functional and nonfunctional genes [2]. The products of these human immune response genes are heterodimeric α-β cell surface molecules which bind fragments of extracellularily derived proteins and activate peptide-specific helper T lymphocytes

known as haplotypes. Thus, the descriptions of class I B locus associations B44, Bw60 and Bw62 are now clearly related to linkage disequilibrium to DR4 [44]. A breakthrough was achieved with the demonstration of a strong association between RA and the mixed lymphocyte culture (MLC) determinant Dw4 [39]. This was rapidly followed by the use of alloantisera which defined a more strongly associated determinant, DR4, that was related but not identical to Dw4 [28, 40]. The convenience of serological as opposed to cellular methods has meant that the majority of studies of the HLA-D or class II region in RA have been carried out with antisera.

Molecular Polymorphism of DR4

HLA-DR molecules are now known to be composed of a nonpolymorphic α chain and a polymorphic β chain. MLC reactivity distinguishes several genetically determined forms of HLA class II molecules each associated with

Table 1. Summary of amino acid and nucleotide polymorphisms in the first domain of DRβ1 DR4 subtypes

Residue contact[a]	Pep	Pep	Pep	Pep	Pep TcR	Pep	Pep	Pep	Reference
Aminoacid	37	57	67	69	70	71	74	86	
Dw4	Tyr TAC	Asp GAT	Leu CTC	Glu GAG	Gln CAG	Lys AAG	Ala GCG	Gly GGT	Gregersen et al. 1986 [14]
Dw14.1	–	–	–	–	–	Arg G	–	Val TG	Cairns et al. 1985 [6]
Dw14.2	–	–	–	–	–	Arg G	–	– TG	Lanchbury et al. 1990 [21]
Dw13.1	–	–	–	–	–	Arg G	Glu A	Val TG	Cairns et al. 1985 [6]
Dw13.2	–	–	–	–	–	Arg G	Glu A	–	Lanchbury et al. 1990 [21]
DwKT2	Ser C	–	–	–	–	Arg G	Glu A	Val TG	Gregersen et al. 1987b [16]
Dw10	–	–	Ile A	–	Asp A G C	Glu G	–	Val TG	Gregersen et al. 1986 [14]
Dw15	–	Ser AGC	–	–	–	Arg G	–	–	Gregersen et al. 1986 [144]

pep, peptide contact residue; pep/TcR, peptide or T cell receptor contact residue
[a] Based on predictions from Brown et al. 1988 [5].

the public DR4 serological specificity. These are the Dw4, Dw10, Dw13, Dw14, and Dw15 and DwKT2 subtypes. The molecular basis for this DR4 associated polymorphism was first shown by biochemical studies using DR- and DQ-specific monoclonal antibodies (MAbs) [24]. The Dw type of a DR4 cell line correlated with electrophoretic mobility of the DRβ1 chain but not the linked DRβ4, DQβ or DQα chains [24, 4]. Confirmation was provided by molecular cloning of class II genes from DR4 haplotypes. Each MLC variant was associated with a unique DR4β1 primary sequence [6, 14]. Table 1 gives nucleotide and corresponding amino acid sequences of the presently defined DR4 alleles. Variation between DR4 subtypes occurs in the first protein domain of the DRβ1 chain with most but not all of it clustered in a portion termed the third hypervariable region (HVR3). The table includes the recently characterized 13.2 and 14.2 alleles which carry a glycine substitution at position 86 and are less common than the previously sequenced 13.1 and 14.1 alleles.

HLA-DR4β1 Chain Polymorphism and RA

The elucidation of the molecular basis of DR4 subtype polymorphism has had important consequences for our understanding of the nature of HLA-DR association with RA. Although most studies confirm the DR4 association with RA, especially among groups of North European descent, several populations show associations with DR1 or no association at all [44]. Taken together with limited data sets from MLC studies among normals of different ethnic groups and among Caucasoid RA patients, it was suggested by Nepom et al. [25] and Gregersen et al. [15] that it was the HVR3 of HLA-DR1β1 and of particular DR4β1 subtypes which was fundamentally associated with RA. Evidence from other sources implicates the existence of a shared epitope in RA. A serological cluster, MC1, has been defined which includes DR1 and DR4 [10] while alloreactive T cell clones primed on Dw14 cells are reactive with DR4 negative targets from normals and RA patients [13]. To generate the volume of data needed to answer this question at the molecular level, biochemical and cDNA cloning techniques were clearly inappropriate. The breakthrough came with the use of synthetic oligonucleotide probes which detect specific nucleotide sequences in polymerase chain reaction (PCR) amplified DNA or restriction enzyme digested genomic DNA. As expected, the sequences of alleles derived from RA patients proved to be no different from the equivalent alleles of healthy individuals. The difference lay in the frequency distribution of alleles between patient groups and controls. RA is associated with the Dw4, Dw14 and Dw15 alleles of DR4 and with DR1, while the DR4 alleles Dw10 and Dw13 are protective or neutral [45, 26, 43, 11]. Table 2 lists the RA associations for which molecular data exist together with the HVR3 amino acid sequence for each allele. The susceptibility alleles are not, however, equivalent and a hierarchy exists with the Dw4 allele exerting by far the greatest influence. In Japanese

Table 2. HLA-DR4 associations with rheumatoid arthritis together with third hypervariable region pentapeptide

DR4 subtype	DR4 allele designation	HVR3 pentapeptide[a]	Association with RA
w4	0401	QKRAA	Positive
w14.1	0404	QRRAA	Positive
w14.2	0408	QRRAA	Unknown[c]
w15	0405	QRRAA	Positive
w10	0402	DERAA[b]	Negative
w13.1	0403	QRRAE	Negative
w13.2	0407	QRRAE	Unknown
wKT2	0406	QRRAE	Unknown

[a] Amino acid sequences are given in single letter code.
[b] Amino acids in bold indicate nonconservative substitutions compared to QRRAA template.
[c] Indicates insufficient population data exist to indicate RA association.

and Jewish populations, in which Dw 4 is relatively uncommon, RA has recently been shown to be associated with the Dw 15 allele [43, 11]. The Dw 15 allele is rare in normal Caucasoids, but our own study found it in 5% of RA patients with a relative risk 5.2 (unpublished data). The QRRAA sequence is also carried by the rare DRw 6 Dw 16 DRβ 1 allele. So far no data exist on whether this allele is implicated in susceptibility to RA. It is likely that the HLA associations found with RA and the incidence of disease will reflect the prevalence of the high and low risk alleles in the gene pools of particular populations.

Controversy exists over whether DQw 7, which is linked to certain subtypes of DR 4, plays an independent role in susceptibility to RA or whether it is related to particular clinical features [20]. More data need to be collected at the molecular level to determine whether any DQ effect is the result of preferential linkage to DR 4 subtypes.

Structural Considerations

The HLA-DR association with RA can be analyzed in terms of an HVR 3 pentapeptide "epitope" which is relatively conserved between susceptibility alleles. Dw 4 carries QKRAA and differs only at position 71 (a conservative lysine for arginine change) from Dw 14, Dw 15 and DR 1 which carry QRRAA (see Tables 1 and 2). Dw 10 and Dw 13, the two DR 4 non-risk alleles, closely resemble Dw 4 and Dw 14 but carry nonconservative acidic substitutions at positions 70 and 71 (Dw 10) and 74 (Dw 13) [45]. The HLA component of susceptibility or protection to RA is probably determined by these few amino acids.

What are the implications of this? Recently, a generalized HLA class II structure modelled on the three-dimensional structure of HLA-A 2 was proposed [5]. This model suggests that the first protein domains of DRα and β fold to provide a platform based on a β pleated sheet structure bounded on two sides by α helices. It is suggested that peptide fragments are held in this "cleft" and that their recognition by T lymphocytes forms the basis of MHC classII restriction. Based on this structure it can be predicted whether individual amino acid residues of DR 4 chains are likely to contact antigenic peptide or T cell receptor. Likely contacts for polymorphic amino acids among DR 4 alleles are given in Table 1. Although the situation for residues at position 70 is ambiguous, all other variable residues are likely to bind peptide. From this, two important points can be drawn. The first is that if the residues which distinguish alloreactive variants of DR 4 are involved in peptide binding, then it is probably differential binding of self peptides which is the basis of the detection of DR 4 Dw types. The second and more important point is that it is peptide binding residues which determine the influence of DR 4 and DR 1 alleles on the development of RA. This would implicate specific HLA binding of a peptide or a structurally related group of peptides in RA.

Non-MHC Genes in RA

Twin concordance and haplotype sharing figures imply that the HLA region contributes around 35% of the total genetic component to RA [8]. This suggests that important genetic factors for development of RA map outside the human MHC. Attractive candidate genes include those encoding chains of the T cell receptor (TcR) and those genes located in the telomeric region of the long arm of chromosome 14 (14q32), which contains the immunoglobulin heavy (IgH) chain genes and the protease inhibitors α1 antitrypsin (A1AT) and α1 antichymotrypsin (A1ACT) genes.

Chromosome 14q32

A role for genes in this region has been suggested from studies of IgH and A1AT protein polymorphisms in RA. The germline organization of IgH chain loci and other chromosome 14 loci under discussion is given in Fig. 1. Studies on γ IgH constant (C) region polymorphisms (Gm allotypes) have given controversial results. A few studies found a weak association with RA or with DR4-positive RA while others found no association [46]. A single study on α2 IgH (A2m allotypes) reported no association [35]. Findings on A1AT phenotypes in RA again have been inconsistent. Some studies showed weak associations with deficiency phenotypes or with other variants, while other studies found no association. A few studies have examined A1AT variants in severe RA or in RA complicated by interstitial lung disease, but no clear picture has emerged [18, 27]. By RFLP analysis, the IgH gene segments that have been investigated in RA include a hypervariable locus 5′ of the JH region and the switch (S) regions of μ (Sμ) and α1 (Sα1) chains. No significant perturbation of allele frequencies was observed. Interestingly, the Sμ and Sα1 RFLP patterns do not correlate with serum Ig [22] or with serum rheumatoid factor levels. Similar RFLP analyses of A1AT, A1ACT and the A1AT related genes which map near the A1AT gene have not been informative in RA [33]. In conclusion, these studies suggest that IgH and protease inhibitor polymorphisms, whether examined at the protein level or by RFLP, are unlikely to have any major effect on the susceptibility to RA. However, some caution is justified since high recombination frequencies have been observed within the IgH loci [19].

In the region between IgH and the A1AT genes few anonymous DNA fragments and hypervariable loci have been mapped thus far. It is conceivable that this region may contain genes important for the immune response, since genes encoding proteins of similar function tend to be organized in clusters. RFLP analysis of the anonymous DNA fragments D14S17 and D14S18 and of the hypervariable loci D14S16 and D14S1 (Fig. 2) revealed an association with the 10.3/10.3 Kb D14S1/*Hin*dIII genotype [31]. The significance of the D14S1 association with RA is unknown, since no clear function has so far been attributed to hypervariable regions in humans. Alternatively, this association

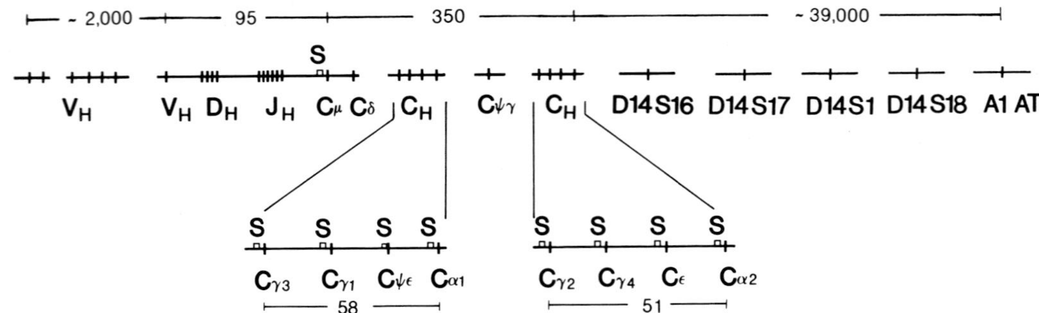

Fig. 2. Genomic organization of immunoglobulin heavy chain (IgH) loci and other relevant genes on human chromosome 14q32. Distances, not to scale, are in kilobases. There are around 200 variable (*VH*), 35 diversity (*DH*) and 6 joining (JH) segments. During the differentiation of B lymphocytes individual segments from the VH, DH and JH regions recombine to form a functional gene for the variable region of the IgH chain. The switch (*S*) regions, which are stretches of tandem repeats, are thought to be involved in the IgH class switch. The IgH-A1AT distance has been estimated from recombination values, but the physical distance is estimated to be less than 10000 Kb. (From [3, 19, 23])

might reflect weak linkage to an uncharacterized RA susceptibility locus. The possibility that this region contains a gene relevant to arthritis susceptibility is strengthened by the fact that the same marker has also been found to be associated with psoriatic arthritis, polymyalgia rheumatica and primary generalized osteoarthritis [33]. RFLP analysis of the IgH-A1AT region is far from complete since the distances separating the analyzed loci are very large and frequent recombination events occur [23]. Additional markers will be necessary before one can evaluate the significance of chromosome 14q32 in the pathogenesis of RA.

T Cell Receptor Genes in RA

The HLA-DR4 association with RA suggests the possibility that the disease may be mediated by particular TcR. The classical TcR is an αβ heterodimer which recognizes processed antigen fragments bound to HLA molecules. A second receptor is composed of a γδ heterodimer but its function is not well characterized. Like the immunoglobulins, variable (V) regions of the TcR α, β, γ and and δ chains are encoded in germline DNA by noncontiguous variable, diversity (D) (β and δ chains only) and joining (J) region segments which rearrange to the C region segments to form functional genes. Past efforts to characterize a TcR component in RA have involved two distinct approaches. The first method has addressed germline polymorphisms of TcR genes and has been largely uninformative. RFLP analysis of TcR α and β C region polymorphisms shows no association with RA [32]. This is not surprising since it is the products of TcR V, D and J regions and their junctions which are likely to contact the HLA-antigen complex. The recombination events observed within the TcR α and β gene loci emphasise the need for RFLP study of V region genes in RA. It is interesting in this context to consider the association reported between RA and a TcR V^β polymorphism [41]. A single analysis of a J^γ germline polymorphism has shown no distortion of genotype frequencies in RA [34]. The interest in this type of approach relates to the potential for identification of linkage to germline TcR segment insertions, deletions or polymorphisms of structural or regulatory sequences.

An alternative approach has involved the analysis of TcR gene rearrangements in synovial fluid or synovial membrane derived T lymphocytes and has yielded controversial results. The claim by some workers to have demonstrated limited T cell rearrangement in synovial populations implies selective involvement of particular TcR [38], but this claim has been refuted by others [9].

Future Directions

It is likely that a complete and highly informative linkage map of the human genome will be established shortly. Allied to well characterized family material and suitable computer analysis, this approach should allow identification of regions of DNA containing novel genes relevant to the development of RA.

The generality of the HLA-DR epitope theory has been based on few independent studies at the molecular level. It is particularly important that more studies are carried out on large numbers of patients especially among different ethnic groups. Genetically homogeneous groups such as Felty's syndrome patients may prove useful in tying genetic associations to specific pathogenetic processes. One major challenge remaining is to identify the axis by which specific HLA structures predispose to or protect from RA. This may involve specific antigen binding to HLA together with recognition by particular TcR. Recent molecular techniques based on PCR have enabled the examination of rearranged TcR sequences from specific disease lesions. Such an approach in RA might identify TcR components which could be correlated with responses to candidate antigens. Approaches such as those outlined above will lead to the dissection of the multifactorial basis of RA and will clarify the relationship between the constituitive, environmental and possible random processes involved.

References

1. Aho K, Koskevuo J, Tuominen J, Kaprio J (1986) Occurrence of rheumatoid arthritis in a nationwide series of twins. J Rheumatol 13:899–902
2. Auffray C, Strominger J (1985) Molecular genetics of the human major histocompatibility complex. Adv Hum Genet 15:197–247

3. Berman JE, Mellis SJ, Polock R, Smith CL, Suh H, Heinke B, Kowal B, Surti U, Chess L, Cantor CR, Alt FW (1988) Content and organization of the human Ig VH locus: definition of three new VH families and linkage to the Ig CH locus. EMBO J 7:727–738

4. Bontrop RE, Schreuder GMT, Mikulski EMA, van Miltenburg RT, Giphart MJ (1986) Polymorphisms within the HLA-DR4 haplotypes. Various DQ subtypes detected with monoclonal antibodies. Tissue Antigens 27:22–31

5. Brown JH, Jardetzky T, Saper MA, Samraoui B, Bjorkman PJ, Wiley DC (1988) A hypothetical model of the foreign antigen binding site of class II histocompatibility molecules. Nature 332:845–850

6. Cairns, JS, Curtsinger JM, Dahl CA, Freeman S, Alter BJ, Bach FH (1985) Sequence polymorphism of HLA DRβ alleles relating to T-cell-recognized determinants. Nature 317:166–168

7. De Jongh BM, van Romunde LKJ, Valkenburgh HA, de Lange GG, van Rood JJ (1984) Epidemiological study of HLA and GM in rheumatoid arthritis and related symptoms in an open Dutch population. Ann Rheum Dis 43:613–619

8. Deighton CM, Walker DJ, Griffiths ID, Roberts DF (1989) The contribution of HLA to rheumatoid arthritis. Clin Genet 36:178–182

9. Duby AD, Sinclair AK, Osborne-Lawrence SL, Zeldes W, Kan L, Fox DA (1989) Clonal heterogeneity of synovial fluid T lymphocytes from patients with rheumatoid arthritis. Proc Natl Acad Sci USA 86:6206–6210

10. Duquesnoy RJ, Marrari M, Hackbarth S, Zeevi A (1984) Serological and cellular definition of a new HLA-DR associated determinant, MC1, and its association with rheumatoid arthritis. Hum Immunol 10:165–176

11. Gao X, Brautbar C, Gazit E, Livneh A, Stastny P (1989) Study of HLA-DR4 subsets in Israeli patients with rheumatoid arthritis. Hum Immunol suppl:51

12. Go RCP, Alarcon GS, Acton RT, Koopman WJ, Vittor VJ, Barger BO (1987) Analyses of HLA linkage in white families with multiple cases of seropositive rheumatoid arthritis. Arthritis Rheum 30:1115–1123

13. Goronzy J, Weyand CM, Fathman CG (1986) Shared T cell recognition sites on human histocompatibility leukocyte antigen class II molecules of patients with seropositive rheumatoid arthritis. J Clin Invest 77:1042–1049

14. Gregersen PK, Shen M, Song Q-L, Merryman P, Degar S, Seki T, Maccari J, Goldberg D, Murphy H, Schwenzer J, Wang CY, Winchester RJ, Nepom GT, Silver J (1986) Molecular diversity of HLA-DR4 haplotypes. Proc Natl Acad Sci USA 83:2642–2646

15. Gregersen PK, Silver J, Winchester RJ (1987) The shared epitope hypothesis. An approach to understanding the molecular genetics of susceptibility to rheumatoid arthritis. Arthritis Rheum 30:1205–1213

16. Gregersen PK, Goyert SM, Song Q-L, Silver J (1987) Microheterogeneity of HLA-DR4 haplotypes: DNA sequence analysis of LD "KT2" and LD "TAS" haplotypes. Hum Immunol 19:287–292

17. Grennan DM, Sanders PA (1988) Rheumatoid arthritis. In: Grennan DM (ed) Genetics of rheumatic diseases. Balliere Tindall, London, pp 585–601

18. Hietala J, Rantala H, Hakala M, Koivisto O (1987) Alpha-1-antitrypsin phenotypes in rheumatoid arthritis. Arthritis Rheum 30:958

19. Hofker MH, Walter MA, Cox DW (1989) Complete physical map of the human immunoglobulin heavy chain constant region gene complex. Proc natl Acad Sci USA 86:5567–5571

20. Lanchbury JSS (1988) Molecular genetics of the HLA-D region component of inherited susceptibility to rheumatoid arthritis. Br J Rheumatol 27:171–175

21. Lanchbury JSS, Hall MA, Welsh KI, Panayi GS (1990) Sequence analysis of HLA-DR4B1 subtypes – additional first domain variability is detected by oligonucleotide hybridization and nucleotide sequencing. Hum Immunol 27:136–144

22. Mayer L, Kwan SP, Thomson C, Ko HS, Chiorazzi N, Waldman T, Rosen F (1986) Evidence for a defect in "switch" T cells in patients with immunodeficiency and hyperimmunoglobulinaemia M. N Engl J Med 314:409–413

23. Nakamura Y, Lathrop M, O'Connell P, Leppert M, Kamboh MI, Lalouel J-M, White R (1989) Frequent recombination is observed in the distal end of the long arm of chromosome 14. Genomics 4:76–81
24. Nepom BS, Nepom GT, Mickelson E, Antonelli P, Hansen JA (1983) Electrophoretic analysis of human HLA-DR antigens from HLA-DR4 homozygous cell lines: correlation between β-chain diversity and HLA-D. Proc Natl Acad Sci USA 80:6962–6966
25. Nepom GT, Hansen JA, Nepom BS (1987) The molecular basis for HLA class II associations with rheumatoid arthritis. J Clin Immunol 7:1–7
26. Nepom GT, Byers P, Seyfried C, Healey LA, Wilske KR, Stage D, Nepom BS (1989) HLA genes associated with rheumatoid arthritis. Identification of susceptibility alleles using specific oligonucleotide probes. Arthritis Rheum 32:15–21
27. Ollier W, Thomson W, Welch S, de Lange GG, Silman A (1988) Chromosome 14 markers in rheumatoid arthritis. Ann Rheum Dis 47:84–848
28. Panayi GS, Wooley P, Batchelor JR (1978) Genetic basis of rheumatoid disease: HLA antigens, disease manifestations and toxic reactions to drugs. Br Med J 2:1326–1328
29. Papiha SS, Lanchbury JS, Pal B (1986) Genetic structure of the population with rheumatoid arthritis in north east England: a genetic approach to define different subtypes. Ann Rheum Dis 45:881–891
30. Read A, Grennan DM, Dyer P, Dodds W, Hamer D, Clague R, Harris R (1983) HLA and blood group markers in multicase rheumatoid families: sibshipand linkage analyses. Dis Markers 1:271–282
31. Sakkas LI, Demaine AG, Vaughan RW, Welsh KI, Panayi GS (1987) The association of DNA variants at or near the IgH locus with rheumatoid arthritis. J Immunogenet 14:189–196
32. Sakkas LI, Demaine AG, Welsh KI, Panayi GS (1987) Restriction fragment length polymorphism for the T cell receptor α and β chain genes in rheumatoid arthritis. Arthritis Rheum 30:231–232
33. Sakkas LI, Macfarlane DG, Bird H, Welsh KI, Panayi GS (1990) Association of osteoarthritis with homozygosity for a 5.8 Kb Taq I fragment of the α1-antichymotrypsin gene. Br J Rheumatol 29:245–8
34. Sakkas LI (1990) Molecular immunogenetic studies in rheumatic diseases. Thesis London University, London
35. Sanders PA, de Lange GG, Dyer PA, Grennan DM (1985) Gm and Km allotypes in rheumatoid arthritis. Ann Rheum Dis 44:529–532
36. Sansom DM, Bidwell JL, Maddison PJ, Campion G, Klouda PT, Bradley BA (1987) HLA DQα and DQβ restriction fragment length polymorphisms associated with Felty's syndrome and DR4-positive rheumatoid arthrits. Hum Immunol 19:269–278
37. Silman AJ, Ollier W, Hayton RM, Holligan S, Smith IL (1989) Twin concordance rates for rheumatoid arthritis: preliminary results from a nationwide study. Br J Rheumatol 28 (suppl 2):95
38. Stamenkovic I, Stegagno M, Wright KA, Krane SM, Amento EP, Colvin RB, Duquesnoy RJ, Kurnick JT (1988) Clonal dominance among T-lymphocyte infiltrates in arthritis. Proc Nathl Acad Sci USA 85:1179–1183
39. Stastny P (1974) Mixed lymphocyte culture typing cells from patients with rheumatoid arthritis. Tissue Antigens 4:571–579
40. Stastny P (1978) Association of the B-cell alloantigen DRw4 with rheumatoid arthritis. N Engl J Med 298:869–871
41. Stastny P, Ball EJ, Khan MA, Olsen NJ, Pinkus T, Gao X (1988) HLA-DR4 and other genetic markers in rheumatoid arthritis. Br J Rheumatol 27 (suppl 2):132–138
42. Walker DJ, Burn J, Griffiths ID, Roberts DF, Stephenson AM (1987) Linkage studies of HLA and rheumatoid arthritis in multicase families. Arthritis Rheum 30:31–36
43. Watanabe Y, Tokunaga K, Matsuki K, Takeuchi F, Matsuka K, Maeda H, Omoto K, Juji T (1989) Putative amino acid sequence of HLA-DRB chain contributing to rheumatoid arthritis susceptibility. J Exp Med 169:2263–2268
44. Woodrow JC (1986) Analysis of the HLA association with rheumatoid arthritis. Dis Markers 4:7–12

45. Wordsworth BP, Lanchbury JSS, Sakkas LI, Welsh KI, Panayi GS, Bell JI (1989) HLA-DR4 subtype frequencies in rheumatoid arthritis indicate that DRB1 is the major susceptibility locus within the human leucocyte antigen class II region. Proc Natl Acad Sci USA 86:10049–10053
46. Zarnowski H, Mierau R, Werdier D, Antons M, Genth E, Hartl PW (1986) Increased frequency of GM(1,2;21) phenotype in HLA-DR4 positive seropositive rheumatoid arthritis. J Rheumatol 13:858–863

Rheumatoid Arthritis in Southeastern Europe

H. M. Moutsopoulos and P. G. Vlachoyiannopoulos

Department of Internal Medicine, School of Medicine, University of Ioannina,
45110 Ioannina, Greece

Introduction

Rheumatoid arthritis (RA) was originally described in nine women by AJ Landre-Beauvais (1772–1840), who suggested that it represented a variant of gout. Jean-Martin Charcot (1825–1893) described gout, rheumatic fever, rheumatoid arthritis and osteoarthritis and pointed out their similarities and differences. In addition, he suggested that it is sometimes difficult to differentiate the various forms of "rheumatism" but that it is possible to show that they all originate from one and the same cause. The term "rheumatoid arthritis" was applied in 1958 by AB Garrod, who thought that "the disease is an arthritic or joint disease and manifests some of the external characters of rheumatism" [1].

The pleomorphic natural history of RA and the difficulties in establishing the diagnosis, especially in the early stages, indicated a need for diagnostic criteria. In 1956 the American Rheumatism Association (ARA) proposed diagnostic criteria for RA [2] that were revised in 1958 in order to increase specificity and sensitivity [3]. The ARA revised criteria for RA were extensively used for nearly 30 years. The diagnostic criteria improved accuracy of diagnosis and produced comparable research results [4]. Nevertheless, many other forms of arthritis, previously included in the spectrum of RA, have been separately classified and our knowledge of the mechanisms of RA pathogenesis and articular damage have been extensively broadened. Later, the ARA established new, more simple and specific criteria for the diagnosis of RA [4]. However, even now, "four conditions [systemic lupus erythematosus (SLE), psoriatic arthritis, mixed connective tissue disease and Reiter's syndrome] appear likely to have substantial numbers of patients who might fullfill the requirements of the new RA criteria and caution should be observed in these circumstances" [4].

A critical point in establishing the diagnosis of RA is the persistence of the clinical features for at least 6 weeks. Nonetheless, even within groups of patients with RA who have been followed for years, many dissimilarities in the clinical picture exist from patient to patient sand possibly from one ethnic group to another. It is generally believed, for instance that RA in Mediterranean

Smolen, Kalden, Maini (Eds.)
Rheumatoid Arthritis
© Springer-Verlag Berlin Heidelberg 1992

countries is less severe than in Northern Europe and the USA. Felty's syndrome and other systemic manifestations are very rare. The dissimilarities of RA constitute a great puzzle and an effort was undertaken to unravel this puzzle through immunogenetics. It was found, for instance, that the serologically defined HLA-DR4 is highly associated with RA and is a marker of more aggressive disease [5]. New studies from several ethnic groups, however, especially those from Southern Europe (Spain, Italy, Greece) and Israel, and from Asian immigrants living in the UK supported an HLA-DR1 association, or no association at all between the disease and HLA class II antigens [6].

It is of great interest to study the immunogenetics of such populations, using techniques of molecular biology, in order to better understand the mechanisms that are possibly important in the pathogenesis of RA. In this chapter we will summarize current knowledge of the clinical, serological and immunogenic profiles of RA patients in different Mediterranean countries.

Clinicoserologic Considerations

In 1984 Moutsopoulos et al. described a high frequency of anti-Ro (SSA) antibodies in Greek RA patients [7]. Ro (SSA) antigen is a complex of two polypeptides with molecular weights of 60 KDa and 50 KDa [8] and small cytoplasmic RNAs (ScRNAs), known as hYRNAs [9]. In addition, it was pointed out that anti-Ro (SSA) positive Greek RA patients experienced a high frequency of D-penicillamine side effects. To further address the question whether Greek RA patients with anti-Ro (SSA) antibodies constitute a disease subgroup, the clinical, laboratory, histological and radiological manifestations of anti-Ro (SSA) positive and anti-Ro (SSA) negative RA patients were investigated [10]. It was noted that anti-Ro (SSA) positive RA patients are primarily females with a articular and extra-articular disease pattern similar to anti-Ro (SSA) negative RA patients. Nevertheless, anti-Ro (SSA) positive RA patients more often had lymphoid infiltrates in labial minor salivary gland biopsies and significantly lower titers of serum rheumatoid factor (t = 2.62; p < 0.01). A high incidence of D-penicillamine side effects in Greek anti-Ro (SSA) positive patients was again demonstrated. This association may be in the same line as Panayi's [11] and Emery's [12] observations that RA patients expressing the HLA-DR3 alloantigen have a greater risk of D-penicillamine side effects. A high HLA-DR3 incidence has been described in anti-Ro (SSA) positive individuals [13]. Subsequently, a large number of Greek RA patients from two medical centers (Ioannina and Athens) were tissue-typed for HLA-A, -B, -DR antigens, regardless of sex, severity of disease, seropositivity and age of disease onset. An association between these variables and any of the HLA alloantigens tested was not found. Only an increased prevalence of the HLA-DR5 antigen in the Ro (SSA) positive RA group was noted, but this did not reach statistical significance [14]. The high frequency of anti-Ro (SSA) autoantibodies and the lack of any HLA antigen association in Greek RA patients prompted us to examine possible differences regarding clinical manifestations in certain RA patient groups of different age at onset and disease duration [15]. The patients were divided in three groups accordingt to the age at disease onset: group A with disease onset age less than 40 years, group B between 40 and 59 years and group C 60 years and above. Each group was further subdivided into two subgroups, 1 and 2, with disease duration below 5 and above 5 years, respectively. The main conclusions drawn from this study were as follows: The highest articular index was observed in individuals with disease duration greater than 5 years and disease onset between the age of 40 and 59 years. Females are more severely affected by RA compared with males but this was not obvious in individuals whose disease started at the age of 60 years and above. The latter observation has not been noted previously [16, 17]. Rheumatoid nodules were observed in 13% of our RA population. Despite the fact that the prevalence of this finding was more common in the younger group of RA patients, this was not of statistical significance. The overall prevalence of rheumatoid nodules in our population is significantly lower than that described in other series [5]. The same is also true for other extra-articular manifestations such as episcleritis, Felty's syndrome and vasculitis. The prevalence of rheumatoid factor in Greek RA patients is similar to that described by others but, in contrast to previous reports [18–20] the prevalence in different age groups did not differ. In this study, Greek RA patients had a higher prevalence of antinuclear antibodies (ANA) compared with patients in other studies [17]. This difference may be attributed to methodological parameters such as the substrate used for the detection of antibodies. Finally, the present study again pointed out the relatively high prevalence of anti-Ro (SSA) antibodies in Greek RA patients.

The work presented here imposed two important questions which needed explanation: (1) Does the anti-Ro (SSA) positive RA group include patients with an overlaping syndrome made up of RA, SLE and Sjogren's (Ss)? What are the implications of the presence of anti-Ro (SSA) antibodies in the sera of these patients? (2) Are there, in addition to anti-Ro (SSA) antibodies, any other predicting factors for D-penicillamine toxicity in RA patients? Do these patients constitute a disease subgroup?

The clinical and serologic findings of 25 patients with anti-Ro (SSA) antibodies and RA of more than 5 years duration were compared with those of 50 RA patients without anti-Ro (SSA) antibodies with similar disease duration [21]. In both groups almost three-fourths of the patients satisfied the 1958 ARA criteria [3] for classical RA and the remaining those for definite RA. According to the 1987 revised criteria (4) all patients fullfilled the diagnosis of RA. The anti-Ro (SSA) positive individuals, compared with the anti-Ro (SSA) negative ones, were younger female patients. In the majority of the anti-Ro (SSA) positive patients the disease started symmetrically in the small joints of the hands, progressed to the larger joints of the upper extremities in 87% and to the small and large joints of the lower extremities in 85% and 63%, respectively. In 80% of the patients, hand X-rays revealed erosive disease. Similar features were seen in the anti-Ro (SSA) negative population. Extra-articular manifestations were observed with similar frequencies in both groups. In contrast, subjective xerophthalmia, positive rose Bengal staining of the cornea and a labial minor salivary gland biopsy compatible with Ss were more prevalent in the anti-Ro (SSA) positive RA patients. Patients from this group were also significantly more often positive for rheumatoid factor (RF) ($p < 0.001$) although in titers lower than the anti-Ro (SSA) negative group [10]; they also more often had positive ANA tests ($p < 0.001$) and D-penicillamine side effects compared with the anti-Ro (SSA) negative group ($p < 0.005$).

In order to answer the question on the prevalence of secondary sS in Greek RA patients we evaluated 143 unselected patients and a 31% prevalence of sS in RA was found. The diagnosis of sS was established when a patient with a positive minor labial salivary gland biopsy ($\geq 2 +$ score) [22] had keratoconjunctivitis sicca (KCS) (positive rose Bengal staining of the cornea and/or the combination of subjective xerophthalmia and positive Schirmer's test) and/or xerostomia (subjective xerostomia and decreased parotid flow rate). Parotid gland enlargement was unusual, and extraglandular manifestations, with the exception of diffuse interstitial lung disease, were very uncommon in all sS patients. Anti-Ro (SSA) antibodies were detected in 23.5% of the patients with sS and 6.4% of patients without. In conclusion, sS in our RA patients is common, benign and subclinical, requiring specific tests for diagnosis [23].

To answer the second question, on the existence of predicting factors, in addition to anti-Ro (SSA) antibodies markers, for D-penicillamine toxicitiy in RA patients, we retrospectively evaluated 62 consecutive RA patients [24]. The clinical picture in both groups was similar, but the group with D-penicillamine was characterized by a high prevalence of anti-Ro (SSA) antibodies ($p < 0.01$) or circulating cryoglobulins ($p < 0.001$).

In conclusion, the Greek RA patients have, in general, a pattern of disease similar to that described by others, but the systemic (extra-articular) manifestations are less often observed. In addition, a subgroup of Greek RA patients with anti-Ro (SSA) antibodies are usually women with disease onset at a younger age, with more frequent sS manifestations and a tendency to develop side effects after D-peniicillamine treatment. These patients, who were initially diagnosed as having RA, continue after 5 years observation to present the same clinical pattern. Most importantly, deformities and erosions characteristic of classical RA are evident in the majority of our RA patients, a finding which argues strongly against SLE or primary Sjogren's syndrome (pSs), a term applied for a chronic autoimmune inflammatory disorder characterized of Ss in the absence of any other connective tissue disease. The arthritis of SLE and pSs is usually a mild transient synovitis, which does not lead to joint destruction [25, 26]. Moreover, the absence of anti-Sm and anti-DNA antibodies argues against the diagnosis of SLE [27]. Antibodies to Sm are directed against the Sm antigen, which is a complex of several small nuclear RNA (SnRNA) species, the URNAs (U_1 to U_6 RNAs), which at least eight polypeptides [9]. Thus, the presence of anti-Ro (SSA) antibodies in patients with a clinical picture of RA should not discourage the diagnosis of RA, at least in Greek patients.

Immunogenetic Considerations

RA is considered to be an autoimmune disease caused by T cell mediated inflammation and damage of articular elements. The activation of T cells involves the recognition of an antigen, coupled to an HLA class II molecule by the T cell receptor [28]. The nature of the antigen is unknown at present. Regarding the MHC gene products implicated in this interaction, studies of several ethnic groups have shown a positive association of RA with the serologically defined specificity HLA-DR4 [29]. HLA-DR4 is also associated with more aggressive disease [5]. Exceptions to this rule exist; for instance, the RA in black Americans [30] and Asian immigrants living in the UK, is associated with HLA-DR1 and not HLA-DR4 antigen [31].

Several reports from Mediterranean countries also argue against a unique association of RA with the serologically defined HLA-DR4 antigen. A report from Spain has suggested a more close association with HLA-DR1 rather than HLA-DR4 specificity [32]. An earlier study of Israeli Jews also suggested an association with HLA-DR1 alloantigen [33], while recently only a weak, nonsignificant association with HLA-DR4 was documented [34]. A report from Greece showed a lack of association of RA with HLA antigens, and only a weak, statistically in significant association was observed with HLA-DR1 and HLA-DR4 [14]. A report from Northern Italy [35] did not show any HLA association, although HLA-DR1 was increased in RA patients without extra-articular manifestations while B8 and DR3 were increased in patients with extra-articular disease features. The latter finding is in agreement with another report correlating HLA-B8, -DR3 phenotype with rheumatoid vasculitis [36]. In another report from Italy, a strong association between HLA-DR4 was found, but no correlation between HLA-DR4 and RF, and consequently no association between HLA-DR4 and articular erosions were seen [37]. A low frequency of HLA-DR2 antigen was also noted in the same report, which is in agreement with the findings concerning other Caucasian populations [12].

All these observations led investigators to ask the following question: Is there any gene product that possibly can be implicated in the pathogenesis of RA? The human HLA class II locus (HLA-D locus) has three major subregions, HLA-DR, HLA-DQ, HLA-DP, encoding a number of highly polymorphic surface glycoproteins. These glycoproteins consist of an α and a β chain which are not covalently linked and together form the serologically defined HLA-DR antigens [38]. In the case of HLA-DR antigens the β chain is the polymorphic one. Two β chains are expressed DRβ1 and DRβ3 [39]. DRβ1 encodes all the known HLA-DR specificities, while DRβ3 encodes HLA-DRW52 and HLA-DRW53 specificities. DNA sequence analysis of the HLA-DR molecules has revealed that most of the polymorphisms are clustered into three hypervariable regions located in the first domain of the DRβ1 gene [39]. Using cellular typing techniques, HLA-DR4 can be subdivided into five subtypes. HLA-DW4, -DW10, -DW14 and -DW15 [40]. Sequence analysis of the above subtypes has shown that all of their differences lie within the third hypervariable region [41].

When the position of this region was examined in the proposed class II structure, it was found that it was located within the peptide binding groove and thus could influence the immune response [39].

The above findings indicate that the HLA-DR 4 specificity (defined serologically in population studies) is based on a particular configuration of amino acids in one of the hypervariable regions of the glycoprotein determined by an allele at the DRβ 1 locus [6]. This specificity however, does not take into account the whole repertoire of DR 4 molecule polymorphisms, and a number of epitopes shared between HLA-DR 4 and other DR molecules [42]. The experience from Mediterranean countries, mentioned previously, strongly supports the idea of Gregersen et al., that susceptibility to RA may be due to a group of related epitopes found in common among some HLA-DR 4 and HLA-DR 1 alleles [43]. The association of RA with HLA-DR 1 in Israeli Jews and with HLA-DR 4, -DW 15 in Japanese was explained by Fathman and colleagues by the fact that both of these genes share the same epitope in the third hypervariable region [39]. Nevertheless, the susceptibility to the disease and its severity on immunogenetic grounds is more complex. A higher incidence of the HLA-DR 4, HLA-DQW 3.1 haplotype has been observed, especially in the more severe forms of the disease [44]. It seems, therefore, that HLA-DQ and HLA-DP alleles can be involved in particular disease patterns.

In the light of the previously mentioned work we concentrated again on the HLA association in Greek RA patients. Using the Taq 1 restriction enzyme and DRβ, DQα probes, the DNAs of 57 Greek RA patients and 37 controls were characterized for restriction fragments length polymorphisms (RFLPs) associated with DR 4. Three DRβ bands, 14.8 kb, 6.1 kb and 5.4 kb, were observed at significantly higher frequency in patients than in controls. A 5.3 kb band that hybridized to a DQα probe (associated with DR 4, DR 7 and DR 9) was found at a higher frequency in RA patients, although this increase did not reach statistical significance [45]. In view of the lack of any HLA association with RA in Greeks, previously documented using serological techniques, the above results suggest that some of HLA class II association with RA may exist in Greeks at the DNA level. Finally, investigators from Italy, using a monoclonal antibody (XI 21.4) for cellular typing, found that this antibody was highly correlated with the HLA-DR 1, -DR 4 and -DRW 10 antigenic specificities [46].

In conclusion, the immunogenetic studies seem to be rather helpful in understanding the mechanisms of initiation of disease and its dissimilarities in different ethnic groups than in discovering its cause. The weak HLA-DR 4 association observed in individuals from Mediterranean countries possibly explains the observed low incidence of extra-articular disease manifestations in our populations. However, in a recent report from Italy, even in patients with extra-articular manifestations, the incidence of HLA-DR 4 was low [35]. It should be stressed also that, in addition to genetic factors, other factors may influence disease expression. This hypothesis is supported by a study from South Africa, which revealed an increasing incidence and severity of RA in rural compared to unrbanzed African populations [47]. Thus, the variability factor influencing disease expression may lie in the environment [6].

References

1. Short CL (1959) Rheumatoid arthritis: historical aspects. J Chron Dis 10:367–387
2. Ropes MW, Bennet GA, Cobb S, Jacox R, Jessar RA (1956) Proposed diagnostic criteria for rheumatoid arthritis. Bull Rheum Dis 7:121–124
3. Ropes MW, Bennett GA, Cobb S, Jacox R, Jessar RA (1958) Revision of diagnostic criteria for rheumatoid arthritis. Bull Rheum Dis 9:175–176
4. Arnett FC, Edworthy SM, Bloch DA, McShane DJ, Fries JF, Healey LA, Kaplan SR, Liang MH, Luthra HS, Medsger TA Jr, Mitchell DM, Neustadt DH, Pinds RS, Schaller JG, Sharp JT, Wilder RL, Hunder GG (1988) The American Rheumatism Association 1987 revised criteria for the classification of rheumatoid arthritis. Arthritis Rheum 31:315–24
5. Bennett JC (1988) Rheumatoid arthrits – clinical features. In: Schumacher RH Jr (ed) Primer on the rheumatic diseases. Arthritis Foundation, Atlanta GA: 88–92, 9th Ed
6. Woodrow JC (1988) Immunogenetics of Rheumatoid Arthritis (Editorial). J Rheum 15(1):1–3
7. Moutsopoulos HM, Giotaki H, Maddison PJ, Mavridis AC, Drosos AA, Skopouli FN (1984) Antibodies to cellular antigens in Greek patients with autoimmunen rheumatic diseases: anti-Ro (SSA) antibody a possible marker of D-penicillamine intolerance. Ann Rheum Dis 43:285–287
8. Rader MD, O'Brien C, Liu Y, Harley JB, Reichlin M (1989) Heterogeneity of the Ro (SSA) antigen. J Clin Invest 83:1293–1298
9. Hardin JA (1988) The molecular biology of autoantibodies. In: Schumacher RH Jr (ed), Primer of the rheumatic diseases, Arthritis Foundation, Atlanta GA: 32–35, 9th Edn
10. Moutsopoulos HM, Skopouli FN, Sarras AK, Tsampoulas C, Mavridis AK, Constanto-poulos SH, Maddison PJ (1985) Anti-Ro (SSA) positive rheumatoid arthritis (RA): a clinicoserological group of patients with high incidence of D-penicillamine side effects. Ann Rheum Dis 44:215–219
11. Panayi GS, Wooley P, Batchelor JR (1988) Genetic basis of rheumatoid disease. HLA antigens, disease manifestations and toxic reaction to drugs. Br Med J ii:1326–1328
12. Emery P, Panayi GS, Huston G, Welsh RH (1984) D-penicillamine induced toxicity in rheumatoid arthritis: The role of sulphoxidation status and HLA-DR$_3$. J Rheum 11(5):626–632
13. Bell DA, Maddison PJ (1980) Serologic in relationship to clinical features of disease and HLA antigens. Arthritis Rheum 25:1268–1274
14. Papasteriades CA, Kappou ID, Skopouli FN, Farla MN, Fostiropoulos GA, Moutsopou-los HM (1985) Lack of HLA-antigen association in Greek rheumatoid arthritis patients. Rheumatol Int 5:201–203
15. Andonopoulos AP, Galanopoulou V, Drosos AA, Moutsopoulos HM (1987) Rheumatoid arthritis in Greece: manifestations in different age groups. Rheumatol Int 7:101–105
16. Tarkeltaub R, Esdaile J, DeCary F, Tannenbaum H (1983) A clinical study of older age rheumatoid arthritis with comparison to a younger onset group. J Rheumatol 10:418–424
17. Deal CL, Meenan RF, Goldenberg DL, Anderson JJ, Sack B, Pastan RS, Cohen AS (1985) The clinical features of elderly onset rheumatoid arthritis: a comparison with younger onset disease of similar duration. Arthritis Rheum 28:987–994
18. Mongan ES, Atwater EC (1968) Comparison of patients with seropositive and seronega-tive rheumatoid arthritis. Med Clin North Am 52:533–538
19. Masi AT, Maldonado-Cocco JA, Kaplan SB, Feigenbaum SL, Chandler RW (1976) Prospective study of the early course of rheumatoid arthritis in younger adults: comparison of patients with and without rheumatoid factor positivity at entry and identification of variables corrleating with outcome. Sem Arthritis Rheum 5:299–326
20. Alarcon GS, Koopman WJ, Acton RJ, Barger BO (1982) Seronegative rheumatoid arthritis: a distinct immunogenetic disease? Arthritis Rheum 50:507

21. Skopouli FN, Andonopoulos AP, Moutsopoulos HM (1988) Clinical implications of the presence of anti-Ro (SSA) antibodies in patients with rheumatoid arthritis. J Autoimmun 3:381–388
22. Tarpley TM, Anderson LG, White CL (1974) Minor salivary gland involvement in Sjogren's syndrome. Oral Surg 37:64–74
23. Andonopoulos AP, Drosos AA, Skopouli FN, Acritidis NC, Moutsopoulos HM (1987) Secondary Sjogren's syndrome in Rheumatoid Arthritis. J Rheum 14:1098–1103
24. Vlachoyiannopoulos PG, Skopouli FN, Drosos AA, Moutsopoulos HM (1991) D-penicillamine toxicity in rheumatoid arthritis patients: anti-Ro(SSA) antibodies and cryoglobulinemia are prediciting factors. J Rheum 18:44–49
25. Castro-Paltronieri A, Alarcon-Segovia D (1983) Articular manifestations of primary Sjogren's syndrome. J Rheum 10:485–488
26. Tsampoulas CG, Skopouli FN, Sartoris DJ, Kaplan P, Kursunoglu S, Pineda C, Resnick D, Moutsopoulos HM (1986) Hand radiographic changes in patients with primary and secondary Sjogren's syndrome. Scand J Rheumatol 15:333–339
27. Moutsopoulos HM, Chused TM, Mann DL, Klippel JH, Fauci AS, Frank MM, Lawley TJ, Hamburger MI (1980) Sjogren's sydrome (Sicca syndrome): current issues. Ann Intern Med 92:212–226
28. Fathman CG, Frelinger JG (1983) T-lymphocyte clones. Ann Rev Immunol 1:633–655
29. Zvaifler NJ (1988) Rheumatoid arthritis – epidemiology, etiology, rheumatoid factor, pathology, pathogenesis. In: Schumacher RH Jr (ed), Primer of the rheumatic diseases, Arthritis Foundation, Atlanta GA: 85–87, 9th Edn
30. Alarcon GS, Koopman WJ, Acton RT (1983) DR antigen distribution in blacks with rheumatoid arthritis. J Rheumatol 10:579–583
31. Woodrow JC, Nichol FE, Zaphiropoulos G (1981) DR antigens and rheumatoid arthritis: a study of two populations. Br Med J 283:1287–1288
32. Nunez-Roldan A, Arguer-Zuazua E, Villechonous-Pineda E, dela Prada-Arroyo M (1982) Estudios de los antigenos HLA-DR en la arthritis rumatoides. Rev Esp Rheum 9:9–11
33. Schiff B, Mizrachi Y, Orgad S (1982) Association of HLA-DW$_{31}$ and HLA-DR$_1$ with adult rheumatoid arthritis. Ann Rheum Dis 41:403–404
34. Brautbar C, Naparstek Y, Yaron M (1986) Immunogenetics of rheumatoid arthritis. Israel Tissue Antigens 28:8–14
35. Ferraccioli GF, Savi M (1988) Association between DR antigens, rheumatoid arthritis with and without extra-articular features and SLE in northern Italy. J Rheum 15:51–53
36. Cunningham TJ, Tait BD, Mathews TD (1987) Clinical rheumatoid vasculitis associated with B8-DR3 phenotype. Rheumatol Int 2:137–139
37. Lulli P, Cappellaci S, Morellini M, Galleazzi M, Schiavetti L, Tuzi T (1983) HLA antigens and rheumatoid arthritis (letter). Arthritis Rheum 26:1053
38. Moller G (1983) Molecular genetics of class I and class II MHC antigens. Immunol Rev 70:193–218
39. Morel AP, Fathman CG (1989) Immunogenetics of rheumatoid arthritis. J Rheum 16:421–423
40. Reinsmoen N, Bach FH (1982) Five HLA-D clusters associated with DR4. Hum Immunol 4:249–258
41. Anderson PK, Shen K, Song Q (1986) Molecular diversitiy of HLA-DR4 haplotypes. Proc Natl Acad Sci USA 83:2642–2646
42. Nepom BS, Nepom GT, Michelson E (1983) Electrophoretic analysis of human HLA-DR antigens from HLA-DR4 homozygous cell lines: correlation between β chain diversity and HLA-D. Proc Natl Acad Sci USA 80:6962–6966
43. Gregersen PK, Silver J, Winchester RJ (1987) The shared epitope hypothesis: an approach to understanding the molecular genetics of susceptibility to rheumatoid arthritis. Arthritis Rheum 40:1205–1213
44. Singal DP, Benson WG, Kasan YB (1988). HLA-DQ polymorphism in rheumatoid arthritis. Lancet i:58–59

45. Cutboush S, Ollier W, Papasteriades C, Awad J, Boki K, Moutsopoulos HM, Festenstein H (To be published) Association of DR4 related RFLP bands and RA in Greeks. J Autoimmunity
46. Cappelaci S, Tuzi T, Mazzilli MC, Morellini M, Lullil P, Galeazzi M (1987) HLA antigens and adult rheumatoid arthritis: a study with a monoclonal antibody. Clin Exp Rheumatol 5:63–66
47. Brighton SW (1987) Studies on populations with high and low prevalence rates of rheumatoid arthritis (abstract). Clin Exp Rheumatol (suppl) 5:186

Pathogenesis

Pathogenesis of Rheumatoid Arthritis: Cellular and Cytokine Interactions

M. Feldmann[1], F. M. Brennan[1], M. Field[2], and R. N. Maini[2]

[1] Charing Cross Sunley Research Centre, Lurgan Avenue, Hammersmith, London, W6 8LW, UK
[2] Kennedy Institute of Rheumatology, 6 Bute Gardens, Hammersmith, London, W6 7DW, UK

Overall Framework

Rheumatoid arthritis (RA) is an inflammatory disease with autoimmune features chiefly affecting synovial joints. In more severe cases there are extra-articular and systemic complications. The basic aetiology of this disease is not known, but there is a clear genetic predisposition. This maps clearly, but not exclusively, to the HLA-DR region; however, genetic predisposition is not sufficient to explain the disease, as identical twins are often ($\sim 50\%$) discordant [25].

Investigation of the cellular composition of RA joints reveals an extensive infiltrate of haemopoietic cells, chiefly T cells, macrophages and plasma cells. Many of these appear to be activated, as judged by morphological criteria and surface markers. One of the most important activaton markers is the expression of HLA class II antigens. These are expressed on a wide variety of cell types: approximately 50% of T lymphocytes, B lymphocytes, monocytes/macrophages, dendritic cells, endothelial cells, and fibroblasts. Augmented expression of HLA class II has functional relevance, as it is essential for antigen presentation. Increased expression of adhesion molecules, such as the intercellular adhesion molecule-1 (ICAM-1), is also of functional relevance since it increases binding of lymphoid cells, augments antigen presentation and may be important for the influx of cells.

Over the past few years, we have established an overall concept of the pathogenesis of autoimmune diseases [4, 15], which has been tested most extensively (due to readier access to tissue) in Grave's disease, i. e. autoimmune hyperthyroidism. The basic premise is that the maintenance phase of the disease is due to continual interactions between autoantigen reactive T lymphocytes and tissue antigen presenting cells. In thyroid disease, it has been shown that thyroid epithelial cells can present antigen, either influenza peptides [27] or surface autoantigens [26]. It is envisaged that the autoantigen reactive cells, upon stimulation by class II expressing thyrocytes acting as antigen presenting cells (APC), release cytokines which maintain thyrocyte class II expression and

Smolen, Kalden, Maini (Eds.)
Rheumatoid Arthritis
© Springer-Verlag Berlin Heidelberg 1992

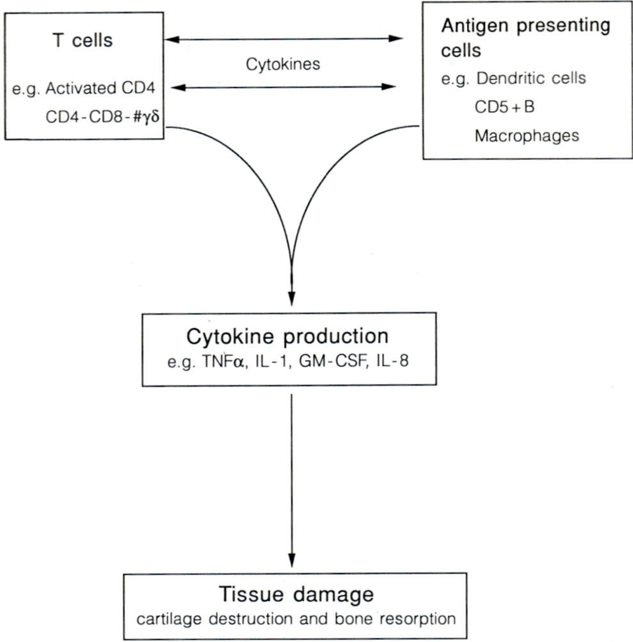

Fig. 1. Scheme of the cellular and cytokine interactions in rheumatoid arthritis

antigen presenting function. Much evidence has been accumulated to support this concept, such as the cloning of thyrocyte specific and stimulatable T cells from the thyroid infiltrate [26, 14], and the demonstration that cytokines such as interferon-γ (IFNγ) and tumour necrosis factor) (TNF) induce thyrocyte class II expression. Cytokines such as IFNγ and TNF, interleukin-1 (IL-1) and IL-6 have been detected in the thyroid [20, 47].

RA would appear to fit into this overall scheme, as there is abundant local antigen presenting capacity [16], autoantigen reactive T cells are demonstrable [28] and cytokines are abundant [11, 6] (Fig. 1).

T Cells in RA

T lymphocytes are one of the most abundant cells in active RA, ranging from 20%–50% of the cells extracted from synovial membrane. Many studies have documented their properties. $CD4^+$ cells are more abundant than $CD8^+$ in the membrane, but not necessarily in the synovial fluid. The $CD4^+$ cells tend to concentrate in perivascular nodules, whereas the $CD8^+$ are more diffusely scattered. $CD4^+$ cells have been subdivided into subsets, depending on their CD45 expression. In normal blood approximaltely half are $CD45RA^+$,

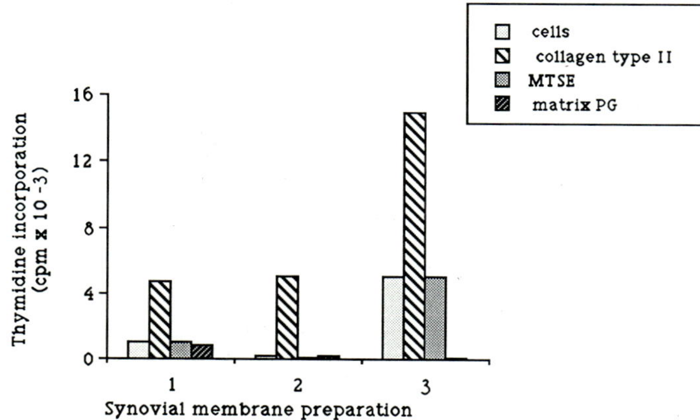

Fig. 2. Proliferative response of collagen type II specific clones. Cloned T cells from three separate synovial membrane preparations from one RA patient were cultured with autologous irradiated cells with or without antigen indicated. *Cells,* T cells with autologous feeders; *collagen type II,* 100 µg/ml; *MTSE,* mycobacterium tuberculosis soluble extract; *matrix PG,* matrix proteoglycan

indicating a "virgin state". Essentially all the cells in the RA joint lack CD45RA and express CD45RO/CD29, indicating a "primed" or "memory" state [32]. This is not surprising since there is evidence for an ongoing immune response, as judged by the expression of T cell activation markers, such HLA class II (in 50%), and IL-2 receptors (2%–12%) [5, 28].

T lymphocytes may also be classified according to their T cell receptor for antigen. In normal blood the great majority ($> 95\%$) express a heterodimer of α and β chains, whereas a minority use γ and δ chains. Of interest was the observation [8] that there was selective enrichment of γδ T cells in active RA joints. This result is discussed in more detail in the chapter by Plater-Zyberk et al. in this volume).

An important question is whether T cells have a critical role in RA. Various lines of evidence support this possibility. First, is the abundance of T cells in RA joints; virtually none are present in normal joints. Second, is their activated status (see above). Third, is the fact that the proportions of different types of T cells present in RA joints are not the same as in blood (as discussed above), indicating that it is not a reflection of passive trafficking due to an inflammatory response. Fourth, is the observation that antigen specific T cells are present, are activated and persist in RA joints. For example, we found that collagen type II specific T cells were present and expressed IL-2 receptors in three operative specimens from an RA patient taken over a period of more than 4 years (Fig. 2) [28]. T cells, including γδ T cells responsive to heat-shock proteins, have also been described in RA joints (see chapter by Plater-Zyberk et al., this volume. Their relevance to the disease process is not clear, as normal individuals and patients with other joint diseases also have them. Clearly much more work is needed in this area.

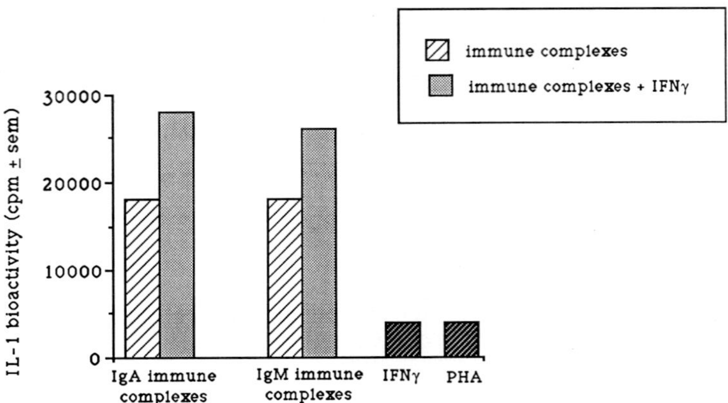

Fig. 3. Induction of IL-1 bioactivity with immune complexes and synergy with interferon-γ. Immune complexes were either IgA or IgM-containing as indicated. *IFNγ*, interferon-gamma; *PHA*, phytohaemagglutinin. IL-1 bioactivity was measured in the mouse comitogenic thymocyte proliferation assays and is indicated as counts per minute thymidine incorporation

In experimental models of arthritis, T cell dependence can be demonstrated directly, either by transfer of T cell lines and clones, which elicits disease, e. g. in collagen arthritis [43], or by T cell depletion [37]. The first of these obviously cannot be attempted in humans, but there are reports that treatment with anti-T cell (e. g. anti CD4) antibodies has an effect in human RA [21]. Taken together, and noting that all known autoimmune diseases are T cell dependent, it is very likely that RA is also T cell dependent.

B Cell Lineage

Plasma cells are abundant in RA. Some, but not all, are involved in the production of rheumatoid factors. Rheumatoid factor immune complexes have been shown to induce the production of cytokines such as IL-1 and TNF (Fig. 3) [13].

The specificity of the antibodies produced in RA joints has been investigated by the cell fusion technique using the human B cell fusion partner, SPAZ4. High frequencies of hybridomas producing IgM and IgG were detected. While a few of these were "polyreactive" and some produced rheumatoid factors and antibody to collagen type II, the majority did not bind to a battery of autoantigens tested. Klareskog and colleagues have recently described that the majority of RA joints contain B cells producing to collagen type II, detected by the ELISA spot technique [40].

Antigen Presenting Cells

There are abundant cells with antigen presenting capacity in human RA joints. Which of these are of major importance is a controversial question. Macrophages and monocytes represent about 30%–50% of the cell pool, and there is evidence for their activation, e.g. augmented HLA-DQ and diminished CD14 expression. Dendritic cells (DC) are present in increased numbers. Regrettably, due to lack of specific markers for human DC, their numbers are not easy to quantitate; however, cell separation studies by several groups have all demonstrated augmented numbers of DC in rheumatoid synovial fluid, comprising of 5%–7% of the mononuclear cells, whereas synovial tissue contained few DC [31, 44]. These DC from RA synovial fluid were shown to be potent APC, but not more so than normal DC.

CD5$^+$ B cells have Fc receptors and many produce rheumatoid factors. These may permit CD5$^+$ B cells to take up immune complexes and present the relevant antigens. The possible importance of CD5$^+$ B cells in antigen presentation in RA has been discussed [30].

Cell Interactions

The importance of cell interactions in the rheumatoid joint can be inferred from immunohistological studies. There are close appositions of T cells and APC in nodules and other sites throughout the synovial membrane. However, there are very few T cells in the pannus [17], suggesting that different interactions may prevail in this specialized site.

Dissociated cultured RA joint cells, in the absence of any extrinsic stimulus, rapidly form aggregates. This suggests that interactions are of critical importance in the disease process. Experimentally, it is possible to demonstrate that cell interactions are of importance in RA using an in vitro model. We have noted that cultured RA synovial cells, in the absence of extrinsic stimulation, retain many features of active RA. Thus, HLA class II expression is found to persist in vitro at both the protein and mRNA levels provided the whole mixture of joint cells is cultured (Fig. 4). If only the adherent cells (chiefly fibroblasts) are cultured, class II expression does not persist in culture [41]. The persistence of cytokine production is discussed below.

The role of T cells in the persistence of class II expression has been studied by depleting T cells using a combination of lysis with antibody and complement, and antibody coated magnetic beads. Even with an incomplete depletion of cells, a marked reduction in class II expression was noted after 6 days in culture. This emphasizes the importance of cell interactions but does not clarify which T cells are of critical importance nor which are the critical APC.

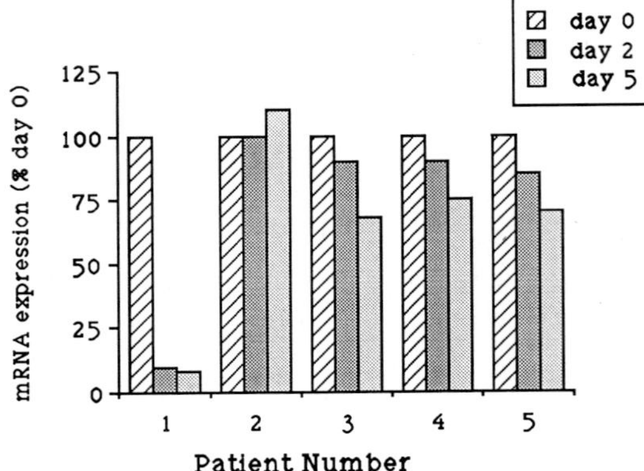

Fig. 4. Expression of DRα mRNA from RA synovial joint cells. Synovial cells from five RA patients were cultured and RNA isolated at times indicated. Amounts of DRα mRNA were determined and are expressed as percentage of basal level

Another cell interaction of critical importance is between blood cells and endothelium in the RA joint. If haematopoietic cells did not enter joints, the RA process could not be sustained. Selective trafficking has been proposed [48].

Cytokine Expression in RA

Since RA is mostly manifest in synovial joints, which are the sites of inflammation and joint destruction, we have chiefly investigated cytokine production in the joints. However, cytokines can also be detected in blood cells by immunostaining, e. g. IL-1α [3]. Whether other cytokines can also be detected in blood cells remains to be established.

Rheumatoid joints contain a wide variety of activated cell types, and so it would be expected that many cytokines would be produced locally in the joint. When we began studies on RA joint cytokine expression, in 1985, slot blotting and cDNA hybridization techniques were used to obtain the maximum amount of data on cytokine expression from a small number of cells. With these techniques, 2×10^6 were used and could provide data on about six or sometimes up to ten cytokines. By densitometry relative quantitation was possible. Further advantages of this technique are its specificity for individual cytokines, ease of performance (same technique for all cytokines), and its resistance to artifacts caused by rheumatoid factors, a problem in binding assays, and "toxic" components of synovial fluid in bioassays [10, 11]. A disadvantage is that cytokine mRNA levels being measured need not always correlate with the levels of cytokine protein produced. This is especially a problem with cytokines known to be post-transcriptionally regulated, e. g. TNFα. If this type of work was initiated again, in 1990, the polymerase chain reaction (PCR) would be used, for its obvious greater sensitivity. Although the use of PCR is not without problems, e. g. quantitation and contamination, the results have been the same as slot blotting, that is, a predominance of IL-1α, abundance of TNFα [9]. In situ hybridization has also yielded analogous results [18].

Table 1. Summary of cytokines produced by RA synovial cells

Cytokine	mRNA	Protein
IL-1α	Yes	Yes
IL-1β	Yes	Yes
TNFα	Yes	Yes
LT	Yes	No
IL-2	Yes	No
IL-3	No	No
IL-4	NA	No
IFNγ	Yes	No
GM-CSF	Yes	Yes
IL-8	Yes	Yes
G-CSF	Yes	NA
M-CSF	No	NA
TGFβ	Yes	Yes
TGFα	Yes	Yes
PDGF-A	Yes	Yes
PDGF-B	Yes	Yes

Due to the wide variety of activated cells it is not surprising that virtually all cytokines sought have been detected. Table 1 summarizes cytokine expression in the RA joint. There are some interesting generalizations that can be made. For example, cytokines which are predominantly macrophage products are abundant at both the mRNA and protein level, e.g. IL-1, TNF, IL-8. In contrast, cytokines produced by T cells are detectable at the mRNA level, but barely detectable at the protein level, e.g. lymphotoxin IFNγ, (LT), IL-2. The reasons for this discrepancy are not yet known, transforming growth factor-β but (TGFβ) which inhibits cytokine production posttranscriptionally, may be responsible. Local consumption of cytokines by cells with high-affinity receptors may also contribute; for example, there are free cell-bound IL-2 receptors in RA joint cells [39].

Cytokines are essential for many processes in RA, such as cell growth and HLA class II expression. However, it is not clear which cytokines are of major importance in different processes. A critical step in the generation of an immune or inflammatory reaction is activation of macrophages and induction of HLA class II expression. IFNγ is potentially the most effective cytokine at inducing HLA class II expression in the absence of other factors [34] However, negligible amounts of IFNγ (or other T cell lymphokines) are produced by rheumatoid synovial cells [19, 6], suggesting that other factors alone or in combination with IFNγ are involved. One possible candidate is the haematopoietic growth factor granulocyte/macrophage colony-stimulating factor (GM-CSF) which induces HLA-DR expression on human monocytes [12] and has been suggested to be both an important macrophage activator and to induce HLA class II expression in the RA joint [1]. Nonetheless, the most significant inhibition of HLA class II expression which we observed in RA synovial cultures was with anti-TNF antibody (unpublished observation) and was greater than with antibodies to IFNγ or GM-CSF. This unlikely to be a direct effect as TNF by itself does not induce HLA class II expression [35]. This suggests that many different cytokines may synergise to induce HLA class II expression or that other as yet undefined molecules may be involved. Alternatively (or in addition) cell-cell interactions through cell adhesion molecules may be necessary to maintain this. Of interest is the observation that TNFα is a potent inducer of many adhesion molecules including ICAM-1 and INCAM-110 (inducible cell adhesion molecule 110 KD – VCAM-1) [33, 38].

The activation and differentiation of B cells is also mediated by cytokines of which IL-4 and IL-6 are the most important. IL-4 is a potent B cell growth factor but is detected in negligible amounts in RA synovial cells (unpublished observation) or in synovial fluid. In contrast, high levels of IL-6 have been detected both in RA synovial fluid and in RA synovial membrane cells [22]. The presence of high levels of IL-6 in RA joints may explain the infiltration of the synovium by large numbers of plasma cells and the production of autoantibodies including rheumatoid factors. LT and TNFα are also known to be capable of acting as B cell growth factors [24]. The presence of rheumatoid factor-containing immune complexes may further contribute to the pathogenesis of rheumatoid by inducing the production of IL-1 [13]. In addition, it has recently been shown that Epstein-Barr virus (EBV)-transformed B cells can use IL-6 as a growth factor [42] and that IL-6 is produced by such cells [46].

T cell growth is clearly controlled by cytokines. For many years, after the discovery of "T cell growth factor" and the purification, cloning and expression of IL-2, it was thought that all T cell growth was IL-2 mediated. Subsequent work has shown that the process is much more complex. IL-4, initially described as a B cell stimulating factor, is also a potent growth factor for many T cells and IL-7, described as a pre-B growth factor, is also highly active [29, 45]. T cell activation is noted in RA, with many cells expressing HLA class II (20%–50%) and a few (2%–12%) expressing IL-2 receptors. However, the mechanism of T cell growth is unclear, since while IL-2 mRNA is found the protein is not readily detectable. This could be due to absorption, IL-2 inhibitors, such as the soluble IL-2 receptor [39] or post-transcriptional regulation. IL-4 is also not readily detectable for possibly the same reasons. The presence of IL-7 is currently unknown, but it is clearly an important candidate. A fourth cytokine with T cell growth promoting activity in the mouse, p40, has been described, but it is not clear whether it is present in RA joints. A synergy between all these cytokines could permit T cell growth in the absence of significant protein levels. This possibility requires investigation using RA joint cells in culture.

Fibrosis is an important component and complication of RA. It participates in deformations of joints, and pulmonary fibrosis can be a damaging systemic complication. Which cytokine drives the fibrosis in the RA joint (or other tissues) is not currently known. There are abundant candidates present in the RA joint, e. g. IL-1α and β and TNFα. These may act indirectly via platelet-derived growth factor (PDGF) induction [36], TGFα, or TGFβ. The presence of members of the FGF family is not known but is likely.

Cytokine Localization

Most cytokine effects are exerted locally over short ranges and only occasionally act at long distances, e. g. IL-1 and IL-6 in the induction of fever. Determining which cells make cytokines, where they are situated, and their neighbouring cells with which they could interact with most effectively are thus questions of importance.

Two techniques have been developed which permit the localization of cells producing cytokines. In situ hybridization allows the detection of cells containing cytokine mRNA. It has the advantage that it unambiguously detects producing cells and not cells having bound cytokine, but suffers from the disadvantage that, like all mRNA studies, there is no evidence that the mRNA is translated into protein.

Immunohistological approaches have the advantage of detecting cyto-kine protein, but whether the cell detected produces cytokines, or has bound cytokines via receptors is not always clear. If staining of the Golgi is noted, it is a producing cell [2]. Cytoplasmic staining usually signifies a producing cell, whilst ring staining could be a cell which has bound cyto-kines. However, the limited number of cytokine receptors and the fact that they are readily internalized makes it unlikely that many cells which exter-nally bind cytokines are easily detected with the existing sensitivity of immunostaining assays.

Cytokine localization techniques are thus a valuable addition to other techniques in obtaining a comprehensive picture of cytokine production. They are particularly useful in defining cytokine production in highly specialized parts of the RA joint, such as the lining layer and the pannus. There is also considerable potential for defining which cells are the predominant sources of various cytokines.

With these techniques, it has been established that the lining layer is a major source of cytokine production – for TNFα and IL-6, for example. Most important has been the observation that the cytokines capable of degrading cartilage and bone, IL-1 and TNF, are found at the cartilage-synovium junction, the pannus [17].

Cytokine Regulation

Our initial results investigating IL-1 expression revealed that all samples contained IL-1 mRNA. Since, following experimental activation in vitro, IL-1 (and other cytokine) mRNA expression is brief, the fact that all RA samples were positive suggested that cytokine production in the RA joint may be relatively stable and persistent. In a chronic disease only persisent features can be relevant to the maintenance of the disease process. The persistence of

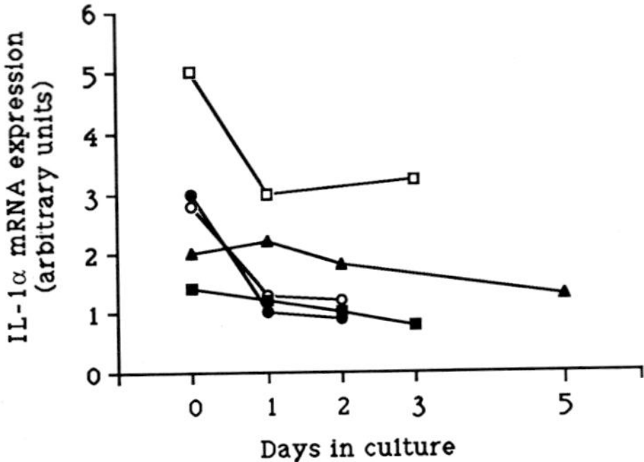

Fig. 5. Levels of IL-1α mRNA in synovial cells. RNA was extracted from synovial cells from five patients at times indicated. RNA was blotted onto nitrocellulose and probed for IL-1α

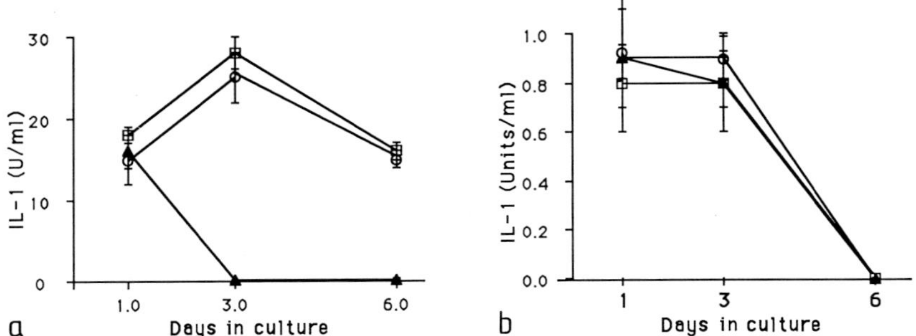

Fig. 6. a Rheumatoid arthritis or b osteoarthritis synovial membrane cells were incubated in culture with polyclonal antibodies to TNFα (△) lymphotoxin (□) or equivalent amount of control rabbit IgG (○). IL-1 levels were measured in the supernatants after 1, 3 and 6 days in culture by the comitogenic thymocyte assay

cytokine production therefore suggested that it was of importance in the pathogenesis [11].

Cytokine persistence was directly tested in vitro by culturing dissociated RA joint cells in the absence of extrinsic stimulation. The initial results showed that both IL-1α andIL-1β mRNA persisted for up to 5 days culture in (Fig. 5) [11]. This indicates that the signals necessary to regulate cytokine production are present in the culture and can be analysed.

Neutralizing antibodies were chosen as the tool to investigate the signals involved in regulating IL-1 production. Since the strongest cytokine signals in the regulation of production were found to be TNFα and TNFβ (LT), neutralizing antibodies to these two cytokines were used in the initial experiments. The results were clear-cut. Anti-TNFα, but not anti-TNFβ or contrl rabbit Ig, inhibited IL-1 production after the first day of culture (Fig. 6a) [7]. Assays at the mRNAlevel showed more rapid kinetics; however, the lack of an early protein effect indicated that already ongoing IL-1 synthesis was not affected, but that subsequent activation was blocked. As a control, the same antibodies were used on cultures of osteoarthritis (OA) joint cells. Despite the presence of immunoreactive TNFα, there was no effect of anti-TNFα on the low IL-1 levels in OA (Fig. 6b). The reasons for this difference are being investigated.

The finding that TNFα was the dominant signal regulating IL-1 production was surprising. It had been anticipated that multiple signals were of importance, including those from immune complexes and perhaps other non cytokines. However, samples from the first seven patients behaved in this way, regardless of the patient's therapy. This led us to investigate what other effects of anti-TNFα on the diseases process may be. It has been postulated that GM-CSF is an important cytokine in RA, as it is an inducer of class II on monocytes and induces cytokine production and macrophage activation [1]. It was thus of interest to determine which cytokine regulates the production of GM-CSF joint cell cultures. Anti-TNFα was found to inhibit markedly the production of GM-CSF, but at a slower rate than inhibition of IL-1, being virtually complete by day 5. We have also found that anti-TNF partially inhibits class II expression and also inhibits the aggregation normally found in these cultures. The effects of TNF in RA joints can be summarized as follows:

1. Induces PGE_2 production and collagenase release causing cartilage destruction
2. Induces activation of osteoblasts which activate osteoclasts
3. Induces synthesis of IL-1 (α and β) causing bone resorption
4. Induces synthesis of GM-CSF which induces HLA class II expression and activates macrophages
5. Induces adhesion molecules such as ICAM-1, INCAM-110 (VCAM-1)
6. Effect on cartilage and bone degradation.

The results obtained in RA are analogous to those recently described in the response to bacteria. Production of TNFα, IL-1 and IL-6 were monitored and peaks of TNFα were found to precede those of IL-1 followed by IL-6. Anti-TNFα abrogated IL-1 and IL-6 production in the animal model. Thus, it seems likely that in RA cultures the dominant position of TNFα merely recapitules the physiological situation.

There are still many interesting issues. Why is TNFα produced in OA without IL-1? Conceivably, the newly described IL-1 or TNF inhibitors may be involved. What controls the production of TNFα in RA? What is the role of potentially inhibitory cytokines in controlling inflammation, e. g. IFNα, TGFβ, oncostatin M, cytokine synthesis inhibitory factor (CSIF)? Investigation of these issues will help to elucidate the mechanisms which contribute to the pathogenesis of RA.

References

1. Alvaro-Garcia JM, Zvaifler NJ, Firestein GS (1989) Cytokines in chronic inflammatory arthritis. Granulocyte/macrophage colony stimulating factor-mediated induction of class II MHC antigen on human monocytes: a possible role in rheumatoid arthitis. J Exp Med 170:865–875
2. Andersson U, Matsuda T (1989) Human interleukin 6 and tumour necrosis factor alpha production studied at a single-cell level. Eur J Immunol 19:1157–1160
3. Barkley D, Feldmann, M, Maini RN (1989) The detection by immunofluorescence of distinct cell populations producing interleukin-1α and interleukin-1β in activated human peripheral blood. J Immunol Meth 120:277–283
4. Bottazzo GF, Pujol-Borrell R, Hanafusa T, Feldmann M (1983) Hypothesis: role of aberrant HLA-DR expression and antigen presentation in the induction of endocrine autoimmunity. Lancet ii:1115–1119
5. Brennan FM, Allard S, Londei M, Savill C, Boylston A, Carrel S, Maini RN, Feldmann M (1988) Heterogeneity of T cell receptor idiotypes in rheumatoid arthritis. Clin Exp Immunol 73:417–423
6. Brennan FM, Chantry D, Jackson AM, Maini RN, Feldmann M (1989) Cytokine production in culture by cells isolated from the synovial membrane. J Autoimmunity 2 (suppl):177–186
7. Brennan FM, Chantry D, Jackson A, Maini RN, Feldmann, M (1989) Inhibitory effect of TNFα antibodies on synovial cell interleukin-1 production in rheumatoid arthritis. Lancet ii:244–247
8. Brennan FM, Londei AM, Jackson A, Hercend T, Brenner MB, Maini RN, Feldmann M (1988) T cells expressing γδ chain receptors in rheumatoid arthritis. J Autoimmunity 1:319–326
9. Brenner CA, Tam AW, Nelson DA, Suzuki N, Fry KE, Larrick JW (1989) Message amplification phenotyping (MAPPing): a technique to simultaneously measure multiple mRNAs from small number of cells. Bio Techniques 7:1096–2003
10. Buchan G, Barrett K, Fukita T, Taniguchi T, Maini RN, Feldmann M (1988) Detection of activated T cell products in the rheumatoid joint using cDNA probes to interleukin 2, IL-2 receptor and interferon γ. Clin Exp Immunol 71:295–301
11. Buchan G, Barrett K, Turner M, Chantry D, Maini RN, Feldmann M (1988) Interleukin-1 and tumour necrosis factor mRNA expression in rheumatoid arthritis: prolonged production of IL-1α. Clin Exp Immunol 73:449–455
12. Chantry D, Turner M, Brennan F, Kingsbury A, Feldmann M (1990) Granulocyte-macrophage colony stimulating factur induces both HLA-DR expression and cytokine production by human monocytes. Cytokine 2 (1):60–67
13. Chantry D, Winearls CG, Maini RN, Feldmann M (1989) Mechanism of immune complex mediated damage: induction of interleukin 1 by immune complexes and synergy with interferon γ and tumour necrosis factor α. Eur J Immunol 19:189–192
14. Dayan CM, Londei M, Corcoran AE, Grubeck-Loebenstein B, James RFL, Rapaport B, Feldmann M (1990) Heterogeneous T cell specificities in Grave's thyroiditis: implications for pathogenesis and immunotherapy of human autoimmunity. Proc Natl Acad Sci 88:7415–7419
15. Feldmann M (1987) Regulation of HLA class II expression and its role in autoimmune disease. In: Autoimmunity and autoimmune disease. Wiley, (Ciba Foundation Symposium 129) Chichester, pp 88–108
16. Feldmann M (1989) Molecular mechanisms involved in human autoimmune diseases: relevance of chronic antigen presentation. Class II expression and cytokine production. Immunology 2 (suppl):66–71
17. Field et al. to be published
18. Firestein GS, Alvaro-Gardia JM, Maki R (1990) Quantitative analysis of cytokine gene expression in rheumatoid arthritis. J Immunol 144:3347–3353

19. Firestein GS, Zvaifler NJ (1987) Peripheral blood and synovial fluid monocyte activation in inflammatory arthritis. II. Low levels of synovial fluid and synovial tissue interferon suggest that γ-interferon is not the primary macrophage activating factor. Arthritis Rheum 30:864–871
20. Grubeck-Loebenstein B, Buchan G, Chantry D, Kassal H, Londei M, Pirich K, Barrett K, Turner M, Waldhäusl W, Feldmann M (1989) Analysis of intrathyroidal cytokine production in thyroid autoimmune disease: thyroid follicular cells produce IL-1α and interleukin-6. Clin Exp Immunol 77:324–330
21. Herzog, C, Walker C, Müller W, Rieber P, Reiter C, Riethmüller G, Wassmer P, Stockinger H, Madic O, Pichler WJ (1989) Anti CD4 antibody treatment of patients with RA: effect on clinical course and circulating T cells. J Autoimmunity 2:627–642
22. Hirano T, Matsuda T, Turner M, Miyasaka N, Buchan G, Tang B, Sato K, Shimizu M, Maini RN, Feldmann, M, Kishimoto T (1988) Excessive production of interleukin 6/B cell stimulatory factor-2 in rheumatoid arthritis. Eur J Immunol 18:1797–1801
23. Holoshitz J, Koning F, Coligan JE, De Bruyn J, Strober S (1989) Isolation of CD4- CD8- mycobacteria-reactive T lymphocyte clones from rheumatoid arthritis synovial fluid. Nature 339:226–229
24. Kehrl JH, Alvarez Mon M, Delsing GA, Fauci AS (1987) Lymphotoxin is an important T cell derived growth factor for human B cells. Science 238:1144–1147
25. Lawrence JS (1970) Rheumatoid arthritis – nature or nurture. Ann Rheum Dis 29:357
26. Londei M, Bottazzo GF, Feldmann M (1985) Human T- cell clones from autoimmune thyroid glands: specific recognition of autologous thyroid cells. Science 228:8–89
27. Londei M, Lamb JR, Bottazzo GF, Feldmann M (1985) Epihelial cells expressing aberrant MHC class II determinants can present antigen to cloned human T cells. Nature 312:639–641
28. Londei M, Savill C, Verhoef A, Brennan F, Leech ZA, Duance V, Maini RN, Feldmann M (1989) Persistence of collagen type II specific T cell clones in the synovial membrane of a patient with RA. Proc Natl Acad Sci 86:636–640
29. Londei M, Verhoef A, Hawrylowicz C, Groves J, De Berardinis P, Feldmann M (1990) Interleukin 7 is a growth factor for mature human T cells. Eur J Immunol 20:425–428
30. Maini RN (1989) Exploring immune pathways in rheumatoid arthritis. Br J Rheumatol 28:466–479
31. March LM (1987) Dendritic cells in the pathogenesis of rheumatoid arthritis. Rheumatol Int 7:93–100
32. Pitzalis C, Kingsley G, Murphy J, Panayi G (1987) Abnormal distribution of the helper-inducer and suppressor-inducer T lymphocyte subsets in the rheumatoid joint. Clin Immunol Immunopathol 45:252–258
33. Pober JS, Gimbrone MA Jr, Lapierre LA, Mendrick DL, Fiers W, Rothlein R, Springer TA (1986) Overlapping patterns of activation of human endothelial cells by interleukin 1, tumour necrosis factor, and immune interferon. J Immunol 137:1893–1896
34. Portillo G, Turner M, Chantry D, Feldmann M (1989) Effect of cytokines on HLA-DR and IL-1 production by a monocytic tumour, THP-1. Immunology 66(2):170–175
35. Pujol-Borrell R, Todd I, Doshi M, Bottazzo GF, Sutton R, Gray D, Adolf GR, Feldmann M (1987) HLA class II induction in human islet cells by interferon-γ plus tumour necrosis factor of lymphotoxin. Nature 326:304–306
36. Raines EW, Dower SK, Ross R (1989) Interleukin 1 mitogenic activity for fibroblasts and smooth muscle cells is due to PDGF AA. Science 243:393–397
37. Range GE, Stiram S, Cooper SM (1985) Prevention of type II collagen – induced arthritis by in vivo treatment with anti-L₃T₄. J Exp Med 162:1105–1110
38. Rice GE, Bevilacqua MP (1989) An inducible endothelial cell surface glycoprotein mediates melanoma adhesion. Science 326:1303–1306
39. Symons JA, Wood NC, Di Giovine FS, Duff GW (1988) Soluble IL-2 receptor in rheumatoid arthritis. J Immunol 141:2612–2616
40. Tarkowski A, Klareskog L, Carlson M, Herberts P, Koopman WJ (1989) Secretion of antibodies to type I and II collagen by synovial tissue cells in patients with rheumatoid arthritis. Arthritis Rheum 32:1087–1092

41. Teyton L, Lotteau V, Turmel P, Arenzana-Seisdedos F, Virelizier J-L, Pujol J-P, Loyau G,
    Piaier-Tonneau D, Auffray C, Charron DJ (1987) HLA DR, DQ and DP antigen
    expression in rheumatoid synovial cells: a biochemical and quantitative study. J Immunol
    138:1730–1738
42. Tosato G, Gerrard TL, Goldman NG, Pike SE (1988) Stimulation of EBV-activated
    human B cells by monocyte products. J Immunol 140:4329–4336
43. Trentham DE, Dyesius RA, David JR (1978) Passive transgene by cells of type II collagen-
    induced arthritis in rats. J Clin Invest 62:359–366
44. Tsai V, Bergroth V, Zvaifler NJ (1989) Dendritic cells in health and disease. In: Feldmann
    M, Maini RN, Woody JN (eds) T cell activation in health and disease. Academic Press,
    New York, pp 33–44
45. Varma C, Chantry D, Brennan F, Turner M, Katz F, Feldmann M (1990) Interleukin-7 and
    interleukin-4 stimulate human thymocyte growth through distinct mechanisms. Cytokine
    1:55–59
46. Yokoi T, Miyawaki T, Yachie A, Kato K, Kasahara Y, Taniguchi N (1990) Epstein-Barr
    virus-immortalized B cells produce IL-6 as an autocrine growth factor. Immunology
    70:100–105
47. Zheng RQH, Abney ER, Grubeck-Loebenstein B, Dayan C, Maini RN, Feldmann M
    (1989) Expression of intercelular adhesion molecule-1 and lymphocyte function associat-
    ed antigen-3 on human thyroid epithelial cells in Graves' and Hashimoto's diseases. J
    Autoimmunity 3:727–736
48. Ziff M (1989) Role of endothelium in chronic inflammation. Springer Semin Immunopa-
    thol 11:199–214

Role of Cellular Adhesion in Rheumatoid Synovitis

M. Ziff

The University of Texas Southwestern Medical Center, Dallas, Texas, USA

The basis for rheumatoid synovitis is a cellular immune response in the sublining tissue of the rheumatoid synovial membrane (RSM). As a consequence of this reaction, cytokines and growth factors are released which mediate a nonspecific amplification of the initial inflammatory focus, proliferation of the synovial tissue, and immunoglobulin and rheumatoid factor synthesis.

It has become known in recent years that the extravascular emigration of the cells which participate in the cellular immune response and their subsequent reactions require a series of adhesive interactions, first of emigrating mononuclear cells with endothelial cells (EC) and subsequently of the extravascular mononuclear cells, reacting either with each other or with connective tissue matrix components. These adhesive events are made possible by receptors and ligands, functioning in the binding of cells to cells and cells to matrix components. It is the purpose of this chapter to describe the role of these adhesion phenomena in the rheumatoid chronic inflammatory reaction.

The Integrin Family of Adhesion Molecules

Emigration of leukocytes from the blood requires initial binding of these cells to the EC of postcapillary venules (PCV). Following emigration, the mononuclear cells adhere to each other and to matrix components. Adhesion of mononuclear cells to matrix proteins facilitates their movement toward inflammatory foci and their retention in such foci. Recognition of these phenome has stimulated intensive study of the role of adhesion molecules in the immune response and in chronic inflammation. From these studies, evidence has emerged for the existence of a supergene family of adhesion molecules, the integrins, which carry out a major portion of the adhesive functions of the leukocytes of the body.

The integrin family, as it occurs on nucleated cells, consists of three subfamilies of glycoprotein heterodimers made up of α and β chains. In each of

Smolen, Kalden, Maini (Eds.)
Rheumatoid Arthritis
© Springer-Verlag Berlin Heidelberg 1992

these, the α chains vary in composition and the β chains are constant [1, 2]. These subfamilies are as follows: (1) CD11/CD18 family, a group of three glycoprotein heterodimers expressed on hematopoietic cells and which contains a common β2 variety of β chain. The latter family is responsible for the binding of leukocytes to EC prior to emigration from the blood and for the adhesive interactions of the extravascular cells which participate in the tissue cellular immune response. (2) VLA receptor family, a group of heterodimers containing a common β1 chain, which is present on a variety of cells, and whose main function is to mediate the adhesion of these cells to extracellular matrix proteins. VLA-4 ($\alpha_4\beta_1$ on lymphocytes also mediates the attachment of these cells to the cytokine-inducible vascular cell adhesion molecule-1 (VCAM-1). (3) vitronectin receptor family, a group of heterodimers containing a common β3 chain, present on a variety of cells, which has the function of attachment of these cells to their surroundings by reaction with proteins in the extracellular matrix.

CD11/CD18 Family

The three glycoproteins in this subfamily share the common CD18 β2 chain, but have different α chains. The members of this group (Table 1) are as follows: LFA-1 (leukocyte function-associated antigen-1, CD11a/CD18); Mac-1 (CR3 receptor, CD11b/CD18); and p150,95 (CD11c/CD18). LFA-1 is present on lymphocytes, monocytes, granulocytes, and NK cells and mediates the adhesion of these cell types. OKM1 and p150,95 are restricted to granulocytes, monocytes, and natural killer (NK) cells, contributing to the adhesion of these cells [3–5]. OKM1 also mediates the adhesion of soluble immune complexes or particles opsonized with iC3b. In addition to adhesion to vascular endothelium [5], the CD11/CD18 family mediates homotypic adhesion of cells to each other, as exemplified by the LFA-1 dependent clustering of activated lymphocytes [6], a phenomenon which could play a role in the aggregation of lymphocytes in the lymhocyte-rich areas of the RSM. Cytolytic T cell killing is also LFA-1 dependent [7].

VLA Receptor Family

The receptors of this family are present on a number of hematopoietic and mesenchymal cell types (Table 1). They are heterodimers which have in common the β1 variety of β chain. In the VLA family, which is present mainly on hematopoietic cells, six VLA antigens have been recognized [8]. Since the first two to be identified, VLA-1 and VLA-2, appeared on activated T cells 2–3 weeks after stimulation, this group has been called the very late activation antigens. Because VLA molecules have the ability to adhere to matrix proteins, they may play a role in the compartmentalization of T cells in inflammatory lesions [9]. VLA-1 has been detected on rheumatoid synovial fluid T cells [10]. In view of the fact that this marker appears to characterize T cells which have

Table 1. Integrin adhesion receptor families[a]

Receptor family	CD11/CD18		VLA	Vitronectin
α Chain	αa (LFA-1) αb (OK-M1) αc (p150, 95)		α_{1-6}	α_V αIIB
β Chain	β2		β1	β3[b]
Cells expressing receptor	LFA-1	Neutrophil Monocyte Lymphocyte NK cell	T, activated B Monocyte Fibroblast EC	EC Fibroblast Smooth muscle Macrophage Platelet
	OK-M1, p150, 95	Neutrophil Monocyte NK cell		
Ligand	ICAM-1 (C+I)[c] ICAM-2 (C)		Fibronectin Laminin Types 1, 4 collagen VCAM-1[d]	Vitronectin Fibrinogen von Willebrand factor Fibronectin
Predominant function	Cell to cell adhesion[e]		Cell to matrix adhesion	Cell to matrix adhesion

[a] As present on nucleated cells.
[b] Identical to GPIIIa, the β chain of the platelet adhesion receptor GPIIb, IIIa.
[c] React with LFA-1. C, constitutive; I, cytokine inducible.
[d] Inducible on EC; reacts with VLA-4 [11].
[e] OK-M1 is CR3 and reacts with C3bi, with protein containing the Arg-Gly-Asp tripeptide, and with cellular ligands.

been through an activation step [9], VLA-1-bearing T cells may be memory cells, a cell type which, as will be seen, predominates in rheumatoid effusions. A recent report has shown VLA-4 to be the lymphocyte receptor which reacts with VCAM-1 (vascular cell adhesion molecule-1), an adhesion ligand on cytokine-activated EC [11]. The VLA receptors react mainly with ligands on fibronectin, laminin, and types 1 and 4 collagen.

Receptors of the β1 subfamily have been identified on EC, fibroblasts, and monocytes in addition to lymphocytes. For these cells, these receptors presumably provide anchorage in the connective tissue by virtue of their capacity to react with matrix proteins.

Vitronectin Receptor Family

These heterodimers (Table 1) are characterized by a common β3 chain, which is identical to the GP IIIa β chain of the platelet receptor for fibrinogen and other proteins. The vitronectin receptor is present on EC, fibroblasts and macrophages. It reacts with fibrinogen, fibronectin, von Willebrand factor, and vitronectin. The receptor molecules appear to react mainly with the arginine-glycine-aspartic acid (RGD) tripeptide in these proteins. By binding with the vitronectin cell receptors in this way, the matrix proteins also provide the cells with "anchorage, traction for migration and signals for polarity, position, differentiation and possibly growth" [12].

Lymphocyte-EC Interaction

Binding of Lymphocytes to EC

The binding of lymphocytes to EC has been measured by two methods. In the first, devised by Stamper and Woodruff, lymphocytes are added to frozen sections of tissue and the lymphocytes bound to the EC of PCV are counted [13]. In the second, lymphocytes are added to confluent monolayers of EC and binding quantitated, either by direct counting or by measuring the radioactivity of labeled cells bound to the monolayer [14]. The method of Stamper and Woodruff has been used mainly to identify lymphocyte receptors and EC ligands involved in the homing of lymphocytes to lymphoid tissues. The EC monolayer method has been used to identify leukocyte receptors and EC ligands. Since it permits incubation of the EC with cytokines, however, it has also been employed to investigate the action of cytokines in stimulating EC to express their ligands.

The use of monoclonal antibodies to inhibit lymphocyte binding and to isolate the binding proteins has demonstrated that the two methods detect different molecules on both the lymphocyte and EC. Nevertheless, antibody to LFA-1, a molecule involved in the binding of leukocytes to EC monolayers, inhibited the binding of both human [15] and mouse [16] T cells to lymph node PCV; antibodies against both LFA-1 and Mel-14, a receptor on lymphocytes for homing to peripheral lymph node PCV, inhibited neutrophil accumulation in inflamed mouse peritoneum [17]. Thus, there is overlap in the adhesive functions of the molecules detected by the two techniques. Furthermore, evidence that the adhesive molecules demonstrated by the Stamper and Woodruff method are involved in the inflammatory process is provided by the observation that peripheral blood lymphocytes (PBL), added to frozen tissue sections of RSM, bound to the PCV endothelium of lymphoid aggregates in a manner similar to that observed in lymph node [18, 19].

Cytokine Up-regulation of Lymphocyte Binding Receptors on EC

Since the initial studies of Gowans and Knight [20], it has been known that lymphocytes emigrate in large numbers from PCV with tall or columnar endothelium. The factors governing the tallness of EC of lymphoid tissue have long been a matter of interest. When afferent lymphatic vessels of lymph node were interrupted, the EC became flattened. However, following injection of antigen, tall EC reappeared [21]. The tallness of the EC appeared to parallel the numbers of macrophages in the tissue, suggesting that a macrophage derived cytokine might be responsible for the hypertrophy of the EC. In dermal delayed hypersensitivity reactions, in which cytokines are secreted, venules surrounded by perivascular mononuclear infiltrates showed striking EC hypertrophy [22]. In recent experiments, human umbilical vein endothelial cells (HUVEC) manifested similar hypertrophy when cultured with either tumor necrosis factor-α (TNF-α) or TNF-β [23]. These observations suggest that cytokines may regulate the tallness of the PCV endothelium.

Chronic inflammation, as exemplified by rheumatoid synovitis, involves the emigration of lymphocytes and monocytes from PCV. The initial binding of these cells requires interaction between a receptor on the mononuclear cell and a ligand on the EC. The baseline binding of T cells to HUVEC monolayers is largely achieved by the LFA-1 receptor, as indicated by blocking experiments in which monoclonal antibodies to the α and β chains of this heterodimer inhibited up to 90% of the binding [24]. Binding was increased following stimulation of the T cell with phorbol ester (PMA), and the majority of the increase was due to heightened expression of LFA-1. The ligand on the EC for LFA-1 is the intercellular adhesion molecule-1 (ICAM-1), a single chain glycoprotein expressed on cells from various sources [25–27].

The cytokines interferon-gamma (IFN-γ) [28], interleukin-1 (IL-1) [14], TNF-α, and TNF-β [29] increased the binding activity of HUVEC and dermal microvascular EC [30].[1] In experiments carried out to identify the ligand on the EC which was responsible for the increase in T cell binding, antibodies to LFA-1, which markedly inhibited lymphocyte binding by unstimulated EC, had little effect on the increased binding induced by IL-1 [24], suggesting that the EC ligand induced was not ICAM-1. Dustin and Springer have also observed increased lymphocyte binding on EC stimulated by cytokines [31] and, in their experiments, this was accompanied by up-regulation of ICAM-1 on the EC (Table 2). However, only a portion of the increase in binding could be attributed to increased expression of this ligand. These results have suggested the presence of other ligands for lymphocyte binding on cytokine-stimulated EC. Recently, in fact, an IL-1 or TNF-α induced EC ligand, vascular cell adhesion molecule-1 (VCAM-1), which binds lymphocytes but not neutrophils, has been described [11]. This molecule, which shares sequence homology with ICAM-1 may also play a role in the recruitment of lymphocytes into inflammatory areas. Finally, a third lymphocyte binding molecule on EC, ICAM-2, which is constitutively expressed but not up-regulated, has recently been cloned [32].

---

[1] IL-4 has also recently been shown to stimulate increased EC adhesiveness for T cells (Thornhill MH, Kyan-Aung U, Haskard DO (1990) IL-4 increases human endothelial cell adhesiveness for T cells but not for neutrophils. J Immunol 144:3060–3065).

Table 2. Cytokine up-regulation of endothelial cell ligands binding T cells

EC ligand	Cytokine	Receptor
ICAM-1 [31][a]	IL-1, TNF, IFN-γ, [31]	LFA-1
VCAM-1 [12]	IL-1 or TNF-α [12]	VLA
ELAM-1[b]	–	–
Unidentified [24, 31]	–	–

[a] A second ligand, ICAM-2, is constitutively expressed but not up-regulated by cytokines [32].

[b] ELAM-1 (endothelial leukocyte adhesion molecule-1) has recently been shown to bind resting memory T cells (Shimizu Y, Shaws, Graber N, Gopal TV, Horgan KJ, Van Seventer GA, Newman W. Activation independent binding of human memory T cells to adhesion molecule ELAM-1 (1991) Nature 349:799–802).

In vivo, immunologically induced chronic inflammatory lesions show evidence of up-regulation of EC adhesion ligands. Agents which enhance lymphocyte binding to EC, e. g., lipopolysaccharide, IFN-γ, and TNF-α, stimulate the migration of these cells into the dermis when injected intradermally [33]. In dermal delayed hypersensitivity lesions, EC display the activation marker, endothelial-leukocyte adhesion molecule-1 (ELAM-1), a ligand ordinarily utilized by cytokine activated EC to bind neutrophils [34, 35] but recently shown to bind T cells (see Table 2). Intracutaneous injection of TNF in the baboon, moreover, induced EC hypertrophy accompanied by increased ELAM-1 and ICAM-1 expression; in combination with IFN-γ, TNF induced the changes of a delayed hypersensitivity reaction [36].

EC-Monocyte Interaction

The monocyte is an important component of the chronic inflammatory infiltrate. Macrophages are more frequent in the immunoglobulin producing areas of the RSM [37, 38]. Monocytes [39] and activated macrophages [40] express the three receptors of the CD11/CD18 group, but TeVelde et al. concluded that the adhesion of these cells to EC monolayers is dependent on the p150,95 (CD11c/CD18) molecule [39], on the basis of evidence that an antibody to the p150,95 α chain inhibited this binding. In addition, antibody to the CD11/CD18 β chain [41] inhibited binding of untreated and PMA activated monocytes to EC monolayers.

IL-1 treatment of EC monolayers stimulated increased binding of monocytes [42, 43]. The relative contribution of ligands to CD11/CD18 and other receptors to this increase is not known. The CD11/CD18 independent ligand ELAM-1 may participate in the increased adhesion of monocytes to cytokine-activated EC. Bevilacqua et al. [42] have identified ELAM-1 on EC incubated with IL-1 or TNF. The expression of this ligand is known to increase the binding of neutrophils [34, 35, 44]. However, because ELAM-1 is expressed on EC in delayed hypersensitivity and other chronic inflammatory lesions [34], this ligand may also be involved in the binding of monocytes [36]. Early induction of ELAM-1 on EC by cytokines may explain why the arrival of monocytes precedes that of lymphocytes in the cellular immune response, in spite of the markedly greater number of lymphocytes in the circulation.

Role of Lymphocyte-EC Interaction in Rheumatoid Synovitis

Relation of PCV Endothelium to Histologic Pattern of Infiltration

In the well-developed rheumatoid synovial inflammatory reaction, two patterns of mononuclear cell infiltration may be recognized. In some specimens, aggregates of lymphocytes (lymphocyte-rich areas) are present [38, 45, 45]. These consist mainly of T4 cells [37, 47], associated with lesser numbers of macrophages and interdigitating cells [48]. At their margins, the lymphocyte-rich areas make a transition to more diffuse infiltrates, consisting of lymphocytes, macrophages, plasma cells, and connective tissue cells. These nonspecific mononuclear cell infiltrates are the most common variety of infiltrate in the inflammatory synovium.

Adhesion of lymphocytes and monocytes to the EC of the PCV has an important influence on the patterns of lymphocyte and monocyte infiltration in the RSM. Lymphocytes migrate rapidly through tall endothelial PCV [20]; consistent with this is the observation that the percentage of lymphocytes in perivascular infiltrates is highly significantly correlated with the tallness of the EC of the vessel involved [38, 49]. Thus, the T cell-rich lymphoid aggregates of the RSM tend to be present around tall endothelial PCV, and the diffuse infiltrates of lymphocytes, macrophages, and plasma cells surround PCV with flatter endothelium [38]. These findings suggest that, though lymphocytes emigrate through endothelium of varying degrees of hypertrophy, the migration of these cells through tall endothelium is sufficiently intense to surround the PCV with a dense lymphocyte-rich population.

Role of Cytokines in Synovial Mononuclear Cell Infiltration

As mentioned, IL-1 [14], TNF-α and TNF-β [29], and IFN-γ [28], all of which have been demonstrated in the rheumatoid joint, stimulate increased binding of lymphocytes to HUVEC monolayers when incubated with the EC. Since these cytokines are liberated by activated T cells (IFN-γ and TNF-β) and macrophages (IL-1 and TNF-α), it is likely that, when released by such cells in the RSM, they stimulate the EC of contiguous PCV to increase the binding and emigration of lymphocytes, thereby amplifying the perivascular inflammatory reaction. By this type of mechanism, cytokines may sustain chronic inflammation as long as they are generated.

Following binding to the EC, lymphocytes migrate through the EC junctions into the basement membrane and surrounding connective tissue. To determine whether a cytokine might play a role in this second stage of emigration, Oppenheimer-Marks and Ziff incubated EC monolayers, which had been grown to confluency over nitrocellulose paper and precoated with T cells, with a group of cytokines [50]. Of these, IFN-γ markedly increased the number of T cells which migrated into the nitrocellulose filter, suggesting that this cytokine may activate the EC to facilitate movement of the lymphocyte through the EC junction.

Role of Chemotaxis in Lymphocyte Migration

Chemotaxis may play a role in the migration of lymphocyts and monocytes through the vessel wall and, subsequently, toward an inflammatory focus. A number of chemotactic agents for lymphocyts [51, 52], including also IL-1 [53], IL-8 [54] and C5a [55], have been described. For monocytes, transforming growth factor-β (TGF-β) [56], TNF-α [57, 58], and granulocyte-macrophage colony stimulating factor (GH-CSF) [59], all of which have been demonstrated in rheumatoid synovial fluid, are potent chemotactic agents. These agents participate in the amplification of the inflammatory focus by virtue of their chemotactic activity.

T Cell Diversity in the Rheumatoid Synovial Infiltrate

Accepting the strong likelihood that the cellular response in rheumatoid synovitis is immunologically induced, it may be assumed to begin with a specific interaction between a reactive T cell clone and an antigen. Though, initially, selective recruitment of immune T lymphocytes may occur in this type of reaction [60, 61], the population of lymphocytes finally assembled is in the main immunologically nonspecific, only a small fraction bearing immunity to the injected antigen [61, 62]. As would be predicted from this, analyses of the T cell receptors of the lymphocytes of rheumatoid synovial fluid and tissue have failed to provide convincing evidence of clonality among the infiltrating T cells (Table 3). In experiments which examined the DNA of rheumatoid synovial fluid T lymphocytes for dominant rearrangements of the β chain of the T cell receptor as an indication of clonality, most reports have concluded that the T cells are polyclonal in nature. Though Stamenkovic et al (63) found β chain rearrangements in 13 of 14 SM T cell cultures which they interpreted as indicating oligoclonality, the rearranged bands were all distinct, raising the possibility of outgrowth of random clones. Savill et al. [64] found dominant β chain rearrangements in only 3 of 11 patients, and concluded that most rheumatoid patients had polyclonal syno-

Table 3. Diversity of T cell receptor of RA synovial T lymphocytes

Author	T cells	T cell receptor
Stamenkovic [63]	SM cultures	Clonal dominance, 13/14
Savill [64]	SF cultures	Polyclonal, 8/11
Keystone [65]	SF T cells	Polyclonal, 15/15
Duby [66]	SF T cell clones	Nondominant rearrangement, 38/40[a]
Dier [67]	SM T cell clones	Nondominant rearrangement
Cush [68]	SM T cell clones	Nondominant rearrangement, 77/79

SM, synovial membrane; SF, synovial fluid

[a] In a recent study (Cooper SM, Dier DL, Roessner KD, Budd RC, Nicklas JA (1991) Diversity of rheumatoid synovial tissue T cells by TcR analysis: oligoclonal expansion in IL-2 responsive cells. Arthritis Rheum 34:537–546), in which T cell clones were obtained by expansion with IL-2 alone, there was sharing of rearranged bands by a number of clones.

vial T cell populations. In four other studies, no evidence of significant clonality was found in rheumatoid synovial T cell populations, obtained both from synovial fluid [65, 66] and synovial tissue [67, 68]. It would appear, therefore, that the major fraction of the synovial T cell population is mobilized by a nonspecific process.

It is likely that a major factor in the development of T cell receptor diversity of synovial T cells is the up-regulation of EC binding of these cells by cytokines in an immunologically nonspecific manner. Consistent with a nonspecific effect of cytokines in this process are observations that intradermal injection of IFN-γ and TNF-α induces mononuclear cell infiltration of the dermis which resembles the delayed hypersensitivity reaction [33] and that repeated intra-articular injection of IL-1 induces a mononuclear cell synovitis [69–72]. Although cytokines up-regulate T cell ligands on EC in an immunologically nonspecific manner, the possibility that the activation state of the circulating T cells may be a factor in the selection of these cells for emigration remains to be considered.

Although DR+ T cells, which may express heightened levels of LFA-1, circulate in markedly increased numbers in RA [73], Gohring et al. noted no difference in the binding of normal and rheumatoid peripheral blood T cells to HUVEC monolayers [4]. Moreover, Cush and Lipsky [75] found no difference in the frequency and intensity of expression of LFA-1 on normal and rheumatoid PBL. These findings suggest that the activation state of circulating T lymphocytes may not be a potent factor in the adhesion of rheumatoid lymphocytes to PCV endothelium. Nevertheless, in experiments carried out to determine whether normal circulating T cells differed in their adhesiveness to EC, subsets of varying binding capacity for EC monolayers were detected [76]. Among these subsets, strongly adherent T cells expressed greater levels of LFA-1 than weakly adherent cells.

Preponderance of Memory Cells in Chronic Inflammatory Lesions

Chronic inflammatory lesions tend to be infiltrated largely by memory T lymphocytes in preference to naive T cells. Memory T cells are cells that have been stimulated by an antigen and preserve immunological memory for this antigen. In contrast, naive lymphocytes have not previously reacted with antigen [77]. Memory T cells, which carry the markers CD45RO, CDw29, 4B4, UCHL1, and CD4, are designated as helper-inducer cells because they provide help for pokeweed mitogen (PWM) stimulated Ig production [78]. Naive T cells, which carry the markers CD45RA, 2H4, and CD4, are designated as suppressor-inducer (SI) cells because they induce CD8+ cells to inhibit PWM stimulated production of Ig [79]. The markers of the naive and memory cells are members of the leukocyte common antigen (LCA) [80] family of high molecular weight glycoproteins. The parent molecule of this family is the leukocyte common antigen (LCM) [80]. Proteins of the LCA family are expressed on all leukocytes and their hematopoietic precursors. Though derived from a single gene, messener RNAs for expression of individual members of the family are produced by alternative splicing of three exons of the parent molecule. The change from naive to memory cell marker occurs, presumably, during the mitotic activity resulting from contact of the naive cell with antigen [81]. Of special interest to the present discussion is the observation that memory T lymphocytes express increased levels of LFA-1 [82], VLA-4, and an ELAM-1 binding EC adhesion receptor.[1]

The T4 cells of the chronic inflammatory synovial membrane and effusion are mainly helper-inducer (HI) memory cells, i.e., CD45RO+, CDw29+CD4+ T cells, which are identified by the 4B4 [83] and UCHL1 antibodies [84]. Only small numbers of the naive SI CD45RA+CD4+ T cell subset, reacting with the 2H4 antibody, are present. Pitzalis et al. [83] found that 93.8% of rheumatoid synovial fluid T cells were 4B4+ and that the memory to naive cell ratio was 16.8. Emery et al. [85] found this ratio to be 9.5. These ratios markedly exceeded the values of approximately 1.3:1 in the peripheral blood. Similar findings have been made by others [86]. In addition, on staining isolated RSM cells, Pitzalis et al. found that 90% of the T cells were UCHL1+ and 7% carried the 2H4 marker [87]. Finally, using immunohistologic techniques to stain rheumatoid synovial tissue, a number of other groups [88, 89] also found an excess of the memory cell subset. Elevated memory to naive T cell ratios have also been observed in nonrheumatoid chronic inflammatory synovial effusions [90, 91], in a miscellaneous group of chronic pleural and peritoneal effusions [83], in the thyroid tissue in Grave's disease [92], in the skin in atopic dermatitis [93], and in the plaques and adjacent white matter of central nervous system tissue in multiple schlerosis [94]. Thus, the

---

[1] Shimizu Y, Shaw S, Graber N, Gopal TV, Horgan KJ, Van Seventer GA, Newman W (1991) Activation independent binding of human memory T cells to adhesion molecule ELAM-1. Nature 349:799–802.

predominance of the CD29+ cell is characteristic of a number of chronic inflammatory lesions.

Is the Elevated Memory to Naive Cell Ratio in Chronic Inflammatory Lesions Related to Intercellular Adhesion Phenomena?

The existence of subsets of normal peripheral blood T cells with varying ability to bind to EC has been mentioned [76]. In these subsets, lymphocytes with greater binding ability expressed higher levels of LFA-1. When Pitzalis et al. [83] compared the EC binding of CD45RO+ (memory) cell and CD45RA+ (naive) cell subsets in rheumatoid synovial fluid, the percent binding of the memory cells was 3.8 times that of the naive cells. They also found that the memory cell population expressed a higher LFA-1 density and a greater capacity to form homotyic aggregates than the naive population. Increased expression of LFA-1 by memory T cells has also been reported by Sanders et al. [82] and increased expression of VLA-4, which mediates binding to VCAM-1 on the EC [11], has also been observed on these cells [95]. The elevated binding activity of the memory T cell would favor the preferential emigration of this cell type, and the increased homotypic aggregation would foster the local sequestration of this subset in the perivascular tissue. Finally, the memory cell marker CDw29 has been identified as the β, chain of the VLA integrin family, suggesting that there may be elevated expression of a number of VLA heterodimers on the memory cell [96]. Because of the ability of VLA molecules to bind to matrix proteins, the heightened expression of these markers would also favor the retention of memory cells in the perivascular space. Thus, increased expression of adhesion molecules may be a very important factor in the development of an excess of memory cells in the RSM and effusion.

An alternative point of view about the preponderance of memory cells in the RSM has been presented by Koch et al. [97]. On immunohistochemical staining of RSM, these authors found different staining patterns in perivascular T cell-rich aggregates (lymphocyte-rich areas) and more diffuse lymphocytic infiltrates where Ig synthesis occurs. While perivascular lymphocyte-rich collections contained both CD45RA+ and UCHL1+ cells, the T cells were mainly UCHL1 in the more diffuse type of infiltrate. To explain these findings, the authors suggested that, as the T cells are immunologically activated in the diffuse infiltrates, they lose the CD45RA marker and gain the UCHL1 marker.

The greater concentration of memory cells in synovial effusions than in the peripheral blood may offer an explanation for the interesting observation that synovial fluid lymphocytes show a greater response than PBL to antigens to which patients might be expected to be immunized in association with their disease, i. e., chlamydia, mycoplasma and enteric bacteria in Reiter's syndrome [98, 99], *Borrelia burgdorferi* in Lyme disease [100, 101], and *Yersinia* organisms in Yersinia arthritis [102].

References

1. Hynes RO (1987) A family of cell surface receptors. Cell 49:549–554
2. Hogg N (1989) The leukocyte integrins. Immunology Today 10:111–114
3 Keizer GD, Borst J, Figdor GD, Spits H, Miedma F, Terhorst C, De Vries JE (1985) Biochemical and functional characteristics of the human leukocyte membrane family LFA-1, Mo-1 and p150,95. Eur J Immunol 15:1142–1147
4. Anderson DC, Miller LJ, Schmalstieg FC, Rothlein RR, Springer T (1986) Contributions of the Mac-1 glycoprotein family to adherence dependent granulocyte function assessments employing subunit-specific monoclonal antibodies. J Immunol 137:15–27
5. Arnoult MA, Lewis LL, Faller DJ (1988) Relative contribution of the leukocyte molecules Mo-1, LFA-1, and p150,95 (LeuM5) in adhesion of granulocytes and monocytes to vascular endothelium is tissue and stimulus specific. J Cell Physiol 137:305–309
6. Rothlein RR, Springer TA (1986) The requirement for lymphocyte function antigen-1 in homotypic leukocyte aggregation stimulated by phorbol ester. J Exp Med 163:1132–1149
7. Krensky AM, Mentzer SJ, Clayberger C, Anderson DC, Schmalstieg FC, Burakoff SJ, Springer TA (1986) Heritable lymphocyte function antigen associated-1 deficiency: abnormalities of cytotoxicity and proliferation associated with abnormal expression of LFA-1. J Immunol 135:3102–3108
8. Hemler ME, Crouse C, Takada Y, Sonnenberg A (1988) Multiple very late antigen (VLA) heterodimers on platelets. J Biol Chem 263:7660–7664
9. Hemler ME, Jacobson JG (1987) Cell matrix adhesion-related proteins VLA-1 and VLA-2: regulation of expression on T cells. J Immunol 138:2941–2948
10. Hemler ME, Glass D, Coblyn JS, Jacobson JG (1986) Very late activation antigens on rheumatoid synovial fluid T lymphocytes. Association with stages of T cell activation. J Clin Invest 78:696–702
11. Schwartz BR, Wayner EA, Carlos TM, Ochs HD, Harlan JM (1990) Identification of surface proteins mediating adherence of CD11/CD18 deficient lymphoblastoid cells to cultured human endothelium. J Clin Invest 85:2019–2022
12. Ruoslahti E, Pierschbacher MD (1987) New perspectives in cell adhesion: RGD and integrins. Science 238:491–496
13. Stamper HB, Woodruff JJ (1976) Lymphocyte homing in lymph nodes: in vitro demonstration of the selective affinity of recirculating lymphocytes for high-endothelial venules. J Exp Med 144:828–833
14. Cavender D, Haskard DO, Joseph B, Ziff M (1986) Interleukin-1 increases the binding of human B and T lymphocytes to endothelial cell monolayers. J Immunol 136:203–207
15. Pals ST, Annelies den O, Miedma F, Kabel P, Keizer GD, Scheper RG, Meijer CJLM (1988) Evidence that leukocyte function-associated antigen-1 is involved in recirculation and homing of human lymphocytes via high endothelial venules. J Immunol 140:1851–1853
16. Hamann A, Jablonski-Westrich D, Duijvestijn A, Butcher EC, Baisch H, Harder R, Thiele H-G (1988) Evidence for an accessory role of LFAQ-1 in lymphocyte-high endothelial interaction during homing. J Immunol 140:693–699
17. Jutila MA, Rott L, Berg EL, Butcher EC (1989) Function and regulation of the neutrophil Mel-14 antigen in vivo: comparison with LFA-1 and Mac-1. J Immunol 143:3318–3324
18. Oppenheimer-Marks N, Ziff M (1986) Binding of normal human mononuclear cells to blood vessels in rheumatoid synovial membrane. Arthritis Rheum 29:789–792
19. Jalkanen S, Steere AC, Fox RI, Butcher EC (1986) A distinct endothelial cell recognition system that controls lymphocyte traffic into inflamed synovium. Science 233:556–558
20. Gowans JL, Knight EJ (1964) The route of recirculation of lymphocytes in the rat. Proc R Soc London (Biol) 159:257–282

21. Hendriks HR, Estermans IL (1983) Disappearance and reappearance of high endothelial venules and immigrating lymphocytes in lymph nodes deprived of afferent lymphatic vessels: a possible regulatory role of macrohages in lymphocyte migration. Eur J Immunol 13:663–669
22. Dvorak AM, Mihm MC, Dvorak HF (1976) Morphology of delayed hypersensitivity of reactions in man. II. Ultrastructural alterations affecting the microvasculature and the tissue mast cells. Lab Invest 34:1079–1191
23. Cavender DE, Edelbaum D, Ziff M (1989) Endothelial cell activation by tumor necrosis factor and lymphotoxin. Am J Pathol 134:551–560
24. Haskard D, Cavender D, Beatty P, Springer T, Ziff M (1986) T lymphocyte adhesion to endothelial cells: mechanisms demonstrated by anti-LFA-1 monoclonal antibodies. J Immunol 137:2901–2906
25. Rothlein R, Dustin ML, Marlin SD, Springer TA (1986) A human intercellular adhesion molecule [ICAM-1] distinct from LFA-1. J Immunol 137:1270–1274
26. Marlin SD, Springer TA (1987) Purified intercellular adhesion molecule-1 [ICAM-1] is a ligand for lymphocyte function-associated antigen 1 (LFA-1). Cell 51:813–819
27. Makgoba MW, Sanders ME, Luce GEG, Dustin ML, Spriner TA, Clark EA, Mannoni P, Shaw S (1988) ICAM-1 ligand for LFA-1 dependent adhesion of B, T and myeloid cells. Nature 331:86–88
28. Yu C-L, Haskard DO, Cavender D, Johnson AR, Ziff M (19859 Human gamma interferon increases the binding of T lymphocytes to endothelial cells. Clin Exp Immunol 62:554–560
29. Cavender D, Saegusa Y, Ziff M (1987) Stimulation of endothelial cell binding of lymphocytes by tumor necrosis factor. J Immunol 139:1855–1860
30. Haskard DO, Cavender D, Fleck RM, Sontheimer R, Ziff M (1987) Human dermal microvascular endothelial cells behave like umbilical vein endothelial cells in T cell adhesion studies. J Invest Dermatol 88:340–344
31. Dustin ML, Springer TA (1988) Lymphocyte function-associated antigen-1 [LFA-1] interaction with intercellular adhesion molecule-1 (ICAM-1) is one of at least three mechanisms for lymphocyte adhesion to cultured endothelial cells. J Cell Biol 107:321–331
32. Staunton DE, Dustin ML, Springer TA (1989) Functional cloning of ICAM-2, a cell adhesion ligand for LFA-1 homologous to ICAM-1. Nature 339:61–64
33. Issekutz TB, Stolz JM (1989) Stimulation of lymphocyte migration by endotoxin, tumor necrosis factor, and interferon. Cell Immunol 120:165–173
34. Cotran RS, Gimbrone MA, Bevilacque MP, Mendrick DL, Pober JS (1986) Induction and detection of a human endothelial cell activation antigen in vivo. J Exp Med 164:661–666
35. Dobrina A, Schwartz BR, Carlos TM, Ochs HD, Beatty PG, Harlan JM (1989) CD11/CD18-independent neutrophil adherence to inducible endothelial-leucocyte adhesion molecules (E-LAM) in vitro. Immunology 67:502–508
36. Munro JM, Pober JS, Cotran RS (1989) Tumor necrosis factor and interferon-γ induce distinct patterns of endothelial activation and associated leukocyte accumulation in skin of *Papio anubis*. Am J Pathol 135:121–133
37. Kurosaka M, Ziff M (1983) Immunoelectron microscopic study of the distribution of T cell subsets in rheumatoid synovium. J Exp Med 158:1191–1210
38. Iguchi T, Ziff M (1986) Electron microscopic study of rheumatoid synovial vasculature: intimate relationship between tall endothelium and lymphoid aggregates. J Clin Invest 77:355–361
39. Te Velde AA, Keizer GD, Figdor CG (1987) Differential function of LFA-1 family molecules (CD11 and CD18) in adhesion of human monocytes to melanoma and endothelial cells and activated macrophages. Immunology 61:261–267
40. Grassman G, Springer TA, Adams DO (1985) Studies on antigens associated with the activation of murine mononuclear phagocytes: kinetics of and requirements for induction of lymphocyte-function-associated (LFA-1) antigen in vitro. J Immunol 135:147–151

41. Wallis WJ, Beatty PJ, Ochs HD, Harlan JN (1985) Human monocyte adherence to cultured vascular endothelium: monoclonal antibody defined mechanisms. J Immunol 135:2323–2330
42. Bevilacque MP, Pober JS, Wheeler ME, Cotran RS, Gimbrone MA (1985) Interleukin 1 acts on cultured vascular endothelium to increase the adhesion of polymorphonucleocytes, monocytes, and related cell lines. J Clin Invest 76:2003–2011
43. Downs EC, Cornwell DG, Proctor VK, Whisler RL (1987) IL-1 and bacterial lipopolysaccharide increase the ability of human endothelial cells to bind peripheral blooc monocytes. Lymphokine Res 6:351–355
44. Bevilacqua M, Stringelin S, Gimbrone MA, Seed B (1989) Endothelial leukocyte adhesion molecule 1: an inducible receptor for neutrophils related to complement regulatory proteins and lectins. Science 243:1160–1165
45. Kobayashi I, Ziff M (1973) Electron microscopic studies of lymphoid cells in the rheumatoid synovial membrane. Arthritis Rheum 16:471–486
46. Ishikawa H, Ziff M (1976) Electron microscopic observations of immunoreactive cells in the rheumatoid synovial membrane. Arthritis Rheum 19:1–14
47. Duke O, Panayi GS, Janossy G, Poulter LW (1982) An immunohistochemical analysis of lymphocyte subpopulations and their microenvironment in the synovial membranes of patients with rheumatoid arthritis using monoclonal antibodies. Clin Exp Immunol 49:22–30
48. Iguchi T, Kurosaka M, Ziff M (1986) Electron microscopic study of HLA-DR and monocyte/macrophage staining cells in the rheumatoid synovial membrane. Arthritis Rheum 29:600–613
49. Freemont AJ (1987) Molecules controlling lymphocyte-endothelial interactions in lymph nodes are produced in vessels of inflamed synovium. Ann Rheum Dis 46:924–928
50. Oppenheimer-Marks N, Ziff M (1988) Migration of lymphocytes through endothelial cell monolayers: augmentation by interferon-γ. Cellular Immunol 114:307–323
51. Center DM, Cruikshank W (1982) Modulation of lymphocyte migration by human lymphokines. I. Identification and characterization of chemoattractant activity for lymphocytes from mitogen-stimulated mononuclear cells. J Immunol 128:2563–2568
52. Van Epps DE, Potter JW, Durant DA (1983) Production of a human T lymphocyte chemotactic factor by T cell subpopulations. J Immunol 130:2727–2731
53. Miossec P, Dinarello CA, Ziff M (1986) Interleukin 1 lymphocyte chemotactic activity in rheumatoid synovial fluid. Arthritis Rheum 29:461–470
54. Larsen CG, Anderson AO, Apella E, Oppenheim JJ, Matsushima K (1989) The neutrophil activating protein (NAP-1) is also chemotactic for T lymphocytes. Science 243:1464–1466
55. El Naggar AK, Van Epps DE, Williams RC Jr (1980) Human B and T lymphocyte accumulation in response to casein, C5a, and f-Met-Leu-Phe. Cell Immunol 56:365–373
56. Wahl SM, Hunt DA, Wong HL, Dougherty S, McCartney-Francis N, Wahl LM, Ellingsworth L, Schmidt JA, Hall G, Roberts AB, Sporn MB (1988) Transforming growth factor-β is a potent immunosuppressive agent that inhibits IL-1 dependent lymphocyte proliferation. J Immunol 140:3026–3030
57. Ming WJ, Bersani L, Montevani A (1987) Tumor necrosis factor is chemotactic for monocytes and polymorphonuclear leukocytes. J Immunol 138:1409–1474
58. Yocum DE, Tobin LM, Suderi P (1988) Tumor necrosis factor-alpha production by synovial fluid mononuclear cells and synovial tissue from inflammatory and degenerative arthritis. Arthritis Rheum 32:S91 (abstr)
59. Wang JH, Colella S, Allavera P, Montevani A (1987) Chemotactic activity of human recombinant granulocyte-macrophage colony-stimulating factor. Immunology 60:439–444
60. Lipscomb MF, Lyons CR, O'Hara RM, Stein-Streilein J (1982) The antigen induced selective recruitment of specific T lymphocytes to the lung. J Immunol 128:111–116
61. McCluskey RT, Benaceraf B, McCluskey JW (1963) Studies on the specificity of the cellular infiltrate in delayed hypersensitivity reactions. J Immunol 90:466–477

62. Scheper RJ, van Dinther-Janssen ACHM, Polak L (1985) Specific accumulation of haptene reaction T cells in contact sensitivity reaction sites. J Immunol 134:1333–1336
63. Stamenkovic I, Stegagno M, Wright KA, Krane SM, Amento E, Gluin RB, Duquesnoy RT, Kurnick JT (1988) Clonal dominance among T cell infiltrates in arthritis. Proc Nat Acad Sci USA 85:1179–1183
64. Savill CM, Delves PJ, Kioussis D, Walker P, Lydyard PM, Colaco B, Shipley M, Roitt IM (1987) A minority of patients with rheumatoid arthritis show a dominant rearrangement of the T cell receptor beta genes in synovial lymphocytes. Scand J Immunol 25:629–635
65. Keystone EC, Minden M, Klock R, Poplonski L, Zalcberg J, Takadera T, Mak TW (1988) Structure of T cell antigen receptor β chain in synovial fluid cells from patients with rheumatoid arthritis. Arthritis Rheum 31:1555–1557
66. Duby AD, Sinclair AK, Osborne-Lawrence SL, Zeldes W, Kan L, Fox DA (1989) Clonal heterogeneity of synovial fluid T lymphocytes from patients with rheumatoid arthritis. Arthritis Rheum 32:B44 (abstr)
67. Dier DL, Roessner KD, Cooper SM (1989) Diversity of rheumatoid tissue T cells by T cell receptor analysis. Arthritis Rheum 32:B43 (abstr)
68. Cush JJ, Duby AD, Lightfoot E, Lipsky PE (1990) The search for oligoclonal T cells in rheumatoid synovium (abstract). Arthritis Rheum 33(suppl 9):516
69. Andreis M, Stastny P, Ziff M (1974) Experimental arthritis produced by injection of mediators of delayed hypersensitivity. Arthritis Rheum 17:537–551
70. Dingle JT, Page Thomas DP, King B, Bard DR (1987) In vivo studies of articular tissue damage mediated by catabolin/interleukin 1. Ann Rheum Dis 46:527–533
71. Pettipher ER, Higgs GA, Henderson B (1986) Interleukin 1 induced leukocyte infiltration and cartilage proteoglycan degradation in the synovial joint. Proc Natl Acad Sci USA 83:8749–8753
72. Gilman SC, Hodge T, Chang J (1987) Articular synovitis in rat knee joints induced by interleukin 1. Arthritis Rheum 30:S29 (suppl)
73. Yu DTY, Winchester RJ, Ru SM, Gibofsky A, Ko HS, Kunkel JH (1980) Peripheral blood Ia-positive cells. Increases in certain diseases and after immunization. J Exp Med 151:91–100
74. Gohring PPA, Burmester GR, Kalden JR (1987) Adhesion of human T lymphocytes to endothelial cells isolated from the umbilical vein: I. Similar binding patterns of normal and rheumatoid T cells. Immunobiol 175:385–393
75. Cush JJ, Lipsky PE (1988) Phenotypic analysis of synovial tissue and PBL isolated from patients with rheumatoid arthritis. Arthritis Rheum 31:1230–1238
76. Cavender DE, Haskard DO, Maliakkal D, Ziff M (1988) Separation and characterization of human T lymphocytes with varying adhesiveness for endothelial cells. Immunol 117:111–126
77. Sanders ME, Melegapuru WM, Shaw S (1988) Human naive and memory cells: reinterpretation of helper-inducer and suppressor-inducer subsets. Immunol Today 7:195–198
78. Morimoto C, Letvin NL, Boyd AW, Hagan M, Brown HM, Kornracki MM, Schlossman SF (1985) The isolation and characterization of the helper inducer T cell subset. J Immunol 134:3762–3769
79. Morimoto C, Letvin NL, Distaso JA, Aldrich WR, Schlossman SF (1985) The isolation and characterization of the human suppressor inducer T cell subset. J Immunol 134:1508–1515
80. Thomas ML (1989) The leukocyte common antigen family. Ann Rev Immunol 7:339–369
81. Akabar AN, Terry L, Timms A, Beverly PCL, Janossy G (1988) Loss of CD45R and gain of UCHL1 reactivity is a feature of primed T cells. J Immunol 140:2171–2178
82. Sanders ME, Makgoba MW, Sharrow SO, Stephany D, Springer TA, Young HA, Shaw S (1988) Human memory T lymphocytes express increased levels of three cell adhesion molecules (LFA-3, CD2 and LFA-1) and three other molecules (UCHL1, CDw29 and Ppg-1) and have enhanced IFN-δ production. J Immunol 140:1401–1407

83. Pitzalis C, Kingsley G, Haskard D, Panayi G (1988) The preferential accumulation of helper-inducer T lymphocytes in inflammatory lesions: evidence for regulation by selective endothelial and homotypic adhesion. Eur J Immunol 18:1398–1404
84. Smith SH, Brown MH, Rowe D, Callard RE, Beverley PCL (1986) Functional subsets of helper-inducer cells defined by a new monoclonal antibody, UCHL1. Immunology 58:63–70
85. Emery P, Gentry KC, Mackay IR, Muirden KD, Rowley M (1987) Deficiency of the suppressor inducer subset of T lymphocytes in rheumatoid arthritis. Arthritis Rheum 30:849–856
86. Gerli R, Bertotto A, Rambotti P, Barbieri P, Ciompi ML, Bombardieri S (1988) T cell immunoregulation in rheumatoid arthritis. Arthritis Rheum 31:1075–1076
87. Pitzalis C, Kingsley G, Murphy J, Panayi G (1987) Abnormal distribution of the helper-inducer and suppressor-inducer T lymphocyte subsets in the rheumatoid joint. Clin Immunol Immunopathol 45:252–258
88. Duke O, Panayi GS, Bofill M, Poulter L, Janossy G (1986) Evidence for a deficiency of the suppressor-inducer T cell subset in the synovial membrane in rheumatoid arthritis. Br J Rheumatol 25:(suppl 65, abstr 38)
89. Hanly JG, Pledger D, Roberts M, Parkhill W, Gross M (1989) Expression of 4B4 (CDw29) and 2H4 (CD45R) by T lymphocytes in rheumatoid synovial membrane (SM). Arthritis Rheum 32:S57
90. Kingsley GH, Pitzalis C, Kyriazis N, Panayi GS (1988) Abnormal helper-inducer/suppressor-inducer T cell subset distribution and T cell activation status are common to all types of chronic synovitis. Scand Immunol 28:225–232
91. Morimoto C, Romain PL, Fox DA, Anderson P, Dimaggio M, Levine H, Schlossman SF (1988) Abnormalities in CD4+ lymphocyte subsets in inflammatory rheumatic diseases. Am J Med 84:817–825
92. Ishikawa N, Eguchi K, Otsubo T, Ueki Y, Fukuda T, Tezuka H, Matsunaga M, Kawabe Y, Shimomura C, Izumi M, Ban Y, Ito K, Nagataki S (1987) Reduction in the suppressor-inducer T cell subset and increase in the helper T cell subset in thyroid tissue from patients with Graves' disease. JClin Endocrinol Metab 65:17–23
93. Lever R, Turbitt M, Sanderson A, MacKie R (1987) Immunopathology of the cutaneous infiltrate and of the mononuclear cells in the peripheral blood in patients with atopic dermatitis. J Invest Dermatol 89:4–7
94. Sobel RA, Hafler DA, Castro EE, Morimoto C, Weiner HL (1988) The 2H4 (CD45R) antigen is selectively decreased in multiple sclerosis lesions. J Immunol 140:2210–2214
95. Shinuzu Y, Shaw S, Graber N, Gopal TV, Horgan KJ, Van Seventer GA, Newman W (1991) Activation independent binding of human memory T cells to adhesion molecule ELAM-1. Nature 349:799–802
96. Hemler ME (1990) VLA proteins in the integrin family: structure, functions and their role on lymphocytes. Annu Rev Immunol 8:365–400
97. Koch AE, Robinson PG, Radosevich JA, Pope RM (1989) Immunophenotyping of rheumatoid (RA) synovial tissue lymphocytes. Arthritis Rheum 32:S59
98. Ford DK, DaRoza D (1986) Further observations on the response of synovial lymphocytes to viral antigens in rheumatoid arthritis. J Rheumatol 13:113–117
99. Ford DK, da Roza D, Shah P (1980) Cell mediated immune responses of synovial mononuclear cells to sexually transmitted, enteric and mumps antigens in patients with Reiter's syndrome, rheumatoid arthritis and ankylosing spondylitis. J Rheumatol 8:220–232
100. Sigal LH, Steere AC, Freeman DH et al (1986) Reactivity to *Borrelia burgdorferi* antigens is greater in joint fluid than in blood. Arthritis Rheum 29:761–769
101. Padula SJ, Pfister RD (1988) Lyme disease synovial fluid cells show significantly greater response to *Borrelia Burgdorferi* antigens than peripheral blood cells. Clin Res 36:535A
102. Gaston JSH, Life PF, Granfors K, Merilahti-Palo R, Bailey L, Consalvey S, Toivanen A, Bacon PA (1989) Synovial T lymphocyte recognition of organisms which trigger reactive arthritis. Clin Exp Immunol 76:348–353

Endothelial Cells and Dendritic Cells in Rheumatoid Inflammation*

Ø. Førre[1], K. Waalen[3], and J. B. Natvig[2]

[1]Oslo Sanitetsforenings Rheumatism Hospital, and
[2]Institute of Immunology and Rheumatology, the National Hospital, Oslo, Norway
[3]Present address: Department of Animal Genetics, Norwegian College of Veterinary
Medicine, Oslo, Norway

Introduction

Endothelial cells (EC) and dendritic cells (DC) play an important role in
rheumatoid inflammation. All types of inflammatory cells seem to emigrate to
the synovial tissue by first binding to the high endothelial venules. Certain
cytokines increase this binding and direct the cell traffic to the inflammatory
sites. Interferon-γ stimulates EC to express HLA class-II molecules and to
become accessory cells for T-cell activation. The dendritic cells are probably the
most important accessory cells for the T-cell responses in the inflamed joint
tissues. This is accomplished by their strong HLA class-II antigen expression,
their large surface area, and their production of cytokines.

Endothelial Cells

Chronic inflammation is accompanied by neovascularization or angiogenesis
[17]. The development of a network of new blood vessels in the synovial
membrane is essential to the development of rheumatoid arthritis. Activated
macrophages from rheumatoid synovial tissue can induce formation of new
blood vessels [34]. This induction appears to be initiated by cytokines such as
class-I and class-II heparin-binding growth factors that manifest site-directed
specificity [16, 17]. Once activated to proliferate, endothelial cells fashion
themselves into blood-carrying tubes and express plasminogen activator [44]
and metalloproteinases [26] which facilitate their invasion of connective tissue
to deliver nutrients to proliferating cells.

* This work was supported by grants from the Norma and Leon Hess Foundation for
Research on Rheumatological Diseases, the Norwegian Women's Public Health Organiza-
tion, the Grethe Harbitz Legacy, the Norwegian Research Council for Science and the
Humanities and Hafslund Nycomed, Norway.

Smolen, Kalden, Maini (Eds.)
Rheumatoid Arthritis
© Springer-Verlag Berlin Heidelberg 1992

High Endothelial Venules
and Lymphocyte Homing to the Synovial Membrane

Pathways of Recirculation

Generally, lymphocytes leave the blood adhering to the endothelium in postcapillary venules that are lined by endothelial cells with particuarly tall walls. These vessels are called high endothelial venules (HEV) and are morphologically distinguishable in tissue sections from venules with flat endothelium [14, 30, 32]. After the first binding to HEV the lymphocytes migrate through the walls of the blood vessels and enter the rheumatoid synovial tissue and peripheral lymphoid organs by mechanisms that are largely unknown.

Efferent lymphathic vessels collect the lymphocytes from lymphoid organs via the thoracic duct and transfer them back to the blood circulation. In the early stages of rheumatoid arthritis the lymphocytes then aggregate around the blood vessels below the synovial surface [11, 32, 33].

Lymphocytes which have not met antigen constitute a freely recirculating pool of lymphocytes. After they have encountered antigen, the migration of lymphocytes seems to be localized to sites of original antigenic stimulation, such as the joint tissue in rheumatoid arthritis. Thus, activated lymphocytes seem to undergo a directed assembly which is responsible for local immune responses in vivo. Helper-inducer T lymphocytes (CD4$^+$, CDw29$^+$ T cells) adhere better to endothelial-adhesive proteins in the synovial membrane than the suppressor-inducer subset (CD4$^+$, CD45RA$^+$ T cells). Thus, the helper-inducer T lymphocytes can enter more easily into the extracellular matrix of the synovial membrane than their suppressor-inducer counterparts [56].

The migration of leukocytes is also essential for their maturation and their distribution in various lymphoid tissues, as well as for their homing to inflammatory sites. Accessory cells such as Langerhans cells and probably other kinds of dendritic cells seem to migrate from the periphery, where they have picked up antigens, to lymphoid tissues to initiate immune responses. During migration and recirculation the cells bind to endothelial cells of the HEV in lymphoid tissues and inflamed joint tissues.

There are proteins in the endothelial cells of the HEV which are anchors for lymphocytes. They are referred to as vascular adressins. The surface structures on the lymphocytes mediating adherence to the endothelium of the HEV are called homing receptors [47]. In man, lymphocyte-HEV interaction is mediated at least partly by a 90-kD protein class of molecules. These homing receptors are defined by the Hermes series of monoclonal antibodies [32, 47]. It is also likely that both monocytes and neutrophils express Hermes-defined homing receptors which control the traffic of these cells to sites of inflammation.

Adhesion Molecules on Endothelial Cells (Adressins)

Two adressin molecules which are involved in lymphocyte binding to HEV have been characterized in the mouse: MECA-367 is an adressin for mouse mucosal homing receptors, while MECA-79 is an adressin for mouse peripheral lymphnode receptors [31, 32]. In man, endothelial adressins are yet to be defined, and little is known about the ligand structures on synovial endothelium for homing receptors. The LFA-1 molecule is also involved in the binding of lymphocytes to HEV. This LFA-1-mediated binding, however, does not seem to use the ICAM-1 molecule as a ligand [14, 24].

The monoclonal antibody HECA-452 detects another interesting antigen which is expressed on HEV and on vessels with HEV-like appearance in chronic inflammation [63]. Interestingly, the HECA-452 antigen has very recently been demonstrated on a subpopulation of DC appearing very early in the rheumatoid synovial inflammation [63]. The influx of HECA-452-positive DC is followed by a morphological change in the endothelial lining of the vessels in the inflamed synovium, from flat to cuboid. These HEV might subsequently facilitate the influx of lymphoid cells into the inflamed synovial tissue, leading to the formation of dense cellular infiltrates so characteristic for rheumatoid inflammation [76].

Endothelial Cells as Antigen-presenting Cells

A prerequisite for a certain cell type being able to present peptides for T cells is surface expression of HLA class-II molecules [6]. Surface expression of class-II molecules is not a constitutive characteristic of endothelial cells [15]. Expression of class-II molecules by endothelial cells can be induced after stimulation with interferon-γ [39, 54]. Both IFN-γ and tumor necrosis factor (TNF) augment the expression of HLA class-I molecules on endothelial cells. Endothelial cells activated in this way have been shown to act as accessory cells for antigen stimulation of T cells in an HLA-restricted manner [39, 40, 45, 54].

HLA class-II molecules on endothelial cells might also participate in lymphocyte-endothelial cell adhesion [53]. Thus, HLA class-II molecules expressing endothelial cells in the synovial tissue might have two important functions: (a) to direct the traffic of CD4$^+$, CDw29$^+$ T helper-inducer cells to the inflamed tissue, and (b) to participate in T-cell activation as accessory cells.

Cytokines Produced by Endothelial Cells

The activated endothelial cells produce many cytokines that are important for the inflammatory response (Table 1). The cytokine production by endothelial cells has been demonstrated partly in biological assay systems and partly using blot hybridization. The cytokines derived from endothelial cells are important regulators of differentiation, proliferation, and activation of T and B lymphocytes and of the recruitment of leukocytes to sites of inflammation. They also regulate the production of leukocytes and erythrocytes, i. e., the hematopoietic

Table 1. Cytokines produced by activated endothelial cells. (Modified from [39])

Cytokine	Stimulus	Function
IL-1	LPS IL-1 TNF IFN-γ	Lymphocyte activation; local and systemic inflammation; acute phase responses; hematopoiesis
IL-6	"spontaneous" LPS IL-1 TNF	Lymphocyte activation; acute phase response; hematopoiesis
CSFs	LPS IL-1 TNF	Leukocyte recruitment and activation; hematopoiesis; EC proliferation
Chemotactic factors (IL-8; MCP-1)	LPS IL-1 TNF	Leukocyte recruitment and activation

Table 2. Endothelial cell responses to cytokines. (Modified from [39])

Cytokine	EC functional response	In vivo significance
IL-1; TNF; LT	Production of PGI2	Vasodilatation
	Production of PCA, PAI, TM, PAF, VW release	Thrombosis
	Increased expression of ICAM-1 and 2; expression of ELAM-1	Leukocyte adhesion and extravasation; virus infection
	Production of chemotactic factors (CFs; IL-8; MPC-1)	Leukocyte recruitment
	Production of CSFs	Hematopoiesis
	Production of IL-1; IL-6	Pleiotropic local and systemic effect
	Production of PDGF	Smooth muscle cell proliferation (atherosclerosis)
IFN-γ	MHC class II antigen and ICAM-1 expression	Antigen presentation
G-CSF; GM-CSF; βFGF; FGF; TGF-β	EC proliferation; migration and PA	Angiogenesis; hematopoiesis. Inhibition of endothelial cell functions

POCA, Propocoagulant; PAI, plasminogen activator; TM, thrombomodulin; VW, von Willebrand's factor; FGF, Fibroblast Growth Factor

system [39]. It can be seen in Table 2 that various agents such LPS (lipopolysaccharides) and cytokines such interleukin-1 (IL-1), TNF, and IFN-γ are important stimuli for cytokine production by the endothelial cells [39]. Recent studies have also shown that IL-1 stimulates endothelial cells to produce cytokines that inhibit leukocyte adherence and chemotaxis. These cytokines probably represent important negative feedback signals of leukocyte recruitment [39]. Cytokines produced by endothelial cells reach the blood circulation early and will therefore probably have more systemic effects than cytokines produced by leukocytes at inflammatory sites. However, cytokines produced by the inflammatory cells, for instance in the rheumatoid synovial tissue, also seem to participate in the regulation of cytokine production by endothelial cells.

Regulation of Endothelial Cell Function by Cytokines

IL-1 is a pleiotropic cytokine. It exists in two forms, IL-1α and IL-1β, which have similar biologic effects [13, 35]. IL-1 is produced by many cell types and has multiple target cells, one of them being the endothelial cell [50]. IL-1 causes leukocyte recruitment to inflamed tissues and upregulates leukocyte adhesion to endothelial cells [30]. Notably, it upregulates the endothelial cell expression of the intercellular adhesion molecules ICAM-1, and ICAM-2 [39]. IL-1 also augments the expression of endothelial leukocyte adhesion molecule 1 (ELAM-1). This molecule has been demonstrated on microvascular EC at inflammatory sites. IL-1 also stimulates EC to produce chemotactic factors such as colony-stimulating factors (CFSs) and interleukin-8 (IL-8). Moreover, IL-1 can cause vasodilatation and thrombosis by stimulating the production by EC of prostacyclin PGI_2 and thrombosis-promoting factors such as procoagulant activity (PCA), plasminogen activator (PAI), thrombomodullin (TM), and von Willebrand's factor (VW).

Tumor Necrosis Factor

There are also two forms of TNF, namely TNF-α and TNF-β (lymphotoxin), which act via the same receptors. From Table 2 it can be seen that TNF has effects on EC similar to those of IL-1, in that it causes vasodilatation, thrombosis, leukocyte adhesion and extravasation, leukocyte recruitment, and hematopoiesis. It also has pleiotropic local and systemic effects [39]. TNF also increases the expression of HLA class I and of HLA class II antigens on endothelial cells.

Interferon γ-(IFN-γ)

The actions of the lymphokine IFN-γ on the endothelial cells are different from those of IL-1 and TNF. IFN-γ induces HLA class-II antigen expression. INF-γ also induces an increase in the expression of the ICAM-1 intercellular adhesion molecule. This cytokine also inhibits endothelial cell growth by reducing the expression of receptors for the fibroblast growth factor (FGF) [39].

Colony-Stimulating Factors, Transforming Growth Factor β, Fibroblast Growth Factor, and Interleukin-8

Granulocyte colony-stimulating factor (GCSF), granulocyte macrophage colony-stimulating factor (GMCSF), transforming growth factor β (TGFβ), and (FGF) fibroblast growth factor have all been shown to induce migration and proliferation of endothelial cells, i. e. angiogenesis [39]. TGFβ has been shown to inhibit such various endothelial cell functions as growth, chemotaxis, and proteinase activity. It also inhibits IL-1- and TNF-induced neutrophil adhesion to endothelial cells [39]. FGF induces chemotaxis of endothelial cells and is therefore involved in angiogenesis. It has very recently been shown that interleukin-8 inhibits leukocyte endothelial interactions [23].

Accessory Cells

An accessory cell is a cell that can present antigens and activate T lymphocytes and/or B lymphocytes. For many years the macrophage was regarded as the main accessory cell for the various immune responses [61, 62]. However, it has become evident that a variety of other lymphoid cells – dendritic cells, resting and immune B cells, B cell lines or tumors and MHC class-II-positive T cells – can also act as accessory cells [70, 71]. Recent observations have also disclosed that other cells, such as human thyroid epithelial cells and vascular endothelial cells expressing MHC class-II molecules, may act as accessory cells which probably have local immunoregulatory function. The accessory functions for activation of T cells involve (a) processing of antigen, (b) binding of processed antigen to MHC molecules, and (c) presentation of antigenic fragments.

Processing of Antigens by Accessory Cells

Induction of antigen-specific cellular immune response among T lymphocytes requires that the antigens (microbes/autoantigens) are fragmented or processed to small peptides via proteolytic processes by the accessory cell [22]. The antigens are usually divided into two groups, i. e., exogenous and endogenous.

Exogeneous antigens are processed in the endosomal compartment and presented for CD4-positive helper of cytotoxic T lymphocytes in association with MHC class-II molecules. Endogeneous antigens, processed in the endoplasmic reticulum, are presented in association with MHC class-I molecules for CD8-positive cytotoxic T lymphocytes (CTL) [22]. However, recent data also indicate that some antigens may enter both processing pathways [49].

The processing of antigens has been studied extensively in macrophages [2]. These cells phagocytose foreign and possibly self-molecules which are fragmented by proteolytic enzymes in the lysosomes [2, 42]. The other types of accessory cells are nonphagocytic and have few lysosomes [74]. Alternative routes for antigen processing have been proposed [2]. By these mechanisms the antigens are either intact, unfolded, or internalized in endosomes and processed by other proteolytic systems than that in lysosomes or by proteolysis of the antigens at the cell membrane surface. Recently it has been shown that lymphoid dendritic cells also process soluble antigens by a nonlysosomal pathway [12]. The presentation of the antigen was in other respects similar or identical to that of macrophages.

The Importance of MHC Molecules for Accessory Cell Function

After processing, the antigenic fragments are transported to the cell surface and are then noncovalently bound to specific cell membrane structures, the MHC molecules, on the accessory cell. The complex consisting of fragmented antigenic peptide and MHC class-I or MHC class-II molecules will constitute a specific ligand for the antigen receptor (TCR) on the responding CD4-positive or CD8-positive T lymphocyte (Table 1) [5, 6]. In addition to the antigen-specific binding between the accessory cell and the T cells via the MHC and the TCR molecules, nonspecific is adhesion molecules are also involved (Table 1) [42].

The MHC molecules are highly polymorphic. This polymorphism is located at the putative site for binding of fragments of processed antigen. Recent X-ray crystallographic studies [5, 22] of the purified MHC class-I molecules HLA-A2 and HLA-Aw68 have revealed that HLA class-I molecules have an antigen-binding cleft consisting of the two N-terminal domains of the α-chain, α_1 and α_2 [5]. It is also evident that these two MHC class-I alleles have very similar overall structures, except for 123 amino acids. These studies also show that the polymorphic sites are mainly located in a groove or pocket, providing a site for binding of the processed antigen. Even an unknown "antigen" was found in this pocket in HLA-A2 crystals. In HLA-A2 and HLA-Aw68, 10 of the 13 amino acid differences faced the putative antigen-binding pocket [21]. From these studies it is assumed that the comparison of the three-dimensional structures of HLA-A2 and HLA-Aw68 provide a representative model of the polymorphic changes within the site for antigen binding in MHC class-I molecules. Based on amino acid sequence homology between MHC class-I and class-II molecules and the general secondary molecular conformations predicted by computer, it is reasonable to assume that the three dimensional structure of the MHC class-II molecules resembles the MHC class-I structure quite closely [7]. It thus appears that the class-II MHC molecules, like the MHC class-I molecules, have an antigen-binding cleft which is built up by the N-terminal parts of the α and β chains, the α_1 and β_1 domain. MHC class-II molecules have also recently been shown to bind small peptides [8–10]. The resultant groove between the two α-helices of the MHC class-I molecule is approximately 1 nm wide, 1 nm deep, and 2.5 nm long and is large enough to bind linear peptides of about eight amino acid residues or α-helices of about 20 amino acid residues [75]. Interestingly, the new information on the role of MHC class-II molecules for antigen presentation may lead to the development of new ways of treating autoimmune diseases by peptide competition for antigen presentation [1].

Accessory Cell Heterogeneity

Accessory cells are widely distributed in lymphoid and nonlymphoid organs and are a heterogeneous population. Among these, dendritic cells and macrophages are regarded as the most predominant accessory cell types, although resting B cells and other MHC class-II-positive cells also can act as accessory cells. MHC class-II molecules can be induced on many different cell types by IFN-γ, TNF, GM-CSF. The accessory cells can be further subdivided based on histological localization, marker expression, function, and degree of activation. The relationship and function of all the different types of accessory cells are still under investigation; however, dendritic cells seem to be required for the activation of resting T cells, while sensitized T cells can be activated by other MHC-class-II-positive cells (macrophages, resting B cells) as well [70–72]. The dominant markers and characteristics displayed by monocytes/macrophages, the various dendritic cell types, and B cells are shown in Table 4. Table 5 shows (CD)- Cluster of Differentiation defined membrane molecules also expressed by accessory cells.

Table 3. Membrane adhesion molecules involved in the specific and nonspecific interaction between accessory cells and T cells during activation of T cells

Molecule	Accessory cell	T cell
Specific:	MHC class-I + antigen	TCR$\alpha\beta$-CD3/CD8
	MHC class-II + antigen	TCR$\alpha\beta$-CD3/CD4
Nonspecific:	CD11a/CD18	CD54 (ICAM1)
	CD54 (ICAM1)	CD11a/CD18
	CD58 (LFA3)	CD2

MHC, Major histocompatibility complex; TCR, T-cell antigen receptor; CD, cluster of differentiation; ICAM-1, intercellular adhesion molecule 1; LFA3, leukocyte functional antigen 3

Monocytes and Macrophages

Monocytes are cells in the circulation derived from bone marrow which develop into macrophages after migration into various tissues [64]. Inflammatory conditions will increase the turnover of monocytes with augmented proliferation of progenitors in the bone marrow. This production has been shown to be regulated by circulating enhancing and inhibitory factors produced at inflammatory sites, while very few activated macrophages will proliferate at the inflammatory sites [19, 64]. Blood monocytes are less mature than tissue macrophages. Macrophages can be divided into subpopulations (e. g., peritoneal macrophages, tissue macrophages) based on localization and properties such as MHC class-II expression and microbicidal capacity. In addition, differences may also exist between macrophages located in different regions of the same lymphoid tissue. Macrophages can phagocytose and degrade foreign material in the lysosomes. This property was previously regarded as a prerequisite for accessory cell function [2, 42]. However, new data indicate that the processing and presentation of antigenic molecules may be regarded as separate processes [42, 74]. Macrophages can produce a large variety of biologically active substances. Among these are cytokines, enzymes, and prostaglandins. In addition, monocytes and macrophages express a large number of the newly defined CD molecules [41], as outlined in Table 3.

Dendritic Cells

Dendritic cells were first described in mouse spleen [46, 58]. DC from many different lymphoid (spleen, lymph nodes, thymus, afferent lymph) and nonlymphoid (blood, skin, heart, liver, kidney, inflamed synovial tissue, synovial fluid) organs and from different species (mouse, rat, man) have since been isolated and characterized [3, 70, 71].

It appears from these studies that dendritic cells comprise a heterogeneous group of cells which in most respects differ from classic monocytes/macrophages [62, 65]. The dendritic cells have an irregular shape both when adhering to glass or plastic surfaces and after culture for 1 day in suspension [19, 58, 59]. Viable, adherent dendritic cells continuously form and retract processes, while nonadherent dendritic cells have active banding and wavelike movements which are quite distinct from the behavior of phagocytic cells [19]. Apart from macrophages, the dendritic cells are mainly nonphagocytic. The only known function of dendritic cells is as accessory and antigen-presenting cells for lymphocytes. The number of dendritic cells in the various compartments are very few ($<1\%$), and they are therefore very difficult to purify and characterize. On the other hand, they are very potent in functional assays, and very few cells ($<1\%$) are usually needed for an efficient accessory function. So far no specific marker for dendritic cells has been described.

Table 4. Markers and characteristics of the various types of dendritic cells, monocytes/macrophages (MO/Mø), and B cells

Marker/characteristic	LDC*	IDC	LC	FDC	MO/Mø	B cells
MHC class I	+	+	+	+	+	+
MHC class II	+	+	+	+/−	+/−	+
T-cell antigens (CD 3)	−	−	−	−	−	−
B-cell antigens (CD 19)	−	−	−	−	−	+
MO/Mø antigens	−	−/+	−/+	−	+	−
CD 11b (CR 3, $C3_{bi}R$)	−	nd	+/−	−	+	−
CD 16 (FcRIII)	−	nd	+	+	+	−
CD 35 (CR 1, C 3bR)	−	nd	+	+	+	+
CD 45	+	nd	+	+	+	+
Birbeck granules	−	(+)	+	−	−	−
Pox/NSE	−	nd	−	nd	+	−
Phagocytosis	−	−	−/+	−/+	+	−
IL-1 production	+/−	nd	+	nd	+	−
Accessory activity	+	nd	+	nd	+/−	+

* Including blood and rheumatoid synovial dendritic cells Pox/NSE, Peroxidase/nonspecific esterase; nd, not demonstrated

Classification of Dendritic Cells

Based on anatomical localization and other features dendritic cells are usually and classified as shown in Table 4.

Lymphoid Dendritic Cells

Lymphoid dendritic cells (LCD) have been identified in suspensions of cells from lymphoid organs, peripheral blood, and chronic inflammatory sites. They strongly express MHC class-I and class-II antigens and the common leukocyte (CD 45) determinant, which indicates that they are derived from bone marrow. The lymphoid dendritic cells lack IgG-Fc receptors (CD 16) and C 3b receptors (CR 1, CD 35) as well as the majority of macrophage-specific surface antigens [36, 62, 65, 67]. The LDC are efficient accessory cells for various T-cell responses [59, 68].

Interdigitating Cells

Interdigitating cells (IDC) can be identified in sections from lymphoid tissues. They are localized primarily in the T-cell-dependent areas (paracortical areas) of the spleen, lymph nodes, and thymus. They express MHC class-II antigens and have some surface determinants in common with macrophages. It is not known whether these cells express the CD 16, the CD 35, or the CD 45 surface determinants [62]. Studies on MHC class-II (HLA-DR)-positive human thymic dendritic cells in culture suggest that these cells are identical with the IDC studied in situ [52]. A monoclonal antibody RFD 1 has been reported to be specific for IDC [55]. It has not yet been clarified whether the IDC have accessory functions for T-cell responses.

Langerhans Cells
Langerhans cells (LC) have been identified in cell suspensions obtained from the epidermis. These cells strongly express MHC class-II antigens and have typical Birbeck granules. They also express the CD16, CD35, and CD45 determinants on their surface and are thus derived from bone marrow. The LC also express the CD1a (T6) thymocyte marker, a property which has been used to purify these cells. The LC have some surface markers in common with macrophages and have been shown to exhibit accessory activities in several types of T-cell-mediated immune responses [4, 62].

Follicular Dendritic Cells
Follicular dendritic cells (FDC), sometimes called dendritic reticulum cells, have been identified in sections of lymphoid follicles. In contrast to the IDC, the FDC are localized in close contact with B cells. The FDC are probably accessory cells for B cells [38] and may exert their function through trapping of immune complexes on their surface [27]. These cells express MHC class-II antigens, CD16, CD21 (C_3d complement receptors, CR2), and CD45 antigens but are negative for macrophage-specific antigens, are nonphagocytic and nonadherent. FDC have also recently been isolated and studied in suspension [57].

Isolation of Dendritic Cells

Traditionally, non-T cells from peripheral blood mononuclear cells have been used as accessory cells in most functional studies. The non-T cell population contains a mixture of B cells, monocytes, and dendritic cells as well as NK cells, null cells, and large granular lymphocytes. For isolation of the various types of accessory cells from peripheral blood the following steps are currently used: (a) isolation of mononuclear cells, (b) isolation of non-T cells from mononuclear cells after removal of T cells rosetted with sheep erythrocytes, (c) adherence step to fractinate adherent cells (monocytes), nonadherent cells (B cells), and 16-h semiadherent cells (dendritic cells), (d) further purification of dendritic cells by depletion of unwanted cells, e. g., by the use of cytotoxic monoclonal antibodies specific for contaminating cells plus complement. By this process 80%–85% pure dendritic cells were obtained. The yield of dendritic cells is 0.6% when isolated from peripheral blood and between 0.8% and 2.6% when isolated from inflamed rheumatoid joints [68, 69].

Enriched populations of dendritic cells can also be obtained by density gradient centrifugation [59]. Highly purified blood monocytes ($<$95% pure) can also be obtained by gradient centrifugation on Nycodenz [67].

Table 5. CD molecules expressed by accessory cells

Molecule	Accessory cell	Other cells	Membrane component
CD1a, b, c	LC, B subset	Thymocytes	gp49, 45, 43
CD9	M	Pre-B cells	p24
CD11a	M	Leukocytes	LFA1 (gp180/95)
b	M	G, NK cells	$C3b_1$ receptor
c	M, B subset	G, NK cells	gp150/95
CD12	M	G, platelets	p(90–120)
CD16	M	NK cells, G	FcRIII, gp50–65
CD18		Leukocytes	β-chain to CD11a, b, c
CD23	M (act.) B subset		$FC_\in RIII$, gp45–50
CDw32	M, B	G	FcRIII, gp40
CD45	M, DC, B	Leukocytes	LCA, T200
CD45RA	M, B	T subset, G	Restricted T200, gp200
CD45RB	M, B	T subset, G	Restricted T200
CD45RO	M, B	T subset, G	Restricted T200, gp180
CDw49	M, LC, B	T, Thymocytes	VLA-α4, gp150
CD58		Leukocytes	LFA-3, gp40–65
CD64	M		FcRI, gp75
CD68	M		gp110
CD71	Mac	Prolif. cells	Transferrin receptor
CD74	M, B		Class-II associated invariant chain

LC, Langerhans cells; B, B cells; M, monocytes; DC, dendritic cells; Mac, macrophages; G, granulocytes; T, T cells

Markers and Characteristics of Dendritic Cells

The most characteristic features of dendritic cells, monocytes/macrophages, and B cells are outlined in Table 4. Dendritic cells strongly express CD45 and MHC class II molecules (HLA-DP, -DQ, -DR), but they otherwise lack most markers expressed by monocytes/macrophages and B cells. Even after 3–5 days in culture, the dendritic cells still express MHC class-II antigens. Dendritic cells lack markers expressed by T cells, NK cells, and fibroblasts, and they do not express receptors for complement (CR1, CD35) or transferrin. In contrast to monocytes/macrophages and B cells, no specific marker for dendritic cells has been described. The markers and characteristics expressed by rheumatoid synovial dendritic cells indicate that, together with blood dendritic cells, they belong to the lineage of lymphoid dendritic cells (Table 4) and are probably different from other bone marrow-derived cells. Synovial and blood dendritic cells also lack the D1 antigen (identified by the RFD1 antibody) and the CD1a antigen, expressed by IDC and by LC respectively [68].

Dendritic Cells in Rheumatoid Inflammation

The chronic inflammatory process in rheumatoid arthritis has been intensively studied with respect to the active involvement of T lymphocyte and B lymphocyte systems [48], but until a few years ago, much less was known about accessory cells in the rheumatoid inflammatory process. In light of the importance of accessory cells for the activation of lymphocytes, such cells could be one of the driving forces of the chronic inflammatory processes seen in rheumatoid arthritis.

In an early study by Klareskog et al. [33] it was shown that MHC class-II (HLA-DR)-expressing adherent synovial cells from patients with rheumatoid arthritis were 20–100 times more efficient than non-T cells from peripheral blood as stimulators in allogeneic mixed leukocyte reactions. This indicated that the synovial tissues contained one or more cell populations with efficient accessory activities.

In a series of studies [67–71], dendritic cells from rheumatoid synovial tissue and synovial fluid as well as from normal peripheral blood have been intensively characterized [28]. When dendritic cells from both compartments are incubated with autologous T cells, characteristic cell clusters are observed. If the clusters are carefully stained with a monoclonal anti-MHC class-II antibody, MHC class-II-positive dendritic cells can be visualized in the center of the clusters. On the other hand, by adding monoclonal anti-MHC class-II (anti-HLA-DR) antibodies to the culture at the start of the incubation the cluster formation is almost completely inhibited. A similar inhibition of the cluster formation is also seen after a monoclonal antibody specific for the CD2 antigen on the T cells has been added. Recent studies have revealed that the CD2 antigen is the receptor for the newly defined membrane molecule CD58 (the LFA-3 molecule). CD58 may therefore also be expressed by blood and synovial dendritic cells. Thus, both MHC class-II molecules (HLA-DR) and, most likely, the CD2 antigen are important for cluster formation and cell-to-cell adhesion between human dendritic cells and T cells (Table 3). The majority of the T cells forming clusters with dendritic cells were CD4 positive, although some CD8-positive cells were also seen [68].

In the mouse system it has been shown that cell clusters between dendritic cells and T cells could be separated from nonclustered cells by centrifugation on a Percoll gradient [29]. Using a similar technique, we were able to separate clusters of rheumatoid synovial and blood dendritic cells and T cells from nonclustered cells [68]. Whether the clustered cells were dissociated or not, these cells had five to ten times greater proliferation ([^{3}H] thymidine incorporation) than nonclustered cells. This observation indicates that adhesion and direct cell-to-cell contact between dendritic cells and T cells are of vital importance for the activation of resting T cells. The observed in vitro clustering phenomenon may thus have its counterpart in the nodular aggregates found in vivo in the inflamed synovial tissue of patients with rheumatic disease and at the inflammatory sites of other autoimmune diseases.

Lymphocyte Activation Induced by Dendritic Cells

In agreement with the potent accessory properties of the dendritic cells for the various T-cell responses, we have also found that dendritic cells are able to induce expression of surface activation antigens on large numbers of T cells during autologous MLR cultures [69–71]. These activation markers include MHC class-II (HLA-DR) molecules, receptors for transferrin (TfR), and receptors for interleukin-2 (IL-2) (Tac, CD25). Interestingly, the number of T cells expressing these activation markers after stimulation by dendritic cells was very similar to the number of T cells from rheumatoid synovial tissue and synovial fluid expressing these markers [70, 71]. In addition, the synovial T cells also express the activation markers TliSA1 and VLA1. Synovial dendritic cells may thus be involved in the activation process of T cells seen in rheumatoid synovitis.

After the accessory cell and the T cells have been become attached to each other by various adhesion molecules, the T cell can react with the antigen/MHC molecular complexes on the accessory cell via their receptor for antigen, the TCR-CD3 complex. CD8-positive T cells react with antigen/MHC class-I molecular complexes, while CD4-positive T cells recognize antigens bound to MHC class-II molecules [51].

The antigen presentation for B cells is less well characterized. B cells localized outside lymphoid follicles are most probably activated by a T-cell-dependent activation pathway, while B cells in the follicles seem to be activated by follicular dendritic cells [39].

In recent studies by Waalen [70] and Waalen et al. [71], purified peripheral blood monocytes and dendritic cells from blood and rheumatoid synovial tissue and fluid were compared for various accessory cell functions. These studies clearly showed the dendritic cells both from normal PB and from rheumatoid synovial compartments were superior to monocytes as accessory cells for antigen (PPD, HSV)- and mitogen (PHA and ConA)- induced T-cell responses and to induce autologous as well as allogeneic T-cell responses (MLR). However, when *Chlamydia trachomatis* particles were used as somewhat different picture was seen. Thus a mixture of monocytes and dendritic cells gave an enhanced T-cell response, indicating a possible cooperation between the monocytes and dendritic cells [70, 71]. Monoclonal antibodies to MHC class-II molecules (HLA-DR and HLA-DQ) also inhibited the specific antigen activation of T cells to PPD, HSV, and *C. trachomatis,* indicating that the sites on the MHC molecules for antigen binding were blocked by these antibodies [70,71]. Interestingly, it has also been shown [72] that dendritic cells can present autoantigens like collagen type II and IgG-Fc fragments to autologous T cells.

Other Dendritic-like Cells at Rheumatoid Inflammatory Sites

Cultures of adherent synovial cells have shown that the majority of these cells may have a dendritic-like or stellate morphology. Hendler et al. [25] claim that in 24- to 48-h culture of crude synovial cells the synovial dendritic cells lose their class-II MHC antigens and are transformed into fibroblasts. In addition, other authors claim that synovial fibroblasts acquire a dendritic morphology after stimulation with Il-1 or mast cell products [20]. The results from these two studies imply that rheumatoid fibroblasts and rheumatoid dendritic cells may represent the same cell at two different stages. These findings are in contrast to other observations: It was recently shown that during 3–5 days of culture, isolated synovial dendritic cells retain high expression of MHC class-II (HLA-DR) antigens, together with an efficient accessory activity. No transformation of rheumatoid synovial dendritic cells into fibroblasts was observed, as analyzed with monoclonal antifibroblast antibodies. These observations indicate that, in the rheumatoid synovium, there may exist at least three types of cells with a dendritic morphology: (a) fibroblasts with passively adsorbed or INF-γ induced MHC class-II molecules, which are lost during culture; (b) MHC class-II (HLA-DR)-negative fibroblasts; and (c) classic, MHC class-II-positive lymphoid dendritic cells, which are distinct from fibroblasts and which retain their MHC class-II molecules and accessory activity during short-term culture [68, 70, 71].

Cytokines Produced by Dendritic Cells

The current interpretation of T-cell activation is that an accessory cell presents antigens to the T cells in the context of class-II MHC molecules [60]. In addition, interleukin-1 (IL-1) is produced by the accessory cell and acts as a co-mitogenic signal in the activation process [43]. These stimuli then trigger the T cells to produce and become responsive to IL-2. The recent data indicates that in the mouse, mainly the T_h2 T cells express receptors for IL-1.

Recent studies [70, 71] have shown that dendritic cells from inflamed synovial tissue probably produce large amounts of IL-1-like activity, both spontaneously and after stimulation with lipopolysaccharide (LPS), while the blood dendritic cells produce some, although much less, of this substance [66]. The enhanced release of IL-1 by dendritic cells thus seems to be restricted to the synovial inflammatory compartment. In addition, it is shown [73] that rheumatoid synovial dendritic cells also express mRNA for both interleukin-1-alpha and -beta as well as for interleukin-6.

Thus, soluble mediators produced by accessory cells have important and essential functions in the specific activation of lymphocytes. In addition, these mediators may have several important effects on other cell types and on

Table 6. Cytokines produced by accessory cells

Cytokine	Accessory cells			Other cells	Detected in RA*
	MO/Mø	DC	B		
Interleukin-1 (IL-1 alfa and beta)	+	+	+	+	+
Interleukin-6 (IL-6)	+	+	−	+	+
Interleukin-8 (IL-8)	+	nd	nd	+	nd
Tumor necrosis factor (TNF-alfa)	+	−	−	+	+
Lymphotoxin (TNF-beta)	+	−	+	+	nd
Interferon (IFN-alfa)	+	−	−	−	+/−
Transforming growth factor (TGF-beta)	+	−	−	+	+
G-CSF	+	−	−	+	nd
M-CSF	+	−	−	+	+

RA, Rheumatoid arthritis; nd, not demonstrated; B, B cells
* Detected in the rheumatoid synovial compartments

biological processes in inflammatory reactions; i. e., a number of these cytokines are produced by inflammatory cells in the rheumatoid synovial compartment [18, 37].

Table 6 shows the cytokines produced by accessory cells (monocytes, dendritic cells, and B cells). Some of these cytokines are produced by these cells only, while others are produced by other cell types as well. IL-1 is a pleiotropic factor with many biological functions, the main ones being T-cell and B-cell activation, cartilage resorption, pyrogenic action, and induction of acute-hase proteins. IL-6 is also pleiotropic, and its main property is its effect on B- and T-lymphocyte growth and differentiation. IL-1 and IL-6 stimulate the production of acute-phase reactants. IL-8 stimulates B and T lymphocytes and the chemotaxis of neutrophils. The production of IL-8 is enhanced by IL-1 and TNF-α. TNF-α is a cytotoxic factor with many important biological functions. Among these are induction of MHC class-II expression, IFN-γ production, B-cell proliferation, and Ig secretion. TNF-β has 50% amino acid homology with TNF-α and seems to have many similar biological functions as well. Interferon-alfa has antiviral and antiproliferative functions. It also upregulates MHC class-II expression and enhances the cytotoxic activities of T cells, NK cells, and macrophages. TGF-β is a potent immunosuppressive cytokine and has, in general, many antagonistic effects to TNF-α, i. e., inhibition of MHC class-II expression, IFN-γ production, B-cell proliferation, and Ig secretion. G-CSF induce neutrophil colony formation and have indirect stimulatory effects on erythroid and mixed colony progenitors. M-CSF stimulates the production of PGE_2, IL-1, and TNF-α by monocytes and macrophages. This cytokine also stimulates the growth of monocyte precursor colonies and shows tumoricidal activity. Most cytokines do not work alone but are members of biological cascades which induce responses by their additive, synergistic, or antagonistic effects. Many of these cytokines are produced by and have effects on endothelial cells.

References

1. Adorini L, Nagy ZA (1990) Peptide competition for antigen presentation. Immunol Today 11:21–24
2. Allen PM (1987) Antigen processing at the molecular level. Immunol Today 8:270–273
3. Austyn JM (1987) Lymphoid dendritic cells. Immunology 62:161–170
4. Bjercke S, Lea T, Braathen LR, Thorsby E (1984) Enrichment of human epidermal Langerhans cells. Scand J Immunol 11:255–254
5. Björkman PJ, Saper MA, Samraoui B, Bennett WS, Strominger JL, Wiley DC (1987) The foreign antigen binding site and T cell recognition regions of class-I histocompatibility antigens. Nature 329:512–518
6. Braciale TJ, Morrison LA, Sweetser MT, Sambrook J, Gething J-J, Braciale VL (1987) Antigen presentation pathways to class-I and class-II MHC-restricted T lymphocytes. Immunol Rev 98:95–114
7. Brown JH, Jardetzky T, Saper MA, Samraoui B, Bjorkman PJ, Wiley DC (1988) A hypothetical model of the foreign antigen binding site of class-II histocompatibility molecules. Nature 332:845–849
8. Buus S, Colon S, Smith C, Freed JH, Miles C, Grey HM (1986) Interaction between a "processed" ovalbumin peptide and Ia molecules. Proc Natl Acad Sci USA 83:3968–3973
9. Buus S, Sette A, Grey HM (1987) The interaction between protein-derived immunogenetic peptides and Ia. Immunol Rev 98:115–142
10. Buus S, Sette A, Colon S, Miles C, Grey HM (1987) The relationship between major histocompatibility complex (MHC) restriction and capacity of Ia to bind immunogenetic peptides. Science 235:1353–1356
11. Cavender D, Hasgard D, Yucl H et al. (1987) Pathways to chronic inflammation in rheumatoid synovitis. Fed Proc 46:113–117
12. Chain BM, Kay PM, Feldman M (1986) The cellular pathway of antigen presentation: biochemical and functional analysis of antigen in dendritic cells and macrophages. Immunology 58:271–277
13. Dinarello CA (1984) Interleukin 1. Rev Infect Dis 6:51–95
14. Duijdvestin AM, Hamman A (1989) Mechanisms and regulation of lymphocyte migration. Immunol Today 10:23–24
15. Duijdvestin AM, Schreiber AS, Butcher IC (1986) Interferon-γ regulates an antigen specific for endothelial cells involved in lymphocyte traffic. Proc Natl Acad Sci USA 83:9114–9119
16. Falkman G, Li W, Carey R (1989) Inflammation and angiogenesis. Prog Immunol 7:761–764
17. Falkman G, Klagsbrun M (1987) Angiogenic factors. Science 235:442–447
18. Feldman M, Kissonergis AM, Buchan G, Brennan F, Turner M, Haworth C, Barrett K, Chantry D, Ziegler A, Maini RN (1988) Role of HLA class-II and cytokines in rheumatoid arthritis. Scand J Rheumatol [Suppl] 76:39–46
19. Førre Ø, Waalen K, Thoen J, Hovig T (1985) Macrophages and dendritic cells in rheumatic diseases. In: Gupta S, Talal N (eds) Immunology of rheumatic diseases. Plenum, New York, pp 543–545
20. Gadher SJ, Woolley DE (1987) Comparative studies of adherent rheumatoid synovial cells in primary culture. Characterization of the dendritic (stellate) cell. Rheumatology Int 7:13–18

21. Garrett TPJ, Saper MA, Bjorkman PJ, Strominger JL, Wiley DC (1989) Specificity pockets for the side chains of peptide antigens in HLA-Aw68. Nature 342:692–696
22. Germain RN (1986) The ins and outs of antigen processing and presentation. Nature 322:687–689
23. Gimbrone MA, Obin MS, Brock AF, Luis EA, Hass PE, Hebert CA, Yip YK, Leung DW, Lowe DG, Kohr WJ, Darbonne WC, Bechtol KB, Baker JB (1989) Endothelial interleukin-8: a novel inhibitor of leukocyte-endothelial interactions. Science 246:1601–1603
24. Haynes BF, Hale LP, Denning SM, Le PT, Singer KH (1989) The role of leukocyte adhesion molecules in cellular interactions: implications for the pathogenesis of inflammatory synovitis. Springer Semin Immunopathol 11:163–185
25. Hendler PL, Lavoie PE, Werb Z, Chan J, Seaman WE (1985) Human synovial dendritic cells. Direct observation of transition to fibroblasts. J Rheumatol 12:660–669
26. Herron GS, Bandba MJ, Clark EJ, Gavrilovic J, Werb Z (1986) Secretion of metallo-proteinases by stimulator capillary endothelial cells. II. Expession of collagenase and stromelysin activities is regulated by endogenous inhibitors. J Biol Chem 261:2814–1818
27. Humphrey JH, Grennan D, Sundarm V (1984) The origin of follicular dendritic cels in the mouse and the mechanism of trapping immune complexes on them. Eur J Immunol 14:859–864
28. Inaba K, Witmer MD, Steinman RM (1984) The clustering of dendritic cells, helper T lymphocytes and histocompatible B cells during primary antibody responses in vitro. J Exp Med 160:858–876
29. Inaba K, Steinman RM (1987) Monoclonal antibodies to LFA-1 and to CD4 inhibit the mixed leukocyte reaction after antigen-dependent clustering of dendritic cells and T lymphocytes. J Exp Med 165:1403–1417
30. Jalkanen S (1989) Leukocyte endothelial cell interaction and control of leukocyte migration into inflamed synovium. Springer Semin Immunopathol 11:187–198
31. Jalkanen S, Bagatse RF, de los Toyos J, Butcher EC (1987) Lymphocyte recognition of high endothelium: antibodies to distinct epitopes of an 85–95 kDa glycoprotein antigen differentially inhibit lymphocyte binding to lymp nodes, mucosal or synovial endothelial cells. J Cell Biol 105:983–994
32. Jalkanen S, Steere AC, Fox RI, Butcher EC (1986) A distinct endothelial cell recognition system that controls lymphocytic traffic into inflamed synovium. Science 233:556–561
33. Klareskog L, Forsum U, Kabelitz D, Pløen L, Sundstrøm C, Nilson K, Wigren A, Wigzell H (1982) Immune functions of human synovial cells. Phenotypic and T cell regulatory properties of macrophage-like cells that express HLA-DR. Arthritis Rheum 25:488–501
34. Koch AE, Palverini PJ, Labovich SG (1986) Stimulation of neovascularization by human rheumatoid synovial tissue macrophages. Arthritis Rheum 29:471–479
35. Koide SL, Steinman RM (1987) Induction of murine interleukin 1: stimuli and responsive primary cells. Proc Natl Acad Sci USA 84:3802–3806
36. Kuntz Crow M, Kunkel HG (1982) Human dendritic cells: major stimulators of the autologous and allogeneic mixed leukocyte reactions. Clin Exp Immunol 49:338–346
37. Lipsky PE, Davies LS, Cush JJ, Oppenheimer-Marks N (1989) The role of cytokines in the pathogenesis of rheumatoid arthritis. Springer Semin Immuno Pathol 11:123–162
38. MacLennon IMC (1989) The cellular basis of antibody production. In: Iversen OH (ed) Cell kinetics of the inflammatory reaction. Springer, Berlin Heidelberg New York (Current topics in pathology, vol 79)
39. Mantovani A, Dejana E (1990) Cytokines as communication signals between leukocytes and endothelial cells. Immunol Today 10:370–375
40. Masuyama J, Minoto N, Kano S (1986) Mechanisms of lymphocytic adhesion to human vascular endothelial cells in culture. T lymphocyte adhesion to endothelial cells through endothelial HLA-DR antigens induced by intereferon-γ. J Clin Invest 77:1596–1603
41. McMichael AJ, Beverly PCL, Cobbold S, Crumpton MJ et al. (1989) Leukocyte typing. III. White blood differentiation antigens. Oxford University Press, Oxford

42. Mills KHG (1986) Processing of viral antigens and presentation to class-II-restricted T cells. Immunol Today 7:260–263
43. Mizel SB (1982) Interleukin 1 and T cell activation. Immunol Rev 63:51
44. Montesano R, Vasalli GD, Beard A et al. (1986) Basic fibroblast growth factor induces angiogenesis in vitro. Proc Natil Acad Sci USA 83:7297–7301
45. Möller G (1982) Structure and function of HLA-DR. Immunol Rev 66:1–187
46. Möller G (ed) (1987) Immunol Rev 106:1–187
47. Möller G (1989) Lymphocyte homing. Immunol Rev 108:1–161
48. Natvig JB, Winchester R (eds) (1988) Immunopathology of rheumatoid inflammation. Springer Semin Immunopathol 10:115–277
49. Nuchtern JG, Biddison WE, Klausner RD (1990) Class-II MHC molecules can use the endogenous pathway of antigen presentation. Nature 343:74–76
50. Oppenheim JJ, Kovacs EJ, Matsushima K, Durum SK (1986) There is more than one interleukin 1. Immunol Today 7:45–47
51. Parnes JR (1986) T cell differentiation antigens: proteins, genes and function. Bioessays 4:255–259
52. Pelletier M, Tautu C, Landry D, Montplaisir S, Chartrand C, Perreault C (1987) Characterization of human thymic dendritic cells in culture. Immunology 58:263–270
53. Pober GS, Collins T, Gimbrone MA Jr, Cotran RS, Gicklin GD, Fierse W, Clayburger C, Crensky AM, Burakoff SJ, Reiss CS (1983) Lymphocytes recognize human vascular endothelial and normal fibroblasts Ia antigens induced by recombinant immune interferon. Nature 305:726–730
54. Pober JS, Gimbrone MA Jr, Cotran RS, Reiss CS, Burakoff SJ, Fiers W, Ault KA (1983) Ia expression by vascular endothelium is inducible by activated T cells and human interferon. J Exp Med 157:1339–1345
55. Poulter LW, Campbell DA, Munro C, Janossy G (1986) Discrimination of human macrophages and dendritic cells by means of monoclonal antibodies. Scand J Immunol 24:351–357
56. Pitzalis C, Kingsley G, Haskard G, Panayi G (1988) Preferential accumulation of helper-inducer T lymphocytes in inflammatory lesions: evidence for regulation selective endothelial and homotypic adhesion. Eur J Immunol 18:3097–1404
57. Schnitzlein CT, Kosco MH, Szakal AK, Tew JG (1985) Follicular dendritic cells in suspension: identification enrichment and initial characterization indicating immune complex trapping and lack of adherence and phagocytic activity. J Immunol 134:1360–1366
58. Steinman RM, Cohn ZA (1973) Identification of a novel cell type in peripheral lymphoid organs of mice. I. Morphology, quantitation and tissue distribution. J Exp Med 137:1142–1162
59. Steinman R, van Voorhis WC, Spanding DM (1986) Dendritic cells. In: Weir DM, Blackwell C, Herzenberg LA (eds) Handbook of experimental immunology, 4th edn. Blackwell, Oxford, pp 491–499
60. Thorsby E (1984) The role of HLA in T cell activation. Hum Immunol 9:1
61. Unanue ER (1984) Antigen-presenting function of the macrophage. Annu Rev Immunol 2:385–428
62. Unkeless JC, Springer TA (1986) Macrophages. In: Weir DM, Blackwell G, Herzenberg LA (eds) Handbook of experimental immunology, 4th edn. Blackwell, Oxford, pp 1181–11817
63. Van Dinther-Janssen ACHM, Pals ST, Scheper R, Breetveld F, Meijer CGLM (1990) Dendritic cells and high endothelial venules in the rheumatoid synovial membrane. J Rheumatol 17:11–17
64. Van Furth (1981) The origin of phagocytic cells in the joint and bone. Scand J Rheumatol [Suppl] 40:13–20
65. Van Voorhis WC, Witmer MD, Steinman RM (1983) The phenotype of dendritic cells and macrophages. Fed Am Soc Exp Biol 42:3114–3118
66. Waalen K, Duff GW, Førre Ø, Dickens E, Kvarnes L, Nuki G (1986) Interleukin-1 activity produced by human rheumatoid and normal dendritic cells. Scand J Immunol 23:365–371

67. Waalen K, Thoen J, Førre Ø, Hovig T, Teigland J, Natvig JB (1986) Rheumatoid synovial dendritic cells as stimulators in allogeneic and autologous mixed leukocyte reactions – comparison with autologous monocytes as stimulator cells. Scand J Immunol 23:233–243
68. Waalen K, Főrre Ø, Pahle J, Natvig JB, Burmester GR (1987) Characteristics of human rheumatoid synovial and normal blood dendritic cells. Retention of class-II MHC antigens and accessory function during short-term culture. Scand J Immunol 26:525–533
69. Waalen K, Főrre Ø, Linker-Israeli M, Thoen J (1987) Evidence of an activated T-cell system with augmented turnover of interleukin-2 in rheumatoid arthritis. Stimulation of human T lymphocytes by dendritic cells as a model for rheumatoid T-cell activation. Scand J Immunol 25:367–373
70. Waalen K (1988a) Lymphoid dendritic cells in rheumatoid inflammation. Thesis, University of Oslo
71. Waalen K, Főrre Ø, Natvig JB (1988) Rheumatoid lymphoid dendritic cells – characteristics and functions. Scand J Rheumatol [Suppl] 76:47–60
72. Waalen K, Főrre Ø, Natvig JB (1988) Lymphoid dendritic cell in rheumatoid tissue and normal blood – characteristics and functions. In: Fossum S, Rolstad B (eds) Histophysiology of the immune system: the life organization and interactions of its cell population. Plenum, New York, pp 761–765
73. Waalen K, Főrre Ø (1990) Rheumatoid synovial dendritic cells spontaneously express mRNA for interleukin-1 and interleukin-6. (to be published)
74. Watts C, Howard JC (1986) Membrane recycling and antigen presentation. Bioessays 4:265
75. Winchester RJ, Gregersen PK (1988) The molecular basis of susceptibility to rheumatoid arthritis: the conformational equivalence hypothesis. Springer Semin Immunopathol 10:119–139
76. Ziff M (1990) Rheumatoid arthritis – its present and future. J Rheumatol 17:2127–2132

Cellular and Humoral Immune Response Against Articular Chondrocytes and Proteoglycans in Rheumatoid Arthritis

G. R. Burmester[1], S. Alsalameh[1], and J. Mollenhauer[2]

[1] Institute of Clinical Immunology and Rheumatology, Department of Medicine III and
[2] Institute of Pharmacology and Toxicology, University of Erlangen-Nürnberg, FRG

Introduction

The hallmark of many inflammatory and degenerative joint diseases is the destruction of cartilage. Normally, cartilage is an immunologically privileged, sequestered tissue that has been shown to possess tissue-specific matrix and cell surface antigens [1]. These antigens may cause autoimmune reactions when exposed to the immune system during traumatic or inflammatory processes. Moreover, HLA class-II (Ia) antigens have been demonstrated on human articular chondrocytes, which normally do not express these surface molecules, in certain joint diseases including rheumatoid arthritis (Fig. 1) [2, 3]. In vitro, HLA class-II antigens can be induced on constitutively Ia-negative human chondrocytes by γ-interferon [4]. An aberrant HLA class-II antigen expression in affected organs is a general phenomenon in autoimmune diseases such as thyroiditis, juvenile diabetes mellitus, lichen ruber planus, and primary biliary cirrhosis [5–7]. It has been suggested that this expression contributes to the initiation of autoimmune reactions [8]. Rabbit articular chondrocytes have been shown to bear Ia antigens constitutively [9]. In this species, chondrocytes are able to stimulate allogeneic and autologous T lymphocytes [9–11]. Furthermore, rabbit articular chondrocytes have been shown to function as antigen-presenting cells [9].

In rheumatoid arthritis (RA), the cartilage is invaded by aggressive tissue elements, ultimately leading to the complete destruction of the joint structures. The reasons for the infiltration by this pannus tissue have not been elucidated. However, the presence of large numbers of activated lymphocytes and macrophages in the surrounding synovial membrane [12–15] strongly suggests an antigen-driven process in inflammatory joint diseases.

Despite intensive research, no autoantigen has been clearly identified. There is evidence for the presence of autoantibodies against collagens, especially type II (see also chapter by Holmdahl, this volume, and references [16–20]), and proteoglycans (see below). Parallel studies investigating the cell-mediated

Smolen, Kalden, Maini (Eds.)
Rheumatoid Arthritis
© Springer-Verlag Berlin Heidelberg 1992

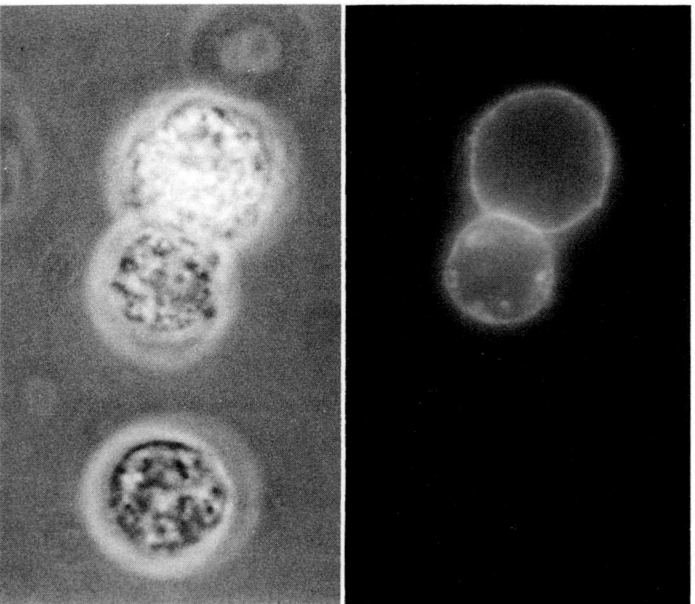

Fig. 1. Expression of HLA-DR molecules on chondrocytes strongly induced by gamma-interferon after 7 days of culture with 200 U/ml gamma-interferon as determined by immunofluorescence

immune response have documented a T-cell responsiveness against these connective tissue elements [21–24].

The degenerative counterpart of RA, osteoarthritis (OA), has been the matter of increasing interest over the recent years. While traditionally believed to be primarily the result of mechanical disruption, it is now evident that the cellular reactions of chondrocytes to various stimuli play an important role in the pathogenesis of OA [for review see 25]. In this disease, normal chondrocytes are frequently displaced by fibrous tissue cells, resulting in cartilage metaplasia. Moreover, a revascularization of the normally avascular cartilage occurs, caused by the penetration of the cartilage tidemark by vessels derived from the subchondral bone [26]. This process may possibly lead to an encounter of the immune system with the normally "immunoprivileged" site of cartilage, thereby resulting in autoimmune phenomena. Therefore, the following chapter will compare findings obtained in RA patients with those seen in the OA population.

Chondrocyte-directed Humoral Immune Reactions

Autoantibodies to Chondrocyte Membranes

In various rheumatic diseases, autoantibodies against tissue elements have been described. These structures include proteins of the extracellular matrix as well

Table 1. Sera from donors with RA, OA, and controls were titrated in ELISA [28] on the indicated membrane species. Values are given as arbitrary photometrical units [28] with the standard deviation

Source of membranes	RA	OA	Control
Cartilage	$4.0 + 1.4$	$2.3 + 0.7$	$1.5 + 0.2$
Fibroblasts	$1.6 + 0.4$	$1.2 + 0.2$	$0.7 + 0.1$
Epithelial carcinoma	< 0.5	< 0.05	< 0.5

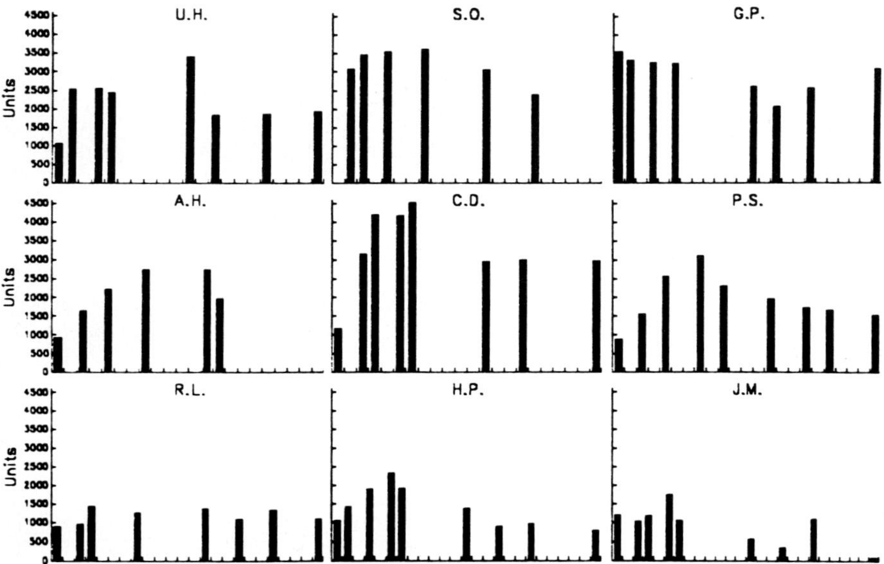

Fig. 2. Time-course study of autoantibody titers against chondrocyte membranes from nine patients with OA. The study began in February 1988 and ended in March 1990. The abscissa is scaled in monthly intervals, the ordinate in photometrical units that were summed up from the titration curves of the ELISA [28]. Months with no bars were not measured

as internal cell compounds: nucleic acids and nuclear, ribosomal, and mitochondrial proteins. In addition, the outer cell membrane compartment has recently been shown to possess proteins with autoantigenic character [27–29]. Thus, patients with RA and OA had significant titers of anti-chondrocyte membrane antibodies that could be measured by an ELISA (Table 1). Over a 2-year period it was demonstrated that patients with OA had relatively stable antibody titers. Patients with low response did not develop higher titers, whereas patients with significant titers conserved these reactions during the whole period (Fig. 2). Interestingly, these data correlated to another possible indicator of joint affection, the cartilage-specific keratan sulfate (KS) [30]. Parallel determinations of the metabolic parameter – KS release – and the

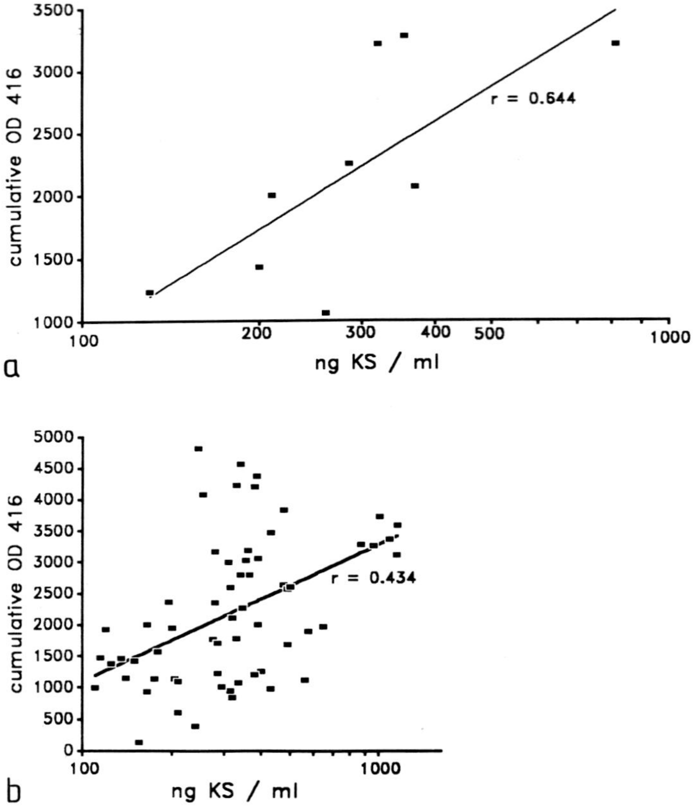

Fig. 3a, b. Correlation analysis between the anti-chondrocyte membrane titers and the keratan sulfate (KS) release [30] in the blood of OA patients. Sera were taken from the study in Fig. 2. **a** Means of all KS values and all antibody values obtained from one patient during the 2-year investigation period, in total from nine patients. **b** Correlation pairs obtained from one single blood sample, in total from nine patients over the 2-year period

immunological parameters – antibody titers – in the patients investigated demonstrated a relatively clear correlation of the two parameters. This correlation was apparent with regard to the mean values for the 2-year period (Fig. 3a), while individual serum samples showed only a weak correlation (Fig. 3b).

Structures of Chondrocyte Autoantigens

The autoantibodies recognized a number of antigens that could be visualized by electrophoretic separation and subsequent blotting of sucrose-density gradient-enriched membrane proteins. Table 2 lists frequently recognized polypeptides. These reactions were absent from membranes prepared from human foreskin fibroblasts or from epithelial tumor cells, but the antibody response was highly

Table 2. Polypeptides from chicken chondrocyte membrane preparations recognized by RA sera in Westernblot. The 135-kD polypeptide corresponds to cell surface-attached collagen type II

M_r (kD)	Control sera	OA sera	RA sera
150	−	+	+
135	(+)	+	+
116	−	+	+
78	−	+	+
76	−	+	+
60–70	−	+	+
52	−	−	+
38	−	−	+
30	−	+	+
29	−	−	+

Table 3. Interspecies cross-reactivity of RA antisera reacting with the 60- to 70-kD polypeptide in Western blot analysis [28] of enriched chondrocyte membrane preparations

Protein	Source of chondrocyte membranes			
	Chicken	Calf	Human, nasal	Human, articular
60- to 70-kD	60%	60%	60%	80%
Collagen type II	30%	20%	20%	n.d.

n.d., Not done

cross-reactive with cartilage cell membranes derived from other species. Table 3 shows the cross-reactivity of the antibodies against the most frequently recognized antigen in RA, a 65-KD polypeptide, in a number of patients, using various sources of cartilage.

Currently, more detailed protein chemical and immunological investigations are being performed to elucidate the nature of this protein. Its possible relationship to hsp 65, a member of the heat-shock protein (hsp) family, is being analyzed, especially since hsp 65 from *Mycobacterium tuberculosis* or *M. butyricum* is thought to play a key role in the initiation of mycobacterial arthritis [31–33]. Since macrophages are able to express a protein homologous to hsp 65 during Il-1-induced activation, such a protein might be involved in the provocation of autoimmune reactions. However, initial data exclude an identity between these two proteins, hsp 65 and the chondrocyte membrane 65-KD polypeptide, despite some interesting structural and immunological correlations (Table 4).

Table 4. Molecular and immunological relationships of the 60- to 70-kD polypeptide with other proteins involved in autoimmune processes in RA patients: hsp 65, the mycobacterial heat-shock protein, cartilage proteoglycan core protein, and type-II collagen

Characteristics	60- to -70-kD protein	hsp 65	Proteoglycan core protein	Collagen type II
Relative molar mass – native (kD)	>300	65	65	300
Relative molar mass – reduced (kD)	60–70	65	65	100 (denatured)
Glycosylation	yes	no	(no)	yes
Distribution	Constitutive outer membranes?	Stress-induced intracellular	Constitutive pericellular cell surface?	Constitutive pericellular interstitial
Tissue types	Cartilage + ?	Widespread	Cartilage	Cartilage
Sequence characteristics	SNP cross-reactive	SNP	Ig superfamily	SNP cross-reactive

SNP, Arthritogenic nonapeptide sequence of hsp 65
Ig superfamily, contains foldings comparable to IgG molecule

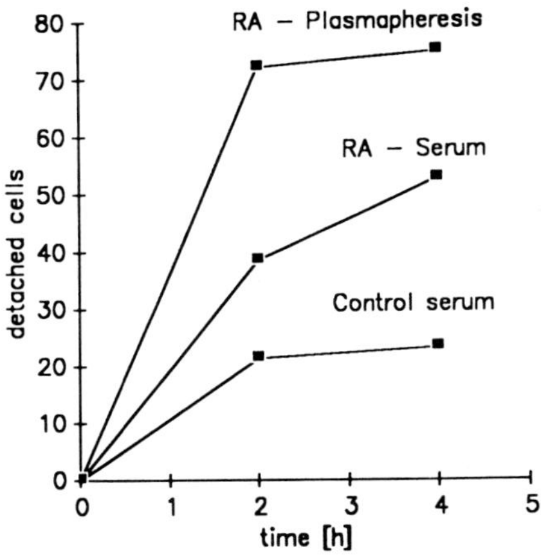

Fig. 4. Detachment of chondrocytes caused by contact with human serum from a normal donor (*control serum*), from one RA serum, and from plasmapheresis fluid obtained from the same RA patient. Values are expressed as the percentage of detached cells on the plates ($100\% = 10^6$ cells) after the indicated incubation times with the sera, at a concentration of 1% serum in culture medium

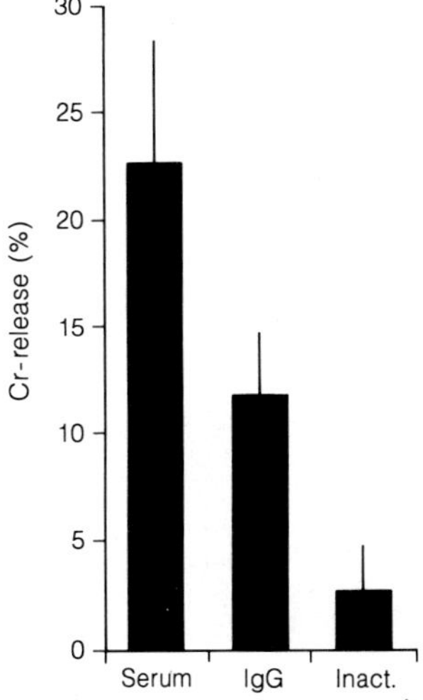

Fig. 5. Cytotoxicity of RA serum in a chromium 51 release assay. Cells were labeled with ^{51}Cr for 2 h, then washed and incubated with 1% RA serum, 1% heat-inactivated RA serum, or the corresponding amount of purified immunoglobulins in culture medium for 1 h. Cells were washed subsequently, and the chromium release was determined by counting the radioactivity in the cell pellet and the medium supernatant. Percent of total radioactivity incorporated by the cells, means of five values

Serum Cytotoxicity

The production of autoantibodies to the cell surface of chondrocytes is not the only impact of the immune system on cartilage cells. Recent investigations [34, 35] revealed that serum itself could damage chondrocytes. A rather mild event is the activation of collagenase in chondrocytes via the adsorption of Fc parts of immunoglobulins on the cell surface [35]. The contact with normal human serum resulted in a much more pronounced effect. Detachment of the cells from the substrate (Fig. 4) and finally cytotoxic destruction of the chondrocytes, as determined by the release of chromium-51, occurred (Fig. 5). Since heat-inactivated serum displayed no cytotoxic activitiy, "spontaneous" complement activation on the chondrocyte surface may cause this destruction (Fig. 5),

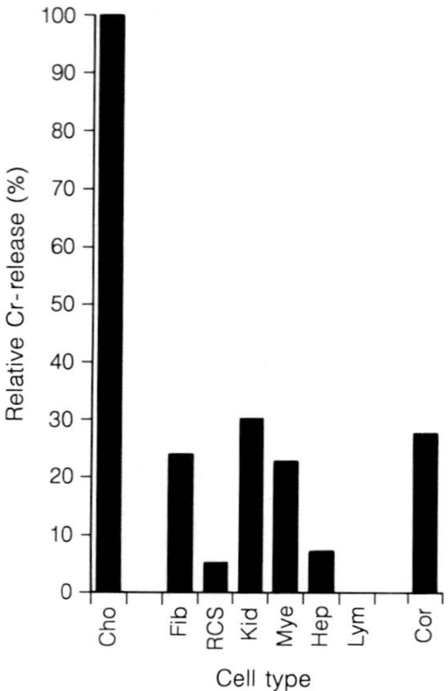

Fig. 6. Cytotoxicity of RA serum to several cell types in vitro. Cells were treated and cytotoxicity was determined as described in Fig. 5. *Cho,* Chicken sternal chondrocytes; *Fib,* human fore-skin fibroblasts; *RCS,* rat chondrosarcoma cell line; *Kid,* epithelial kidney cells; *Hep,* rat hepatoma cell line (H4IIE); *Mye,* mouse myeloma cell line; *Lym,* human peripheral lymphocytes; *Cor,* chicken corneal epithelium (intact layer)

despite a demonstrable influence of purified immunoglobulins derived from RA patients. This phenomenon was shown to be tissue specific, since other cell types, even such bradytrophic cells as in corneal epithelia, did not react like chondrocytes (Fig. 6).

These humoral phenomena again underline the concept of "immunological privilege" of the hyaline cartilage tissue. Their complexity, however, implies that the basic causes of the immune phenomena in patients with arthritic diseases are still poorly understood.

Chondrocyte-directed Cellular Immune Reactions

Chondrocytes Are only Weak Stimulators in Mixed Leukocyte-Chondrocyte Cultures

The antigenicity of native and cultured human chondrocytes was investigated in co-culture experiments. Freshly isolated, native chondrocytes were co-cultured with allogeneic peripheral blood mononuclear cells from normal donors and from patients with RA at different stimulator/responder ratios. Table 5 shows the maximum responses obtained at the ratios of 1:100 or 1:1000. It demonstrates that in both normal donors and RA patients there was only a weak response. In similar experiments, chondrocytes cultured for one or two passages were used as stimulator cells. Four of six chondrocyte samples were stimulatory for allogeneic lymphocytes, again with low net values. Additional stimulation experiments were performed with HLA class-II-positive chondrocytes. For this purpose, parallel cultures were incubated with recombinant

Table 5. Mixed leukocyte chondrocyte cultures: stimulation of allogeneic peripheral blood mononuclear cells by short-term cultured human chondrocytes

Chondrocyte sample no.	Ia-negative chondrocytes			Ia-positive chondrocytes*		
	PBM + Ch	PBM × Ch	Δdpm	PBM + Ch.	PBM × Ch.	Δdpm
3	2500	17000	14500	2500	10500	8000
8	21000	30000	9000	19000	19000	0
8	12000	20000	8000	11000	14000	3000
7	3000	9500	6500	2500	6000	3500
6	3500	9500	6000	4000	9000	5000
5	15000**	14000	n.s.	n.d.	n.d.	–
9	39000	28000	n.s.	39000	32000	n.s.
PBT	23000	16000	n.s.	23000	18000	n.s.

* HLA class-II antigens induced by gamma-interferon (7 days, 200 units/ml; 90% DR$^+$)
** ^{3}H-thymidine uptake in dpm (mean of triplicate determinations)
Δdpm = (PBM × Ch) – dpm (PBM + Ch); PBM, peripheral blood mononuclear cells (10^5 cells/well); PBT, peripheral blood T lymphocytes (isolated by E-rosetting, 10^5 cells/well); Ch, chondrocytes derived from articular human cartilage (10^2–10^4 cells/well: the maximum responses at optimum concentrations of stimulator cells have been indicated); n. d., not done; n. s., no stimulation

γ-interferon for 5–7 days, resulting in 80%–95% HLA-DR-positive cells. These Ia-positive chondrocytes showed only a low stimulatory effect on allogeneic lymphocytes. In contrast, even lower values resulted compared with their Ia-negative counterparts, despite the presence of large amounts of HLA class-II antigens as demonstrated by flow cytometry.

In further experiments, autologous purified T lymphocytes were used as responder cells. Their responses against Ia-positive and Ia-negative chondrocytes were lower (2000 and 5000 Δdpm) compared with the corresponding autologous mixed leukocyte reaction of these individuals (13000 Δdpm).

Reactivity of T Cells Against Cell Membrane Constituents

As outlined above, there was only a weak stimulatory capacity of whole isolated chondrocytes in cellular immune reactions, which seems to be in contrast to the presence of significant levels of autoantibodies to cartilage cell surface structures. Therefore, the peripheral blood cell activation induced by chondrocyte membranes was studied in patients with RA. The data revealed that there was a very high response to chondrocyte-derived materials, with a maximum in the membrane preparation at a concentration of 1.4 to 14 μg/ml at days 7–9 [36]. In contrast, there was no significant response against membranes from fibroblasts or the epithelial tumor cells (Fig. 7).

Experiments were performed to study the cellular nature of the anti-chondrocyte membrane response. Upon incubation of mononuclear cells with

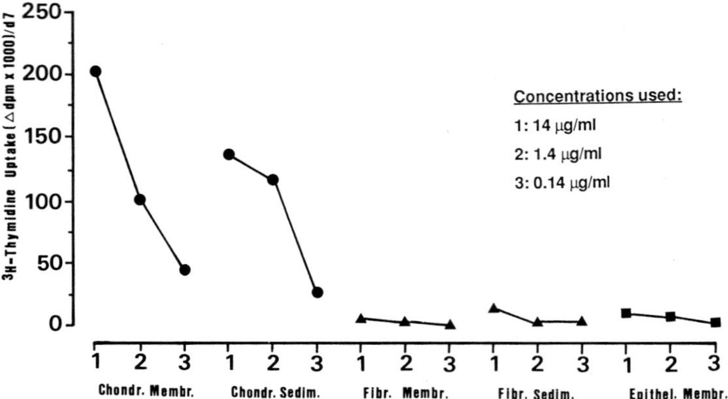

Fig. 7. Dose-dependent T-cell reactivity toward cell membrane preparations of various sources in a patient with rheumatoid arthritis after 7 days of culture as determined by ^{3}H-thymidine incorporation. The highest degree of proliferation was reached with 14 µg/ml of either chondrocyte membrane or sediment preparations (50% cell surface membranes) while there was no significant response to membranes of other sources

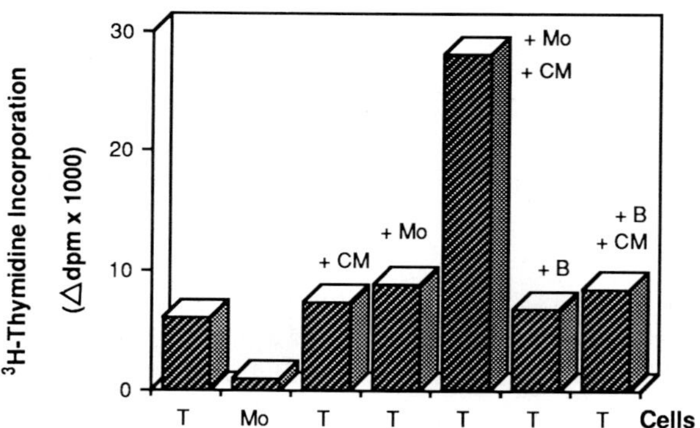

Fig. 8. T-cell proliferation to chondrocyte membranes is dependent on the presence of monocytes. T cells (*T*) were used at a concentrations of 1×10^5/well, monocytes (*Mo*) at 5×10^3/well, and B (*B*) cells at 5×10^3/wel. Chondrocyte membranes (*CM*) were used at a final concentration of 14 µg/ml. Δ dpm values are ^{3}H-thymidine uptake of cultures containing antigen minus controls without antigen

plasma membrane vesicles from all cell types, monocytes accumulated in aggregates (foci) in the culture wells after 3–4 days. Subsequently, after 1–2 additional days of culture, T lymphocytes appeared to migrate toward these monocyte aggregations, finally surrounding them. Phase-contrast microscopy revealed that the cytoplasm of the monocytes was abundantly filled with apparently phagocytosed/pinocytosed material. Similar phenomena were not observed after the incubation of isolated T or B cells alone, or in the presence of other antigens such as tetanus toxoid.

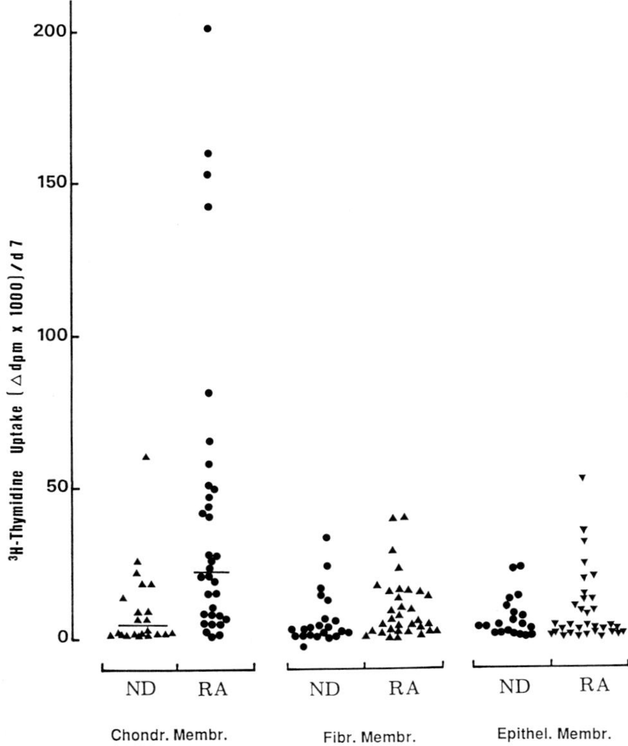

Fig. 9. Blood mononuclear cell response to membrane preparations from various sources as determined by ³H-thymidine incorporation. There was a significantly higher reactivity toward chondrocyte membranes ($p < 0.02$) in patients with rheumatoid arthritis (*RA*) than in normal donors (*ND*)

T cells alone were not reactive against chondrocyte membranes, while the addition of blood monocytes, but not B cells, to T cells incubated in the presence of chondrocyte membranes resulted in a marked proliferation of T cells (Fig. 8). In patients with RA and four normal donors, T cell reactivity against chondrocyte vesicles was studied on a clonal level. In the patients with RA the T cell precursor frequencies were 1:700, 1:770, 1:850, 1:980, and they were $<1:20000$ in additional three patients, while in all normal donors the corresponding frequencies were less than 1:20000.

Figure 9 demonstrates that there was a high stimulatory response to chondrocyte membranes in approximately 50% of RA patients while there was no or only a marginal reactivity towards membranes from other sources. The normal donor cells generally were not stimulated by either membrane preparation. The differences in reactivity towards chondrocyte membrane preparations between patients and normal donors were significant at the level of $p < 0.02$ (chondrocyte membranes).

Table 6. T Cell reactivity cartilage cell membrane constituents in intra-articular sites of RA patients

Patient	Cell source	Human cell membranes						Xenogeneic membranes	
		PaTuII	HFF	SFBl	Adult Ch	Fetal Ch	Infant Ch	Chicken Ch	Rat Ch
RA 1	ST	4.340*	6.445	15.053	39.703	8.749	15.280	34.007	22.771
RA 2	ST	0.844	1.315	8.999	35.165	5.784	6.053	n. d.	n. d.
RA 3	ST	3.205	8.639	n. d.	13.914	n. d.	n. d.	17.453	7.185

* ^{3}H-thymidine incorporation (Δdpm)

Ch, chondrocytes; HFF, human foreskin fibroblasts; SFBI, synovial fibroblasts; PaTuII, pancreatic tumor cell line; n.d., not done

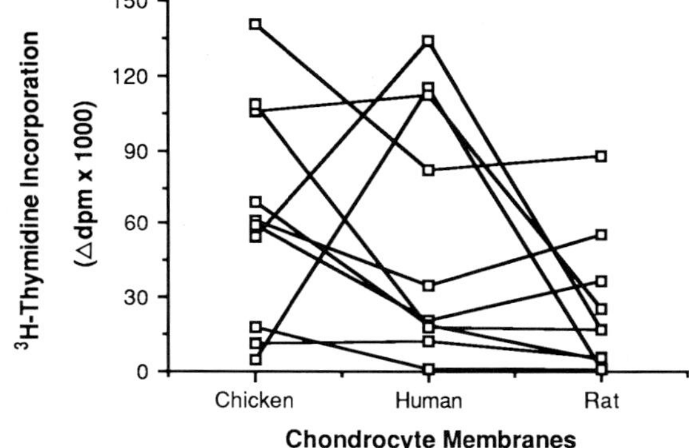

Fig. 10. Reactivity of rheumatoid arthritis blood mononuclear cells toward chondrocyte membrane preparations of human, rat, and chicken origin demonstrating the intraindividual response in each patient

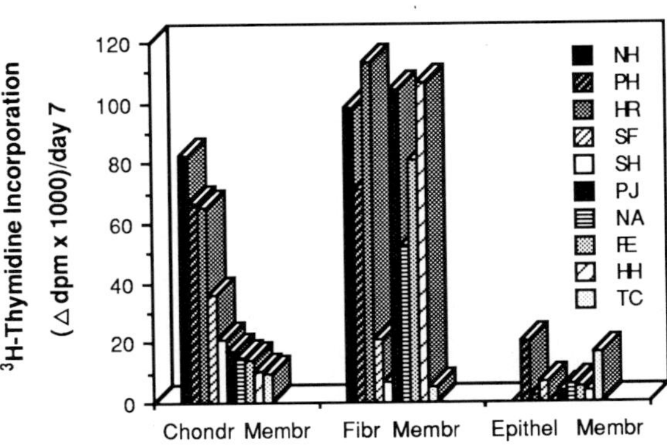

Fig. 11. Blood mononuclear cell responses to membrane vesicles in ten patients with osteoarthritis as determined by ^{3}H-thymidine uptake on day 7 of culture. There were strong responses to both chondrocyte and fibroblast membranes. The intraindividual comparisons demonstrate that in the majority of patients fibroblast reactivity even exceeded the stimulation induced by chondrocyte membranes

Table 6 shows the proliferative responses of synovial tissue mononuclear cells toward membranes from various types of mesenchymal cells. The highest T cell proliferation was measured with human adult chondrocyte membranes, whereas human infant and fetal chondrocyte membranes were less effective in enhancing T-cell proliferation. Xenogeneic membranes from chicken chondrocytes greatly stimulated T-cell proliferation.

Figure 10 shows the intraindividual responses against chondrocyte membranes obtained from various species in ten patients with RA. These data indicate that the patterns of reactivity differ from individual to individual; some patients showed similar responses to all preparations, while some reacted preferentially to membranes obtained from human and chicken sources. In general, chicken membranes elicited the highest responses, followed by human material, while the reactivity against rat membranes was usually the lowest.

Since cellular immunity may play a significant role in the pathogenesis of OA, the reactivity of T cells from patients with severe OA was investigated

(Fig. 11). In contrast to mononuclear cells obtained from patients with RA, there was a significant response not only to membranes of chondrocyte origin, but also to fibroblast membranes. However, epithelial cell membranes were not stimulatory at any concentration tested. The overall data indicated that in the majority of patients the proliferative response to fibroblast membranes even exceeded the reactivity obtained with chondrocyte membranes. In all instances tested, epithelial cell membranes elicited only a marginal responsiveness.

Antigen-presenting Capability of Chondrocytes

The following set of experiments was designed to investigate the antigen-presenting capability of cultured chondrocytes expressing HLA class-II molecules induced by γ-interferon. Since most of the chondrocyte donors lacked vigorous cellular responsiveness against tetanus toxoid due to their immunization status, in most experiments HLA-matched allogeneic T lymphocytes of normal blood donors were used. Therefore, HLA typing of non-T cells or Ia-positive chondrocytes was performed, either conventionally or by immunofluorescence, utilizing monoclonal antibodies against polymorphic epitopes on HLA class-II antigens of the DR and DQ families [37]. The accessory cells (monocytes or chondrocytes) and T lymphocytes shared at least one HLA restriction element.

The response of normal resting peripheral blood T lymphocytes to tetanus toxoid using first-passage allogeneic or autologous chondrocytes as accessory cells was very low. Although the chondrocyte preparations pretreated with γ-interferon contained 70%–90% cells intensely expressing Ia antigens, they were generally only weakly capable of inducing an antigen-driven T cell response, and autologous peripheral blood monocytes proved to be far better accessory cells in the assay system used.

Since resting and preactivated T lymphocytes require different activation signals, T cell lines were raised which were specifically reactive to tetanus toxoid using peripheral blood mononuclear cells as autologous antigen-presenting cells. Using an autologous restimulation system, significant responses of T cell lines were obtained (Fig. 12). The T-cell proliferation was dependent on the number of co-cultured HLA class-II-positive chondrocytes as antigen-presenting cells. The initially Ia-negative chondrocytes also induced T-cell proliferation. However, parallel experiments (not illustrated) demonstrated that Ia-negative chondrocytes expressed HLA-DR antigens on up to 40% of the cell populations within 2 days of co-culture with the T cell lines. The addition of exogeneous recombinant IL-2, but not IL-1, to either chondrocyte preparation significantly increased the T-cell responsiveness. Treatment of chondrocytes with chloroquine, a nonspecific antigen-processing inhibitor which acts in lysosomes, totally inhibited the presentation of tetanus toxoid to T cells. In contrast, chondrocytes fixed with glutaraldehyde after 6 h of tetanus toxoid pulsing showed an increased antigen-driven T-cell response.

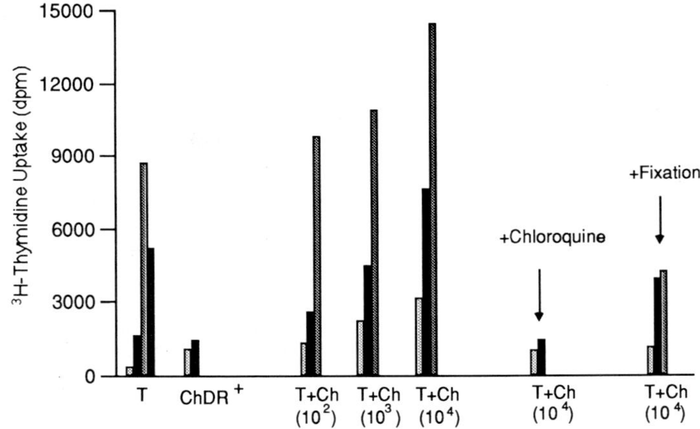

Fig. 12. Antigen presentation of tetanus toxoid (TT) to a TT-reactive T-cell line (*T*) by autologous chondrocytes. ^{3}H-thymidine uptake was measured after 72 h of co-incubation of 5×10^4 T cells/well with 10^2–10^4 HLA-DR-positive ($> 25\%$) chondrocytes (ChDR$^+$, 5 days preincubated with γ-interferon 200 U/ml). The first six bars show the background of ^{3}H-thymidine incorporation of T cells and chondrocytes and the remaining T cell responsiveness to IL-2 (10 U/ml). The antigen-induced T-cell response was dependent on the concentration of chondrocytes added. The addition of exogenous IL-2 (10 U/ml) to the co-cultures significantly increased the T-cell response. Pretreatment with chloroquine ($10^{-5} M$) 30 min after pulsing with TT inhibited totally the TT presentation to T cells by chondrocytes. The last three bars show that fixed chondrocytes (0.1% solution of glutaraldehyde for 5 min at room temperature) after TT pulsing were able to significantly present antigen to TT-reactive T cells. (▨ cells only, ■ cells + TT, ▨ cells + TT + IL-2, ▨ cells + IL-2)

Immune Reactivity Against Cartilage Proteoglycan Components in Animal Models of Arthritis and Human Inflammatory Joint Diseases

Cartilage proteoglycans (PGs) are found within the extracellular matrix in the form of multimolecular aggregates associated with a network of collagen fibrils. They contain polysaccharides covalently linked to a core protein. The saccharides consist of a large number of highly polyanionic chondroitin sulfate and keratan sulfate glycosaminoglycan chains. A peptide region located near the N-terminal of the core protein can specifically interact with hyaluronic acid to permit the formation of aggregates. The binding of hyaluronic acid is stabilized by the link protein. PGs are constantly degraded and resynthesized by chondrocytes with turnover rates between 14 and 30 days.

It has been suggested that autoimmunity to cartilage proteoglycan components plays a role in the etiology of arthritis, particularly in animal models. An intraperitoneal injection of human fetal cartilage PG (depleted of chondroitin sulfate) in Freund's complete (CFA) or incomplete adjuvant induced a chronic erosive polyarthritis and spondylitis in all female BALB/C mice [38]. The occurrence was strain specific but not haplotype specific, and it was sex related. The development of arthritis was associated with the presence of cellular immunity to the immunizing antigen and to chondroitinase ABC-related mouse cartilage PG [39]. Interestingly, associated with the arthritis was the development of cytotoxicity to human and mouse chondrocytes in the presence of complement. In arthiritc rabbits a preferentially humoral immune reactivity was observed in the majority of sera against hyaluronic acid and/or chondroitin sulfate bound to the core protein [40]. Spleen cells from arthritic rabbits responded to both native and degraded PGs. These in vitro blastogenic responses were shown to be completely dependent on the presence of T lymphocytes in the cultures. Some rabbits injected with homologous PGs demonstrated T-cell-dependent cellular, but not humoral immunity to the injected antigens [41]. In contrast, rabbits injected with heterologous human PGs developed cellular and humoral immunity to the immunizing PGs, but they failed to mount a cellular immunity to rabbit PGs. The induction of immunity to PGs was not accompanied by any demonstrable synovitis in these rabbits. A strongly arthritigenic T-lymhocyte clone specific for *M. tuberculosis* antigens in adjuvant arthritis in rats also recognized antigens present in PGs purified from cartilage, human synovial fluid, and medium of chondrocyte cultures, indicating that target epitopes for the arthritigenic clone may be present in PG components of cartilage [42]. The development of this arthritis was accompanied by the expression of cell-mediated and humoral immunity to the immunizing antigen.

In a model of chronic IgG-induced immune synovitis, there were reactive antibodies towards purified rabbit PG monomers in rabbits with immune synovitis. Inhibition studies with PG tryptic peptides showed that peptides which had a poor content of chondroitin sulfate were strong inhibitors of binding of the polyclonal antibodies to the PG substrate [43]. In rats, i. v. injection of PG synergizes with CFA in the induction of adjuvant arthritis, accompanied by both humoral and cellular immunity to PG. Immunity induced by PG alone was not sufficient for the induction of arthritis. Rats immunized with PG had high titers of anti-PG and strong delayed-type hypersensitivity to PG, which was also enhanced by pretreatment with PG intravenously, although none of these animals developed arthritis [44].

In the human situation, in patients with RA or OA [45] peripheral blood lymphocytes did not exhibit a significant proliferative response to homologous cartilage PG. Furthermore, both autologous and heterologous peripheral blood lymphocyte proliferation in patients with RA, OA, and ankylosing spondylitis was unaltered by the addition of cartilage fragments and purified bovine articular PHs [46]. Analysis of arthritic articular cartilage failed to demonstrate the presence of antigen(s) stimulating peripheral blood lymphocytes.

It has been suggested that serum antibodies to the "PG link protein" may be more common in patients with rheumatic disorders than in healthy controls. Antibodies against highly purified cartilage link protein were found in sera of only approximately 25% of patients with RA, using an enzyme-linked immunosorbent assay. No statistically significant differences existed between the non-arthritic control population and the RA patient group with regard to either prevalence or mean titer of anti-link protein antibodies [47].

Since intact non-degraded PGs did not produce arthritis in animals, in contrast to chondroitinase-digested PGs, it is likely that the putative arthritigenic protein epitopes on PGs must be sterically masked from the immune system or expressed as new determinants after modifications of the tertiary structure of the core protein by removal of the negatively charged chondroitin sulfate side chain. In human subjects PGs have not been shown conclusively to induce a marked humoral or cellular immunity.

Perspectives

In rheumatoid arthritis, the articular cartilage is one of the central targets of tissue destruction. Traditionally, the main interest in the search for a possible autoantigenic structure has focused on constituents of the intercellular matrix. However, frequently these reactions did not reach very high stimulation levels [16–24]. The cellular elements of cartilage, the chondrocytes, have also been investigated as possible targets. Again, using whole chondrocytes as stimulators in rodents, but also in the human system, only moderate T-cell reactivities have been described [48]. However, chondrocytes have the capacity to take part in immunological reactions, as shown by their ability to present antigens [9, 48]. Upon inflammation, striking changes occur in cartilage cells, mediated especially by interleukin-1 and tumor necrosis factor-α, resulting in the release of enzymes destructive to the surrounding matrix [49, 50].

Additional evidence for the hypothesis of the involvement of chondrocytes in immunological reactions has recently been provided by the demonstration of autoantibodies against chondrocyte cell surface membrane antigens in destructive joint diseases [28]. These observations prompted us to extend these studies to an examination of the cellular reactivity against chondrocyte membranes. In agreement with the humoral data, a strong T-cell response against these antigens was found in patients with RA.

Of particular importance, as in the spectrum of autoantibodies, this reactivity was obtained against chondrocyte membranes from other species, including chickens and rats. Interestingly, T-cell reactivity was obtained to a significantly less degree using neonatal or newborn human chondrocyte material. This may indicate that a maturation process has to occur in chondrocytes, resulting in a different spectrum of antigen expression. Overall, the findings of both humoral and cellular immune response to chondrocyte material from different species are in good agreement with data obtained for other autoimmune diseases such as juvenile diabetes, demonstrating human autoantibodies against islet cells of rats and of other species [51].

In view of the weak T-cell response found in the mixed leukocyte-chondrocyte reactions, the high response to isolated chondrocyte membranes in patients with RA was remarkable. These high responses surpassed by far T-cell reactivities found against other cartilage constituents, including collagen type II and proteoglycans [21–24]. A possible explanation for these results may be an effective antigen processing. The massive accumulation of whole membrane vesicles in lysosomes or storage granules of blood monocytes present in the in vitro cultures during the T-cell activation experiment speaks in favor of enhanced macrophage phagocytosis. Apparently, the cells readily take up this material and present it to the surrounding T cells. It is very likely that either efficient antigen processing occurs in monocytes [52, 53] and/or additional signals are provided by these cells [54], which then stimulate the T-cell repertoire reactive toward chondrocyte membranes in patients with RA. Similar mechanisms of antigen processing and presentation may be effective in other autoimmune diseases accompanied by macrophage infiltration.

Of particular interest was the observation that T cells from the majority of patients with OA expressed not only a reaction towards chondrocyte membranes, but – even higher – to fibroblast membranes. Since autoantibodies against chondrocyte membranes had already been demonstrated in this disease [28], chondrocyte membrane reactivity was not unexpected. It is attractive, however, to speculate that the unexpected T-cell reactivity toward fibroblast membranes in patients with OA – absent in RA patients and normal donors – is caused by the contact of immune cells with possibly activated and/or altered fibroblastoid cells of chondrogenic cell lineage which have been demonstrated in osteoarthritic joints [for review see 26, 55]. Thus, the surface antigens of possibly dedifferentiated fibroblastoid chondrocytes may be targets recognized by T cells from patients with OA, even though a humoral reaction against the fibroblast membranes was not demonstrated in OA.

The specificity of the T-cell response found in the two groups with destructive joint diseases has not yet been defined. Our previous work [28] indicated that, with regard to autoantibodies, different immunoreactive peptides separated by SDS-PAGE are responsible for the immune reaction detected in Western blot analysis. The significance of the biological phenomenon – the immune response to chondrocyte antigens – requires further investigation. Especially in RA, however, this immune reaction could substantially contribute to the inflammatory process and be a major factor in the pathogenesis of joint destruction in addition to more non-specific processes such as the cytotoxicity of serum, immune complexes, or inflammatory, macrophage-driven degradative processes. Thus, chondrocyte antigens will have to be recognized as potential autoantigens possibly involved in the pathogenesis of destructive joint diseases.

References

1. Glant T, Mikecz K (1986) Antigenic profiles of human bovine and canine articular chondrocytes. Cell Tissue Res 244:359–369
2. Burmester GR, Menche D, Merryman P, Klein M, Winchester RJ (1983) Application of monoclonal antibodies to the characterization of cells eluted from human articular cartilage: expression of Ia antigens in certain diseases and identification of an 85-KD cell surface molecule accumulated in the pericellular matrix. Arthritis Rheum 26:1187–1195
3. Matzkin E, Winchester RJ (1984) Heterogenicity of cell populations in osteoarthritic cartilage as detected by monoclonal antibodies. Arthritis Rheum [Suppl 4]:S 36
4. Jahn B, Burmester GR, Schmid H-J, Weseloh G, Rohwer P, Kalden JR (1987) Changes in cell surface antigen expression on human articular chondrocytes induced by gamma-interferon. Induction of Ia antigens. Arthritis Rheum 30:64–74
5. Bottazzo GF, Path MRC, Dean BM, McNally JM, MacKay EH, Swift PGF, Gamble DR (1985) In situ characterization of autoimmune phenomena and expression of HLA molecules in the pancreas in diabetic insulitis. N Engl J Med 313:353–360
6. Tjernlund UM (1980) Ia-like antigens in lichen planus. Acta Derm Venereol (Stockh) 60:309–314
7. Ballardini G, Bianchi F, Doniach D, Mirakian R, Pisi E, Bottazzo GF (1984) Aberrant expression of HLA-DR antigens on bile duct epithelium in primary biliary cirrhosis: relevance to pathogenesis: Lancet 2:1009–1013
8. Editorial (1985) What triggers autoimmunity? Lancet 1:78–79
9. Tiku ML, Liu S, Weaver CW, Theodorescu M, Skosey JL (1985) Class II histocompatibility antigen-mediated immunologic function of normal articular chondrocytes. J Immunol 135:2923–2928
10. Gertzbein SD, Lance EM (1976) The stimulation of lymphocytes by chondrocytes in mixed cultures. Clin Exp Immunol 24:102–109
11. Gertzbein SD, Tait JH, Devlin SR, Argue S (1977) The antigenicity of chondrocytes. Immunology 33:141–145
12. Burmester GR, Yu DTY, Irani A-M, Kunkel HG, Winchester RJ (1981) Ia$^+$ T cells in synovial fluid and tissues of patients with rheumatoid arthritis. Arthritis Rheum 24:1370–1376
13. Cush JJ, Lipsky PE (1988) Phenotypical analysis of synovial tissue and peripheral blood lymphocytes isolated from patients with rheumatoid arthritis. Arthritis Rheum 10:1230–1238
14. Burmester GR, Dimitriu-Bona A, Waters SJ, Winchester RJ (1983) Idenfification of three major synovial lining cell populations by monoclonal antibodies directed to Ia antigens and antigens associated with monocytes/macrophages and fibroblasts. Scand J Immunol 17:69–82
15. Janossy G, Panayi G, Duke O, Bofill M, Poulter LW, Goldstein G (1981) Rheumatoid arthritis: a disease of T-lymphocyte/macrophage immunoregulation. Lancet:839–842
16. Goldberg VM, Kresina TF (1987) Immunology of articular cartilage. J Rheumatol [Suppl] 14:73–76
17. Trentham DE, Kammer GM, McCune WJ, David JR (1981) Autoimmunity to collagen. A shared feature of psoriatic and rheumatoid arthritis. Arthritis Rheum 24:1363–1369
18. Choi EKK, Gatenby PA, McGill NW, Bateman JF, Cole WG, York JR (1988) Autoantibodies to type-II collagen: occurrence in rheumatoid arthritis, other arthritides, autoimmune connective tissue diseases, and chronic inflammatory syndromes. Ann Rheum Dis 47:313–322
19. Morgan K, Clague RB, Collins I, Ayad S, Phinn SD, Holt PJL (1987) Incidence of antibodies to native and denatured cartilage collagens (types II, IX, and XI) and to type-I collagen in rheumatoid arthritis. Arthritis Rheum 46:902–907
20. Wooley PH, Luthra HS, O'Duffy JD, Bunch TW, Moore SB, Stuart JM (1984) Anti-type II collagen antibodies in rheumatoid arthritis. The influence of HLA phenotype. Tissue Antigens 23:263–269

21. Stuart JM, Postethwaite AE, Townes AS, Kang AH (1980) Cell-mediated immunity to collagen and collagen alpha chains in rheumatoid arthritis and other rheumatic diseases. Am J Med 69:13–18
22. Trentham DE, Dynesius RA, Rocklin RE, David JR (1978) Cellular sensitivity to collagen in rheumatoid arthritis. N Engl J Med 299:327–332
23. Sigal LH, Johnston SL, Philips PE (1988) Cellular immune response to cartilage components in rheumatoid arthritis and osteoarthritis: a review and report of a study. Clin Exp Rheumatol 6:59–66
24. Golds EE, Stephen IBM, Esdaile JM, Strawczynski H, Poole AR (1983) Lymphocyte transformation to connective tissue antigens in adult and juvenile rheumatoid arthritis, osteoarthritis, ankylosing spondylitis, systemic lupus erythematosus, and a nonarthritic control population. Cell Immunol 82:196–209
25. Hamerman D (1989) The biology of steoarthritis. N Engl J Med 320:1322–1330
26. Kuettner KE, Pauli BV (1983) Vascularity of cartilage, vol. 1. In: Hall BK (ed) Cartilage, Academic, New York, pp 281–312
27. Mollenhauer J, Brune K (1988) Detection of autoimmune reactive antibodies against cartilage cell surface proteins in the blood of rheumatic patients. Agents Actions 23:48–49
28. Mollenhauer J, von der Mark K, Burmester G, Glückert K, Lütjen-Drecoll E, Brune K (1988) Serum antibodies against chondrocyte cell surface proteins in osteoarthritis and rheumatoid arthritis. J Rheumatol 15:1811–1817
29. Enzmann H, Mollenhauer J, Brune K (1990) Humoral autoimmunity to cartilage in rheumatoid arthritis? Agents Actions 29:114–116
30. Sweet MBE, Coelho A, Schnitzler CM, Schnitzler TJ, Lenz ME, Kuettner KE, Thonar EJMA (1988) Serum keratan sulfate levels in osteoarthritis. Arthritis Rheum 31:648–652
31. Van Eden W, Hogervorst EJM, Hensen EJ, van der Zee R, van Embden DA, Cohen IR (1989) A cartilage-mimicking epitope on a 65-K mycobacterial heat-shock protein: adjuvant arthritis as a model for human rheumatoid arthritis. Curr Top Microbiol Immunol 145:27–43
32. Kaufmann SHE, Schoel B, Wand-Württemberger A, Steinhoff U, Munk ME, Koga T (1990) T cells, stress proteins, and pathogenesis of mycobacterial infections. Curr Top Microbiol Immunol 155:125–141
33. Karlsson-Parra A, Söderström K, Ferm M, Ivanyi J, Kiessling R, Klareskog L (1990) Presence of human 65-kD heat-shock protein (hsp) in inflamed joints and subcutaneous nodules of RA patients. Scand J Immunol 31:283–288
34. Maeda M, Cooke TDV (1984) Destruction of rabbit knee hyaline cartilage associated with surface antigen-antibody interaction during the Arthus reaction of antigen-induced arthritis. Clin Orthop 190:287–291
35. Uno K, Cooke TDV, Scudamore RA (1989) Interaction of cultured chondrocytes with heat aggreated immunoglobulin (Abstr). Trans Orthop Res Soc 14:581
36. Alsalameh S, Mollenhauer J, Hain N, Stock K-P, Kalden JR, Burmester GR (1990) Cellular immune response towards human articular chondrocytes. T cell reactivities against chondrocyte and fibroblast membranes in destructive joint diseases. Arthritis Rheum 33:1477–1486
37. Burmester GR, Jahn B, Rohwer P, Zacher J, Winchester RJ, Kalden JR (1987) Differential expression of Ia antigens by rheumatoid synovial lining cells. J Clin Invest 80:595–604
38. Mikecz K, Glant TT, Poole AR (1987) Immunity to cartilage proteoglycans in BALB/C mice with progressive polyarthritis and ankylosing spondylitis induced by injection of human cartilage proteoglycan. Arthritis Rheum 30:306–318
39. Glant TT, Mikecz K, Arzoumanian A, Poole AR (1987) Proteoglycan-induced arthritis in BALB/C mice. Clinical features and histopathology. Arthritis Rheum 30:201–212
40. Poole AR, Reiner A, Roughley PJ, Champion B (1985) Rabbit antibodies to degraded and intact glycosaminoglycans which are naturally occurring and present in arthritic rabbits. J Biol Chem 260:6020–6025
41. Champion BR, Sell S, Poole AR (1983) Immunity to homologous collagens and cartilage proteoglycans in rabbits. Immunology 48:605–616

42. Van Eden W, Holoshitz J, Nevo Z, Frenkel A, Klajman A, Cohen IR (1985) Arthritis induced by T-lymphocyte clone that responds to *Mycobacterium tuberculosis* and to cartilage proteoglycans. Proc Natil Acad Sci USA 82:5117–5120
43. Yoo Ju, Kresina TF, Malemud CJ, Goldberg VM (1987) Epitopes of proteoglycans elicited an anti-proteoglycan response in chronic immune synovitis. Proc Natl Acad Sci USA 84:832–836
44. Van Vollenhoven RF, Soriano A, MacCarthy PE, Schwartz RL, Garbrecht FC, Thorbecke GL, Siskind GW (1988) The role of immunity to cartilage proteoglycan in adjuvant arthritis. J Immunol 141:1168–1173
45. Golds EE, Stephan IB, Esdaile JM, Strawczynski H, Poole AR (1983) Lymphocyte transformation to connective tissue antigens in adult and juvenile rheumatoid arthritis, osteoarthritis, ankylosing spondylitis, systemic lupus erythematosus, and a nonarthritic control population. Cell Immunol 82:196–209
46. Schurman DJ, Palathumpat MW, DeSilva A, Kajiyama G, Smith RL (1986) Biochemistry and antigenicity of osteoarthritic and rheumatoid cartilage. J Orthop Res 4:255–262
47. Austin AK, Hobbs RN, Anderson JC, Butler RC, Ashton BA (1988) Humoral immunity to link protein in patients with inflammatory joint disease, osteoarthritis, and in non-arthritic controls. Ann Rheum Dis 47:886–892
48. Alsalameh S, Jahn B, Kalden JR, Burmester GR (1991) Antigenicity and accessory cell function of human articular chondrocytes. J Rheumatol 18:414–421
49. McGuire-Goldring MB, Meats JE, Wood DD, Ihrie EJ, Ebsworth NM, Russell GG (1984) In vitro activation of human chondrocytes and synoviocytes by a human interleukin-1-like factor. Arthritis Rheum 27:654–662
50. Saklatvala J, Sarsfield SJ (1988) How do interleukin-1 and tumor necrosis factor induce degradation of proteoglycan? In: Glauert AM (ed) The control of tissue damage. Elsevier, New York, pp 97–108
51. Bach J-F (1988) Mechanisms of autoimmunity in insulin-dependent diabetes mellitus. Clin Exp Immunol 72:1–8
52. Unanue ER (1984) Antigen-presenting function of the macrophage. Annu Rev Immunol 2:395–402
53. Ziegler K, Unanue ER (1981) Identification of a macrophage antigen-presenting event required for I-region-restricted antigen presentation to T lymphocytes. J Immunol 127:1869–1875
54. Rosenthal AS, Shevach EM (1973) Function of macrophages in antigen recognition by guinea pig T lymphocytes. I. Requirement for histocompatible macrophages and lymphocytes. J Exp Med 138:1194–1212
55. Von der Mark K (1986) Differentiation, modulation, and dedifferentiation of chondrocytes. Rheumatology 10:272–317

Role and Regulation
of Synovial MHC Class II Antigens
in Rheumatoid Arthritis and Related Diseases*

L. Klareskog

Department of Clinical Immunology, Uppsala University Hospital, 75185 Uppsala, Sweden

Introduction

Class II major histocompatibility complex (MHC) transplantation antigens constitute, in addition to a processed antigen and the T cell receptor, the trimolecular complex which governs most T cell-dependent immune reactions [1]. Evidence that MHC class II-dependent T lymphocyte activation is critically involved in the pathogenesis of rheumatoid arthritis (RA) as well as in other inflammatory arthritides derives from a series of indirect but – taken together – convincing findings. Genetic data suggest that the linkage between RA and human leukocyte antigen (HLA) genes can be traced back to structural differences in distinct MHC class I subunits [2]. A massive increase in class II expressing cells as well as in activated T cells in the inflamed synovial tissue indicate that local class II-dependent T cell activation can take place in synovial tissue [3–5]. Treatment with human immunoglobulin fractions enriched for anti-class II antibodies [6] as well as with mouse anti-CD4 monoclonal antibodies [7] may diminish disease activity in RA.

Given that the involvement of class II antigens on synovial cells in inflammatory arthritis is one of the few as yet molecularly defined features of these diseases, the question would be how to use this information both to gain further insight into the pathogenesis of RA, and perhaps also to understand why the joints are so often subject to a variety of inflammations, with enhanced local class II expression as a common feature. The present short review will aim at discussing which particular features of the joint and joint inflammation may make synovial class II molecules so prone to elicit these chronic inflammatory reactions. As many of the basic features of MHC class II distribution and functions and the general mechanisms of MHC class II induction have been

* Experimental studies from our laboratory that are discussed in this article were supported by grants from the Swedish Medical Research Council, from King Gustaf V:s 80-years foundation, from the Swedish Association against Rheumatism and from the Swedish Agency for Technical Development.

Smolen, Kalden, Maini (Eds.)
Rheumatoid Arthritis
© Springer-Verlag Berlin Heidelberg 1992

discussed at length in several recent reviews [8, 9], I will here emphasize my personal views on MHC class II expression within the joint, and how these molecules might confer some tissue-specific characteristics of inflammatory joint disease.

Class II-Expressing Cells
Within the Normal and Inflamed Joint

Normal synovial tissue contains at least two different kinds of MHC class-II-expressing cells, the dendritic cells, which are present in the loose connective tissue of the synovium and of other organs, and the specialized type A cells of the synovial intima [10, 11]. Both types of class II-expressing cells have been shown in the mouse to be derived from the bone marrow [11, 12].

In the normal joint, type A intimal cells can be assumed to be involved in a first line of defense against infectious pathogens; they are phagocytic, express Fc receptors, and also have a capacity to mediate class II-dependent T cell activation [10]. As the presence of infectious living organisms in the joint may lead very rapidly to irreversible destruction, it is reasonable to believe that type A intimal cells are associated with a capacity for rapid and efficient responses to such microorganisms. Thus these cells are probably active in unspecific phagocytosis, the breakdown of pathogens, and in specifically activating local T lymphocytes [10]. A possible side effect of such capacities would be, however, that immune reactions may also be particularly easily triggered in the joint against noninfectious molecules such as fragments from bacteria in reactive arthritis or autoantigens in other chronic inflammatory diseases (see below).

Cellular composition and the distribution and function of MHC class II-expressing cells in inflamed joints have so far only been extensively studied for those chronic arthritides where surgical interventions are undertaken. For other types of joint inflammations and for early stages of chronic diseases such as RA, the data are mainly limited to those derived from immunomorphological investigations on small, arthroscopically obtained biopsies.

A common pattern in arthritides of many different etiologies including osteoarthritis, traumatic synovitis, and crystal-induced arthropathy is an extravasation of T lymphocytes as well as a thickening and increase in the numbers of class II-expressing cells in the intima [4, 5, 13, 14]. In many of these cases, there is also an increase in the numbers of subsynovial MHC class II-expressing cells, out of which some carry macrophage markers and others show similarities to lymphoid dendritic cells [4, 5, 13, 15].

This picture suggests that T cells as well as certain potentially antigen-presenting cells extravasate in response to a variety of different stimuli, including nonimmunological ones, as part of an unspecific surveillance function. Once an immunogenic molecule is available in this environment, prerequisites would exist for rapid and specific T cell activation, for example against invading microorganisms. Thus, an unspecific attraction of T cells into the synovium by trauma, crystals, and a variety of other stimuli would constitute a predisposing factor for the putative subsequent local T cell activation that is assumed to take place in chronic inflammatory joint diseases like RA [3–5]. The situation may be compared with the situation in the skin where the unspecific local extravasation of T cells that is seen in irritant dermatitis is assumed to predispose for a subsequent development of allergic contact dermatitis if a relevant contact allergen is introduced at the irritated site (see [16]).

It also appears that a certain thickening of the synovial lining and an increase in numbers of synovial class II-expressing cells can result from a variety of different stimuli [13], and thereby further contribute to the degree of readiness within the synovial tissue for specific, class II-dependent local T cell activation.

Aspects of the Regulation of MHC Class II Expression in Joints and in the Nerve System

Basic questions that arise from these mainly descriptive studies are how and why the increase in MHC class II expression in synovial tissue occurs, and which functional consequences follow from this increase.

As far as mechanisms are concerned, it is well known that a number of cytokines released from activated T lymphocyts – γ-interferon (IFN-γ) and others [17–19] – may themselves or in synergy with each other induce MHC class-II expression on previously class II-negative cells such as fibroblasts, endothelial cells, and certain macrophages in the synovium (see [4, 5, 18–21]) as well as on chondrocytes within the cartilage [22]. These cytokines would also be able to further enhance class II expression on cells that express class II in the normal joint. Cytokines released from activated T cells and from activated macrophages may also play a part in attracting various circulating leukocytes and in leading resident cells in the synovium to proliferate. For fibroblasts and for cells of the vasculature of at least, we have recently proposed that platelet-derived growth factor (PDGF), which is released from a number of synovial cells including activated macrophages, would constitute one such stimulant [23].

While an enhancing loop encompassing class II induction on the one hand and T cell activation on the other can easily be appreciated in the pathogenenesis of inflammatory joint diseases, it is more difficult to address the "chicken and egg" question, i. e., which of the events in such a loop is triggered first. There are some strong arguments, however, that at least some of the pronounced macrophage activation may occur without being caused only by previous T cell activation at least in RA. Thus messenger ribonucleic acid (mRNA) coding for cytokines released from macrophages has been shown to be abundant from both Northern blot analyses [24] and in situ hybridization [25] on inflamed RA synovium. As will be discussed more extensively for RA, the cartilage and the cartilage fragments released to the synovium in destructive arthritides might, by virtue of their capacity to bind immune complexes and auto-anti-cartilage antibodies [26–28], constitute an element in such a local macrophage activation. Indirect evidence that such humorally mediated activation of synovial intimal cells may occur in vivo is provided from studies in experimental collagen II-induced arthritis, where activation of cells within the synovial intima is seen days before the infiltration of T cells in the synovium, probably as a resultof binding of anticollagen II antibodies to the cartilage [29].

Other contributions to the pronounced synovial macrophage activation of inflammatory arthritis such as viral infections have as yet no empirical support, but cannot be excluded, and altogether, there is a need for more experimental data on the possible background to the pronounced synovial macrophage activation seen in many arthritides.

A quite different line of experiments that may also deserve some attention in conjunction with non-T cell-mediated regulation of MHC class II expression is the influence of nerve functions. There are several indications that the nervous system may in some way influence arthritis development, contributing both to the symmetrical character of diseases like RA, and to the decreased tendency for arthritis in paralytic limbs [30]. We observed during our studies on MHC class II expression in the central nervous system that an induction of class II antigens was seen around a nerve cell that had been subject to peripheral axotomy [31]. Furthermore, this nerve cell also began to express MHC class I antigens. Most interestingly, these observations led to the finding that production of IFN-γ (or molecules very similar to IFN-γ) was induced in the axotomized nerve [32]. Furthermore, it was demonstrated that some IFN-γ (or IFN-γ-like molecules) were also present in normal nerves both in the peripheral and central nervous system [33]. The data also indicated that the axotomy – and possibly the induced IFN-γ production – was of functional importance in inflammation, since experimental allergic encephalitis (EAE) was more easily triggered on the axotomized than on the nonaxotomized side [34]. The implications of these findings for the joint are not yet clear. We have demonstrated, however, that some nerve cells in the synovium also contain (IFN-γ-like molecules (S. Kleinau, L. Klareskog et al., manuscript in preparation), and it is thus possible that various external nonimmunological stimuli may affect the tendency for class II-dependent T cell activation in joints also via the nervous route.

Prospects for Aberrant T Cell Activation in Joints

The fact that joints are subject to longstanding inflammation more often than many other tissues may indicate particular proneness for T cell activation –

which may be called aberrant – for example in conjunction with a diverse array of infections. The joint thus possess certain particular features that favor the elicitation of a variety of immune reactions. If this is so, these features might also be of relevance in explaining why chronic inflammatory joint diseases like RA are so relatively common.

One possibility put forward early in the debate was that an in vivo counterpart to the autologous mixed lymphocyte reaction (MLR) in vitro might be active in synovitis, possibly because of the large number of dendritic cells in the RA joint [5, 35, 36]. Although such a generalized enhancement of T cell reactivity might be less likely to occur in MHC-linked diseases like RA, it is still feasible that the accumulation of the large amounts of dendritic cells with a high capacity for T cell activation (see also [35, 36]) in some way mirror a high degree of "alertness" for immunoreactivity in joints. A more specific feature of the joints is, however, the appearance of intimal macrophage-like cells in immediate association with the cartilage surface. As will be discussed in more detail below, there are indications that immune complexes tend to bind to cartilage surface, a feature that might enhance a subsequent binding, processing, and presentation to T cells of antigens within these complexes.

There are at least two obvious ways via which a local T cell activation confined to joints would then occur. One possibility is the transport of "foreign" molecules to the joint, for example, those derived from microorganisms, and and another is the elicitation of autoimmune reactions against the molecules preferentially available in joints. The first possibility may be exemplified by events recently characterized in reactive arthritis, where molecular fragments of *Chlamydia trachomatis* and *Versinia enterocolitica* have been demonstrated within the joints of patients suffering from corresponding reactive arthritides [37, 38]. It is not yet known in detail how these fragments are transported to the joints from the urinary tract and intestine, but one attractive possibility is that immune complexes encompassing these fragments may have migrated to the joint, and, as a result of their subsequent association with class II-expressing synovial cells, trigger T cell reactivity to these fragments. An interesting issue in this context is that we still do not know to what extent the current bacterial fragments localize selectively to joints, or whether they ay also be found elsewhere in the body. Indirect evidence, for example from experiments in streptococcal cell wall arthritis induced in rats [39], suggest that bacterial fragments may indeed occur all over the body, but still give rise to the most active inflammation in the joints. If this is so for reacive arthritis as well, this would further strengthen the notion of a particular alertness for T cell reactivity in joints.

The possibility that as yet undefined bacterial or viral antigens in the joint may also elicit the more chronic inflammatory diseases like RA can by no means be excluded, particularly as the bacterial fragments of well-known etiologic agents in chlamydia- and yersinia-associated arthritis have only recently been detected. Since there are currently no clues to this kind of reactions in RA, class II-dependent synovial T cell activation in this diseases will be discussed in association with known autoimmune phenomena.

Prospects for Local Autoimmune Reactions in RA

One major characteristic of RA is the erosive character of the joint inflammation [40]. The site of erosion, i.e., the cartilage-pannus junction, is characterized by the presence of large numbers of class II-expressing cells in the infiltrating pannus [21]. Some of the chondrocytes in the vicinity of the erosions most probably also express class II antigens [41]. As discussed above, the class II-expressing cells within the thickened lining layer and the dendritic cells in the sublining layer are also a common feature of other types of synovitis. Finally, an important and, for RA, relatively specific feature is the abundance of synovial B cells/plama cells, a high proportion of which express anti-immunoglobulin-binding antibodies [42], while others produce antibodies which react with cartilage-derived collagen II [43].

The elicitation of autoimmune reactions to cartilage components would – from the APC point of view – be feasible from a number of these cells. The chondrocytes may present molecules present in cartilage in a way similar to that discussed for many other types of autoimmunity [43], and the class II-expressing cells that penetrate the cartilage in the pannus are by immunohistology at least seen to contain collagen fragments [41]. Furthermore, the dendritic cells would have a similarly high capacity to present autoantigens as dendritic cells elsewhere [45]. Anticollagen antibody-expressing cells might obviously very efficiently bind collagen released in the environment, process the antigen, and present it to synovial T cells. Anti-immunoglobulin-expressing B cells may bind immune complexes in the same way. These complexes, in turn, can be assumed to contain collagen as well as other autoantigens, which may thus also be particularly efficiently presented to synovial T cells in a way similar to that described as being very efficient in the follicular areas of normal lymph nodes during secondary immune responses [46].

The occurrence of these hypothetical events in vivo is obviously also dependent on events within the thymus. It can be assumed that T cells can escape being tolerized against certain cartilage antigens because of their relatively low concentrations in the circulation and within the thymic microenvironment. The existance of mechanisms for very efficient uptake, processing, and presentation to T cells of the same autoantigens in joints might subsequently be a decisive event in triggering autoreactive T cells against joint-specific autoantigens that might otherwise escape being seen by the immune system due to their being present in too low concentrations.

Evidence that this kind of autoreactive and potentially arthritogenic T cells are indeed present in the periphery and thus escape tolerization in the thymus has been obtained from experiments in collagen II-induced arthritis in both mice and rats, where immunization with mouse or rat autologous collagen can give rise to T cell-dependent, and MHC class II-restricted chronic arthritis [47, 48].

Concluding Remarks

Synovial MHC class II-expressing cells and their potential role in the activation of T cell reactions that will ultimately contribute to arthritis development have been reviewed here under the assumption that MHC expression on cells within the joint is regulated according to principles similar to those for equivalent cells in other tissues. Thus, the preferential activation of T cells in the joint that appears to occur in RA and several other arthritides will depend either on the unique availability of certain antigens in the joint, a unique potential for efficient presentation of certain antigens to T cells, or a combination of these two possibilities. The particular properties of the functional unit consisting of cartilage and synovial membrane offer, in this respect, both possibilities for a rapid and strong immune response against invading microorganisms, and potential for T cell reactions against self-antigens, for example from the cartilage.

The most interesting question for research in RA – the putative specificity of arthritogenic immune reactions – will possibly also be best tackled if class II-expressing cells of the joint such as chondrocytres, synovial intimal cells, or synovial B lymphocytes are used as antigen-presenting cells in our assays. If combined with appropriate structural determination of the MHC class II molecules of the analyzed patients, we might in this way use our current knowledge of class II antigens in RA to acquire knowledge of the specificity and T cell receptor structure of those T cells which may be arthritogenic and which we can immunomanipulate using methods that are now refined in experimental animal systems for autoimmune disease [49, 50].

References

1. Davies M, Bjorkman P (1988) T cell antigen receptor genes and T cell recognition. Nature 334:395
2. Winchester R, Gregersen PK (1988) The molecular basis of susceptibility to rheumatoid arthritis: the conformational equivalence hypothesis. Springer Semin Immunopathol 10:119
3. Burmester GR, Yu DTY, Irani AM, Kunkel HK, Winchester RJ (1982) Ia$^+$ T cells in synovial fluid and tissue of patients with rheumatoid arthritis. Arthritis Rheum 24:1370
4. Klareskog L, Forsum U, Malmnäs Tjernlund U, Kabelitz D, Wigren A (1982) Evidence in support of a self-prerpetuating HLA-DR dependent delayed type cell reactions in rheumatoid arthritis. Proc Natl Acad Sci USA 79:3632
5. Janossy G, Panayi GS, Duke O, Bofill M, Poulter LW, Goldstein G (1981) Rheumatoid arthritis: a disease of T lymphocyte/macrophage immunoregulation. Lancet ii:839
6. Sany J, Clot J, Bonneau M, Anday M (1982) Immunmodulating effect of human placenta-eluted gamma globulins in rheumatoid arthritis. Arthritis Rheum 25:17
7. Herzog C, Walker C, Ichler W, Aeschlimann A, Wassmer P, Stockinger H, Knapp W, Rieber P, Muller W (1987) Monoclonal anti-CD4 in arthritis. Lancet ii:1461

8. Solheim BG, Möller E, Ferrone S (eds) (1986) Human class II transplantation antigens. A comprehensive review. Springer, Berlin Heidelberg New York
9. Kappes D, Strominger J (1988) Human class II major histocompatibility complex gene and proteins. Ann Rev Biochem 57:991
10. Klareskog L, Forsum U, Kabelitz D, Plöen L, Sundström C, Nilsson W, Wigren A, Wigzell H (1982) Immune functions of human synovial cells. Phenotypic and T cell regulatory properties of HLA-DR expressing macrophage-like cells from normal and rheumatoid synovial tissue. Arthritis Rheum 25:488
11. Klareskog L, Forsum U, Wigzell H (1982) Murine synovial intima contains I-A, I-E/C positive bone-marrow derived cells. Scand J Immunol 15:508
12. Edwards JC, Willoughby DA (1982) Demonstration of bone marrow derived cels in synovial lining by means of giant intracellular granules as genetic markers. Ann Rheum Dis 41:177
13. Lindblad S, Klareskog L, Hedfors E, Forsum U, Sundström C (1983) Phenotypic characterization of synovial cells in situ in different kinds of synovitis. Arthritis Rheum 26:1321
14. Soden M, Rooney M, Cullen A, Whelan A, Feighery C, Bresnihan B (1989) Immunohistopathological features in the synovium obtained from clinically uninvolved knee joints of patients with rheumatoid arthritis. Br J Rheumatol 11:137
15. Duke O, Panayi GS, Janossy G, Poulter LW (1983) An immunohistological analysis of lymphocyte subpopulations and their microenvironment in the synovial membranes of patients with rheumatoid arthritis using monoclonal antibodies. Clin Exp Immunol 49:22
16. Scheynius A, Fischer T, Forsum U, Klareskog L (1984) Phenotypic characterization in situ of inflammatory cells in allergic and irritant contact dermatitis in man. Clin Exp Immunol 55:81
17. Benoist C, Mathis D (1990) Regulation of major histocompatibility complex class II genes. X, Y and other letters of the alphabet. Ann Rev Immunol 8:681
18. Amento EP, Bhan A, McCullagh K, Krane S (1985) Influences of gamma interferon on synovial fibroblastlike cells. Induction and inhibition of collagen synthesis. J Clin Invest 76:837
19. Alvaro-Gracis J, Zvaifler NJ, Firestein G (1989) Cytokines in chronic inflammatory arthritis IV. Granulocyte/macrophage colony-stimulating factor mediated induction of class II MHC antigen on human monocytes. A possible role in rheumatoid arthritis. J Exp Med 170:865
20. Burmester GR, Dimitriu-Bona A, Waters S, Winchester RJ (1983) Identification of three major synovial lining cell populations by monoclonal antibodies directed to Ia antigens and antigens associated with monocytes/macrophages and fibroblasts. Scand J Immunol 17:69
21. Klareskog L, Johnell O, Hulth A (1984) Expression of HLA-DR and HLA-DQ antigens on cells within the cartilage-pannus junctions in rheumatoid arthritis. Rheumatol Int 4:11
22. Jahn B, Burmester GR, Schmid H, Weseloch G, Rohwer P, Kalden JR (1987) Changes in cell surface antigen expression on human articular cartilage induced by gamma-interferon. Arthritis Rheum 30:64
23. Rubin K, Terracio L, Rönnstrand L, Heldin CH, Klareskog L (1988) Induction of receptors for platelet derived growth factor (PDGF) on mesenchymal cells in chronic inflammatory arthritis. Scand J Immunol 27:1988
24. Buchan G, Barrett K, Turner M, Chatry D, Maini RN, Feldmann M (1988) Interleukin-1 and tumour necrosis mRNA expression in rheumatoid arthritis: prolonged production of Il-1a. Clin Exp Immunol 73:449
25. Firestein GS, Alvaro-Garcia JM, Maki R (1990) Quantitative analysis of cytokine gene expression in rheumatoid arthritis. J Immunol 144:3347
26. Jasin HE (1985) Autoantibody specificities of immune complexes sequestered in articular cartilage of patients with rheumatoid arthritis and osteoarthritis. Arthritis Rheum 28:241

27. Nordling C, Klareskog L (1988) Interactions between the immune system and connective tissue in arthritis. Possible significance of an affinity between IgG and native collagen type II. Scand J Rheumatol 74:73
28. Klareskog L, Holmdahl R, Nordling C, Tarkowski A, Rubin K (1987) Synovial class II antigen expresion and immune complex formation in rheumatoid arthritis. Acta Med Scand 715:85
29. Caulfield JP, Hein A, Dynesium-Trentham R, Trentham DE (1982) Morphological demonstration of two stages in the development of type II collagen-induced arthritis. Lab Invest 46:321
30. Fitzgerald M (1989) Arthritis and the nervous system. Trends Neurosci 12:86
31. Maehlen J, Scroeder HD, Klareskog L, Olsson T, Kristensson K (1988) Axotomy induces MHC class I expression on rat nerve cells. Neurosci Lett 92:8
32. Olsson T, Kristensson K, Ljungdahl Å, Maehlen J, Holmdahl R, Klareskog L (1989) Gamma-interferon-like immunoreactivity in axotomized rat motor neurons. J Neurosci 9:3870
33. Ljungdahl Å, Olsson T, van der Meide R, Holmdahl L, Klareskog L, Höjeberg B (1989) Interferon-gamma-like immunoreactivity in certain neurons of the central and peripheral nervous system. J Neurosci Res 24:451
34. Maehlen J, Olsson T, Zachau A, Klareskog L, Kristensson K (1989) Local enhancement of class I and class II expression and cell infiltration in experimental allergic encephalomyelitis around axotomied motor neurons. J Neuroimmunol 23:125
35. Waalen K, Thoen J, Förre Ö, Hovig T, Teigland J, Natvig JB (1986) Rheumatoid synovial dendritic cels as stimulators in allogeneic and autologous mixed leucocyte reactions – comparisons with autologous monocytes as stimulator cells. Scand J Immunol 23:233
36. Zvaifler NJ, Steinman RM, Kaplan G, Lau LL, Rivelis M (1985) Identification of immunostimulatory dendritic cells in the synovial effusions of patients with rheumatoid arthritis. J Clin Invest 76:789
37. Keat A, Thomas B, Dixey J, Osborn M, Sonnex C, Taylor-Robinson D (1987) Chlamydia trachomatis and reactive arthritis: the missing link. Lancet i:72
38. Granfors K, Jalkanen S, von Essen R, Lahesmaaa-Rantla R, Isomäki O, Pekkola-Heino K, Merilahti-Palo R, Saario R, Isomäki H, Toivanen A (1989) Yersinia antigens in synovial-fluid cells from patients with reactive arthritis. N Engl J Med 320:216
39. Eisenberg R, Fox A, Greenblatt J, Anderle S, Cromartie W, Schwab J (1982) Measurement of bacterial cell wall in tissues by solid-phase radioimmunoassay: correlation of distribution and persistance with experimental arthritis in rats. Infect Immun 38:127
40. Arnett F et al (1988) The American Rheumatism Association 1987 revised criteria for the classification of rheumatoid arthritis. Arthritis Rheum 31:315
41. Klareskog L, Jonell O, Hulth A, Holmdahl R, Rubin K (1986) Reactivity of monoclonal anti-collagen II antibodies with cartilage and synovial tissue in rheumatoid arthritis and osteoarthritis. Arthritis Rheum 29:730
42. Munthe E, Natvig JB (1972) Immunoglobulin classes, subclasses and complexes of IgG rheumatoid factor in rheumatoid plasma cells. Clin Exp Immunol 12:55
43. Tarkowski A, Klareskog L, Carlsten H, Herberts P, Koopman WJ (1989) Secretion of antibodies to types I and II collagen by synovial tissue cells in patients with rheumatoid arthritis. Arthritis Rheum 32:1087
44. Hanafusa T, Pujol-Borrell P, Ciovato L, Russell RCG, Doniach D, Bottazzo GF (1983) Aberrant expression of HLA-DR antigen on thyrocytes in Graves disease: relevance for autoimmunity. Lancet ii:1111
45. Metley JP, Puré E, Steinman RM (1989) Control of the immune response at the level of antigen-presenting cells: a comparison of the function of dendritic cell and B lymphocytes. Adv Immunol 47:45
46. Szakal AK, Kosco MH, Tew JG (1989) microanatomy of lymphoid tissue during humoral immune responses. Structure function relationships. Ann Rev Immunol 7:91

47. Holmdahl R, Jansson L, Rubin K, Larsson E, Klareskog L (1986) Chronic and progressive arthritis induced in mice with homologous collagen II. Arthritis Rheum 29:106
48. Larsson P, Kleinau S, Holmdahl R, Klareskog L (1990) Autologous collagen induced arthritis in rats. Demonstration of clinically distinct forms of arthritis in two strains of rats after immunization with the same collagen preparation. Arthritis Rheum 33:693
49. Cohen I (1986) Regulation of autoimmune disease. Physiological and therapeutic. Immunol Rev 94:5
50. Acha-Orbea H, Steinman L, McDevitt HO (1989) T cell receptors in murine autoimmune diseases. Ann Rev Immunol 7:371

CD5$^+$ B Cells and Double-Negative T Cells in Rheumatoid Arthritis

C. Plater-Zyberk[1], R. N. Maini[1], F. M. Brennan[2],
and M. Feldmann[2]

[1] Kennedy Institute of Rheumatology, 6 Bute Gardens, London, W67DW, UK
[2] Charing Cross Sunley Research Centre, Lurgan Avenue, London, W6 8LW, UK

Introduction

The presence of autoantibodies such as rheumatoid factor (RF) in patients with rheumatoid arthritis (RA) prompted the concept that abnormalities in the immune system may be important in the development of the disease [70]. This in turn led to intensive studies on the cells involved and their interactions and homing to the site of local inflammation. In RA, the synovial membrane is characterized by the presence of lymphoid aggregates, local production of cytokines and secretion of immunoglobulins, of which a proportion shows autoantibody specificity (see Feldmann et al., this volume). In fact, the synovial membrane effectively functions as an ectopic lymphoid organ actively involved in an immune response.

The high expression in this tissue of molecules such as MHC class II antigens and the adhesion molecule intercellular adhesion molecule-1 (ICAM-1) further support this concept [37, 18]. MHC class II antigens are essential in antigen presentation to T cells, and adhesion molecules direct lymphocyte trafficking and localisation to extravascular sites [10, 73]. Another important function of adhesion molecules is their role in antigen presentation mediated by increasing the intercellular contacts and providing activation signals. In addition to the local immune response and tissue destruction, circulating autoantibody and immune complexes induce systemic complications which further worsen the outcome of the disease [12].

Given this background, the need to identify the origin and characteristics of autoreactive T and B lymphocytes becomes imperative in understanding the immunopathology of RA. In this chapter, we concentrate on the significance of the observation that T and B subpopulations, with characteristics seen in early stages of ontogeny or differentiation from stem cells, occur with an increased frequency in RA and in systemic connective tissue diseases such as primary Sjogren's syndrome (SS). These subsets are composed of both B cells expressing CD5 (CD5$^+$ B) and T lymphocytes which lack CD4 or CD8 double-negative and which bear either the usual α/β antigen receptor or the alternative γ/δ

Smolen, Kalden, Maini (Eds.)
Rheumatoid Arthritis
© Springer-Verlag Berlin Heidelberg 1992

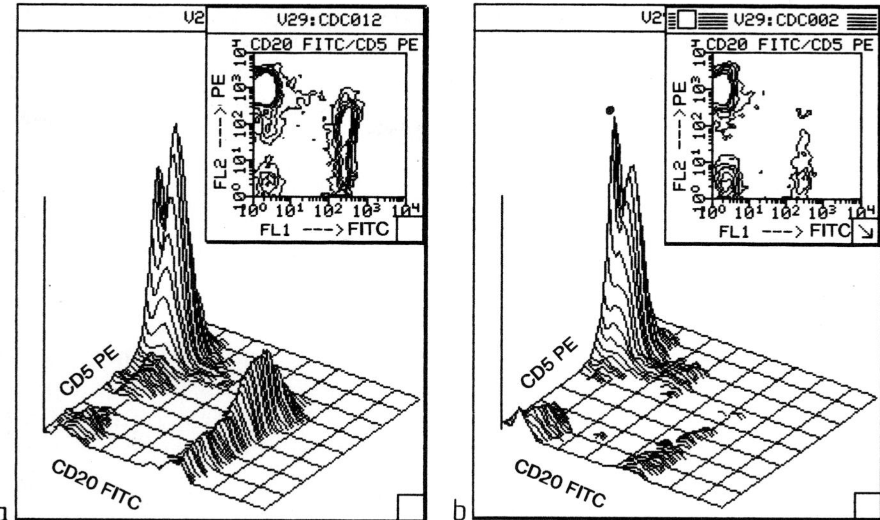

Fig. 1a, b. Flow cytometry profile of the peripheral blood lymphocytes from **a** a "high" and **b** "low" CD5$^+$ B donor. The cells were stained with CD20 FITC (pan-B cell marker) and CD5 PE (marker for T cells and CD5$^+$ B cells

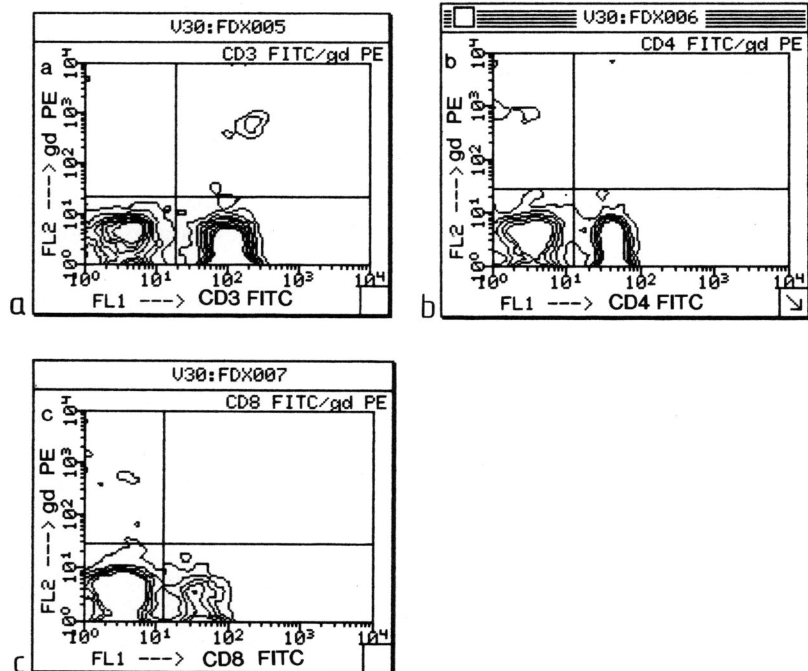

Fig. 2a–c. Flow cytometry profile of $\delta\gamma^+$ T cells showing that **a** $\gamma\delta^+$ T cells coexpress CD3 but **b** are CD4 and **c** CD8 double-negative

receptor (Figs. 1 and 2). An increase in $CD5^+$ B cells was discovered by our group in 1985 [54] and confirmed by several other groups [20, 67, 8, 35]. Double-negative α/β T cells are characteristically increased in systemic lupus erythematosus (SLE) and γ/δ^+ T cells are elevated in RA blood and joints [3].

$CD5^+$ B Cells

The $CD5^+$ B Subset: A Distinct Lineage

The human B cell population can be divided into two subsets, one expressing the CD5 antigen ($CD5^+$) and one negative (conventional) for this surface marker. Similarly, murine B cells can also be divided into $CD5^+$ and conventional B cell subsets according to the expression of Ly-1, a molecule homologous to CD5. A "sister" population with the same surface immunoglobulin phenotype but lacking CD5 has also been described [21]. Murine $CD5^+$ B cells (previously referred to as $Ly-1^+$ B cells) express surface IgM at higher levels and IgD at lower levels than conventional B cells and, when isolated from the peritoneal cavity, express the macrophage associated marker Mac-1. In contrast to murine $CD5^+$ B cells, the differential expression of IgM and IgD is not apparent in humans, although Mac-1 is found on a proportion of $CD5^+$ cells [35].

Flow cytometric analysis has demonstrated that the epitope density of CD5 is much lower on B than on T cells, making the identification of $CD5^+$ B cells dependent on the sensitivity of instrument used [55]. In addition, the CD5 molecule appears to be distributed in variable density on most if not all human B cells (see below), and a separation into $CD5^+$ and conventional B populations can thus be defined only operationally. Consequently, the question has arisen as to whether CD5 expression discriminates between two subsets of B lymphocytes or delineates cells at different stages of differentiation/activation.

In mice, reconstitution experiments have demonstrated that both subsets are distinct and represent two different lineages of B lymphocytes [22]. In the foetus the stem cells for $CD5^+$ B cells are localized in the liver, the omentum and the peritoneal cavity, whereas in adult mice they are found exclusively in the peritoneal cavity but not in the bone marrow which contains stem cells for the conventional B cells. Furthermore, in contrast to conventional B cells which are replenished from bone marrow stem cells throughout adult life, $CD5^+$ B cells appear to be self-renewing and long-lived in adult mice [22, 23, 13, 31]. This implies that the $CD5^+$ B cell repertoire is less diverse than that derived from conventional B cells.

Whether human $CD5^+$ B cells represent a distinct lineage is still a matter of debate. Longitudinal examination and family studies suggest that the levels of circulating $CD5^+$ B cells in each individual is stable and under genetic control, supporting the distinct lineage hypothesis [33, 40, 72]. However, treatment with phorbol esters (PMA) induces expression of CD5 on B cells, making CD5 a marker of activated B cells rather than (or as well as) a marker for a distinct subpopulation. It has not proved possible to demonstrate clearly the expression of CD5 on all activated B cells and the use of other activation stimuli, such as anti-Ig either on its own or with conditioned medium, pokeweed mitogen, purified and recombinant interleukins, or Epstein-Barr virus (EBV), does not result in increased CD5 expression [35]. Therefore, the data obtained in PMA do not preclude the hypothesis that, in humans as in mice, CD5$^+$ B cells belong to a distinct lineage. Furthermore, these findings highlight the need for other more reliable markers of these possible two lineages of B cells.

The CD5 Antigen on T and B Lymphocytes

CD5 is a 67 KD$^\alpha$ glycoprotein expressed very early on the surface of T cells during thymic development. Expression of CD5 is maintained throughout the different stages of T cell differentiation and nearly all mature T lymphocytes are CD5$^+$ with the exception of a very minor population of peripheral CD8$^+$ T cells. CD5 was thought to be exclusively associated with lymphocytes of the lineage up to 1980 when Boumsell et al. observed that, in a high proportion of patients with chronic lymphocytic leukeamia (CLL), the malignant B cell population was also CD5 surface positive. Since then, it has been realized that CD5-expressing B cells define a major proportion of the B population in normal foetal lymphoid organs and cord blood at birth. By adult life, largely due to the increase in absolute numbers of conventional B cells, the proportion of B lymphocytes expressing CD5 is reduced and constitutes 15%–20% of the B cell population in peripheral blood [16, 40, 8].

The cDNA encoding human CD5 has been cloned and the protein sequenced [29]. Structural analysis shows that CD5 has a large extracellular domain of 347 amino acid residues, a short transmembrane portion of 37 residues and a long intracytoplasmic tail of 93 residues. These features makes CD5 a member of the immunoglobulin supergene family and its structure shares characteristics of cell surface receptors which are involved in signal transduction. The natural ligand for CD5 has not yet been determined. Owing to similarities in the in vitro effects of interleukin-1 (IL-1) and anti-CD5 monoclonal antibody on T cell activation, it has been postulated that CD5 could be the receptor for this cytokine. Like IL-1, treatment of preactivated T cells with anti-CD5 increases the concentrations of cytoplasmic free calcium, induces IL-2 production and membrane expression of the IL-2 and also the release of growth and helper factors. However, some differences in the functional effects of anti-CD5 and IL-1, such as their additive effect on in vitro proliferation of T cells, and differences in the cellular distribution of the CD5 antigen and the IL-1 receptor that these two molecules are distinct [35]. In addition, the recent cloning of the IL-1 receptor has allowed direct comparison of its sequence with that of CD5 and has definitively proved that the two molecules are not identical.

Nevertheless, the IL-1 receptor and CD5 are functionally related, and the expression of CD5 appears necessary for the binding of IL-1 to its receptor.

Nishimura et al. [51] demonstrated that a Jurkat mutant which had lost surface expression of CD5 did not bind IL-1. The binding of IL-1 was restored after infection with the retrovector which induced membrane CD5 expression. These elegant experiments demonstrate the importance of the CD5 molecule in IL-1 controlled cell activation.

Human splenic B lymphocytes stimulated by PMA have been used to compare the CD5 molecules expressed on B and T lymphocytes. Experiments have shown that PMA induced CD5 mRNA in splenic B cells was complementary to the T cell derived CD5 cDNA, demonstrating that both B and T lymphocytes use the same gene to encode this protein [15]. This was further confirmed in Northern blot analysis showing that RNA extracted from $CD5^+$ B cells from CLL and several EBV cell lines was similar in size to that of lymphomas [46].

The function of CD5 on B cells may be analogous to its proposed function on T cells where it transduces signals. It has been reported that addition of CD5 monoclonal antibodies (Mabs) to cultures of RA B lymphocytes containing high proportions of $CD5^+$ B cells results in cell proliferation. Furthermore, addition of both anti-CD5 Mab and IL-1 α results in enhanced synthesis of IgM. In these experiments, however, the production of RF was not increased suggesting that some other costimulator may be necessary for its up-regulation [19]. If confirmed, these findings, that CD5 can act as a signal transducer for B cell proliferation and differentiation, may be important in situations where the $CD5^+$ B subset is expanded.

B cells expressing CD5 share phenotypic features with conventional B cells. Both subsets express CD19, CD20, CD21, heavy and light immunoglobulin chains [55]. Experiments using anti-CD5 and anti-CD21 Mabs have demonstrated that CD5 and CD21 (the receptor for C3d) are linked on the surface of leukaemic B cells and that modulation of one antigen results in comodulation of the other [1]. This association of CD5 with the receptor of a complement fragment and the expression of both molecules as a complex receptor may have important implications for the physiology of $CD5^+$ B cells in situations such as inflamed RA joints, in which concentrations of complement fragments are present.

$CD5^+$ Cells in Repertoire Development

In normal human development, the $CD5^+$ B subset represents the major population of B cells in the foetus, at a time when only self-antigens are encountered by the immune system. Studies in mice showed that antibodies secreted in foetal life are mainly of the IgM class with specificity for self-antigens. They often react with each other, displaying characteristic interconnectivity [69]. It has been suggested that these antibodies are important in repertoire development and establish a primordial network of idiotype anti-idiotype reactivity. Anti-idiotypic antibodies can influence the immune system by either suppressing or enhancing specific antibody production [31]. For example, neonatal administration of anti-idiotype Mab, specific for known germline encoded idiotypes (J558 and TEPC-15), permanently depletes the adult repertoire of B cells expressing this idiotype and results in depressed antigenspecific responses. In contrast, in the A48 Id-levan system, administration of the idiotype promotes the development of B cell clones which are normally silent, resulting in production of antibody.

In the T15 dominated anti-phosphorylcholine system, reconstitution of irradiated adult BALB/c mice with bone marrow cells gives rise to an anti-phosphorylcholine response utilizing the dominant T15 idiotype only if purified peritoneal B lymphocytes are also transferred [9]. This has been explained by the absence of an appropriate network interaction selecting for this idiotype, but it could also be due to the absence of B cells synthesizing idiotype positive antibodies. To discriminate between the two possibilities. Masmoudi et al. [45] have transferred bone marrow and peritoneal cells that are congenic for heavy and light chain allotypes. They have demonstrated that the idiotype positive antibodies are exclusively synthesized by peritoneal CD5$^+$ B cells and cannot be induced in bone marrow derived B cells.

The generation of the T cell repertoire for antigen can also be influenced by injection of anti-idiotypic antibody as demonstrated with the TNP F6(51) idiotype system. Mice depleted of B cells by anti-μ treatment from birth lack T cells expressing this major idiotype [43]. This "suppression" of id+T cells remains permanent if the anti-μ antibody is administered at least for the first 3 weeks of life. Interruption of treatment at this time allows a rapid reconstitution of the B population but not of the id+T population [44]. In later experiments, the same group demonstrated that expression of the idiotype on T cells can be restored by transfer of peritoneal CD5$^+$ B cells to the "suppressed" animal [42]. These data illustrate the role of B-T cell interactions early in life in the expression of the idiotype on T cells.

Taken together, these data illustrate the paramount importance of the idiotype expressed by CD5$^+$ B cells in T and B cell-mediated immunity as it appears to influence both the post-thymic maturation of T cell receptor and the synthesis of antibody.

Immunoglobulin V Gene Usage by CD5$^+$ Cells

The Ig heavy chain variable genes (VH gene) used by human CD5$^+$ B cells were analysed in EBV transformed CD5$^+$ B cells from healthy peripheral blood [61]. The antibody produced by these lines displays, the multispecific binding to unrelated antigens typical of "natural" antibodies. Analysis of the VH genes encoding these antibodies has revealed a bias towards usage of genes belonging to the VH4 family expressed in a virtually unmutated configuration. Usage of restricted unmutated genes provides a structural explanation for the high degree of idiotypic cross reactivity characteristically seen in products of normal CD5$^+$ B cells and suggests that VH4 genes may be important in the generation of polyspecificity. As result of binding to a variety of cellular antigens, "natural" polyspecific autoantibodies are thought to play a physiological role in antigen clearance following cell death.

Usage of restricted VH genes with little or no somatic mutations is characteristic of the early B cell population which is also enriched for $CD5^+$ B cells. A study of the B cell development in human foetal liver revealed restriction of the antibody repertoire with a significant limited usage of VH genes [62, 63]. These genes are closely related to the VH genes most proximal to the constant region genes which are preferentially expressed in murine foetal B cells [52]. Such bias suggests that, in humans as in mice, VH rearrangements follow a developmental programme imposed by proximity to the constant locus. However, the organization of the human VH genome has yet been characterized as fully as the mouse and further work is required to substantiate this hypothesis.

Similarly, in CLL, the malignant $CD5^+$ B cells also show usage of $V_\varkappa$ and 3' end VH genes with little diversity from the germline [34, 26, 46]. Whether the restricted usage of Ig VH genes in unmutated configuration by CLL $CD5^+$ B cells will also be the feature of nonmalignant adult $CD5^+$ B cells in health and autoimmune diseases remains to be determined.

$CD5^+$ B Cells and Autoimmunity

An increase in circulating $CD5^+$ B cells is seen in many autoimmune diseases in addition to RA, including primary SS [11, 56, 8], Hashimoto's thyroiditis [66], hyperthyroid Grave's disease [27], primary biliary cirrhosis [71] and insulin-dependent diabetes mellitus [50]. $CD5^+$ B cells are found in the cerebrospinal fluid of patients with multiple sclerosis [48]. In contrast, most patients with SLE do not show elevated proportions of $CD5^+$ B cells in their peripheral blood. The findings in SLE are unexpected as the equivalent population is expanded in some murine models of SLE, especially in the $NZB \times NZW$ strain. Many hypotheses can explain such findings, including the depletion of $CD5^+$ B cells from blood due to localization in lymphoid organs, reduction due to the therapy used in active SLE, or downregulation of CD5 expression to undetectable levels on the activated B lymphocytes found in the circulation of SLE patients. Support for the latter two possibilities is provided by the observation that treatment with corticosteroids decreases the levels of circulating $CD5^+$ B cells and that expression of CD5 becomes undetectable on activated B lymphoblasts and differentiated plasma cells [33, 55, 11, 71].

$CD5^+$ B cells from normal human blood secrete low-affinity, nonpathogenic, polyspecific immunoglobulins reacting with more than one antigen when stimulated in vitro with EBV or *Staphylococcus aureus* Cowan I (SAC). In contrast, $CD5^+$ B cells from RA patients give rise to lines producing monospecific high-affinity RF in addition to the low-affinity polyreactive autoantibody, suggesting a more specific role for $CD5^+$ B cells in the autoantibody secretion in RA. However, in diseases such as insulin-dependent diabetes mellitus and SLE the pathogenic high-affinity IgG are produced by B cells which are CD5 negative [8, 35]. These data support the notion that not all autoantibodies are secreted by CD5$^+$ B cells.

In normal strains of mice, the CD5$^+$ B population is enriched in the peritoneal cavity and is the main source of antibodies recognizing the polar headgroup of phosphatidyl choline, a phospholipid commonly found in cellular membranes and unmasked by enzymatic treatment of red blood cells [47]. CD5$^+$ B cells from autoimmune mice spontaneously secrete IgM autoantibodies reacting with bromelain-treated autologous red blood cells and also with single-stranded DNA and thymocytes [23]. As previously suggested for "natural" antibodies in humans, these autoantibodies may be involved in clearance of intracellular and membrane antigens released following cell damage.

Immunohistological examination of RA synovial membrane has shown that the major population of infiltrating lymphocytes is composed of T cells (see Feldman et al., this volume). High numbers of plasma cells are also found, whereas B lymphocytes are rare [40, 32]. This makes it difficult to identify CD5$^+$ B cells using histological techniques because CD5 is expressed at low levels on B cells and its detection can be masked by the high epitope density of CD5 on the numerous T cells. Nevertheless, small numbers of CD5$^+$ B cells can be observed in RA membrane, but due to the rarity of B cells the absolute numbers of CD5$^+$ B cells are low and their quantification subject to technical inaccuracy.

The lack of an appropriate fusion partner for somatic cell hybridization of human B cells has been a barrier for expanding monoclonal B lymphocytes which would allow the study of B cells at a clonal level. We used a mouse $\times$ human heteromyeloma fusion partner (SPAZ4) and succeeded in immortalizing human B lymphocytes by somatic cell hybridization of lymphocytes extracted from RA synovial membrane [6]. As only activated B lymphocytes are immortalized in this technique, it has permitted a detailed analysis of the activated B cells localized at the site of the disease. By fusing the mononuclear cells extracted from two RA synovia, we obtained a total of 34 hybridomas secreting high levels of IgG (26 hybridomas) and IgM (8 hybridomas); no IgA producing hybridomas were isolated. Surprisingly, most of our hybridomas did not react with a large panel of autoantigens used for screnning. Only a small proportion of hybridomas displayed defined specificity: three recognized IgG-Fc (RF), one bound to collagen type II and one displayed restricted polyspecificity binding to cytoskeletal antigens and phospholipids (Fig. 3).

These findings are in contrast with results obtained by other investigators, who used the ELISPOT technique to detect antibody-producing cells at the single cell level directly from the membrane. The results showed that a high proportion of synovial membrane plasma cells secrete anti-collagen type II antibodies and RF [68]. Their findings, similar to results obtained with synovial T cell clones [39] suggest that cartilage derived collagen type II is an important antigen in the local immune response in RA. However, despite the low number of hybridomas with defined specificity, the data obtained with the immortalized B cells also suggests that a selective mechanism is involved in the expansion of

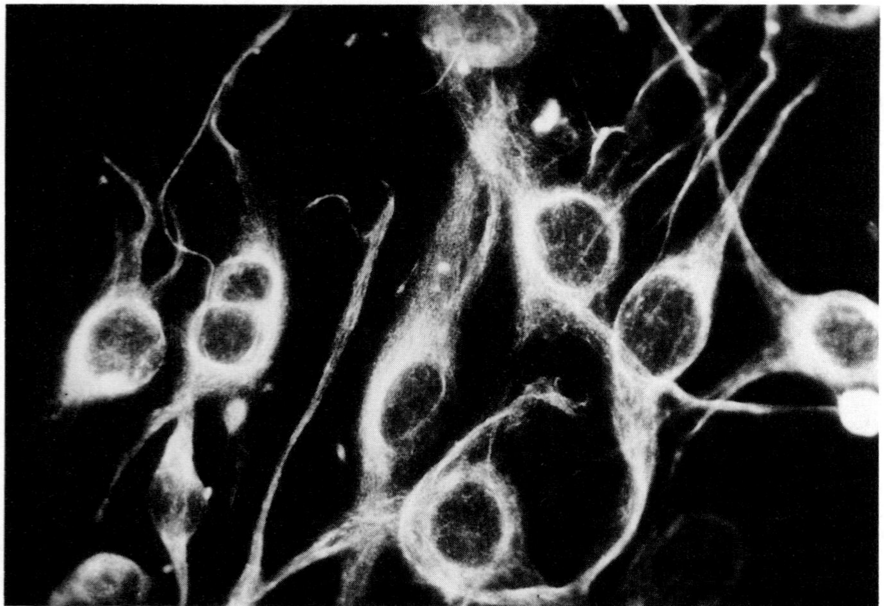

Fig. 3. Indirect immunofluorescent staining of 3T3 mouse fibroblasts with an IgM monoclonal antibody secreted by a hybridoma derived from RA synovial membrane. Reactivity with cytoskeletal filaments is shown

B cells in the RA synovium, since 96% of our IgG hybridomas secrete immunoglobulin belonging to the IgG_1 subclass with a predominance of lambda light chains. The positive selection of the B cells in the synovium could be determined by antigens in the joint or by idiotypes. A possible role for idiotypes is supported by the finding that 9 out of 20 synovial hybridomas expressed cross-reactive idiotypes and/or CD5 antigens [57]. This phenotype is found in primary B cell follicles of human foetal spleen where idiotypic interactions are thought to play an important role in expanding the B cell population [35]. Taken together, these data give rise to the hypothesis that the activated B cell population in RA synovium derives from a subset displaying features normally associated with immaturity whose expansion is controlled by the idiotypic network.

Double-Negative T Cells

γ/δ TCR⁺ T Cells

T cell progenitors migrate initially from foetal liver and later from bone marrow into the thymus where they undergo differentiation and maturation before emigrating into peripheral lymphoid organs. At different stages in this maturation process the T cells express on their surface membrane a variety of surface membrane antigens including receptor for antigen. Early in development T lymphocytes do not express either CD4 or CD8 double-negative. Later, they are thought to go through a CD4$^+$/CD8$^+$ (double-positive stage) before expressing only one or the other of these accessory molecules which point they colonize the secondary lymphoid organs. The T cell antigen receptors (TCR) are heterodimers noncovalently associated with the CD3 complex. Most T lymphocytes in the periphery ($\sim$90%) express a TCR composed of an α and a β polypeptide chain which is necessary and sufficient for recognition of antigen in the context of MHC restriction. A minor population of T cells which are CD4- and CD8 express the alternative form of the TCR consisting of a γ and δ chain [5].

Although the TCR γ/δ uses similar recombination processes to the conventional TCR, the repertoire is potentially very limited with only eight functional variable and five functional joining segments on the γ gene and with an even smaller number of V, D and J segments defining the δ locus [59]. However, further diversity is generated by deletion and/or addition of nucleotides to the junctional regions (N regions) during rearrangement of the γ and δ loci [65].

Three distinct form of the TCR γ/δ T cell have been described: a disulphide-linked heterodimer composed of Vγ9-JγP-Cγ1 elements coupled to the Vδ2 element (preferentially used in peripheral blood), and both disulphide-bonded and nondisulphide-bonded heterodimers which express Vγ1 coupled to either Cδ1 or Cδ2 [38]. These latter forms represent only minor population in peripheral blood but represent the majority in the thymus.

The proportion of γ/δ TCR$^+$ T cells in normal human adult peripheral blood is low (1%–10%) but has been shown by us to be expanded in patients with RA and primary SS with elevated numbers of CD5$^+$ B cells [4]. This expansion in both subsets of lymphocytes may imply some interconnection between CD5$^+$ B cells and γ/δ+ T cells, as both subpopulations are found early in ontogeny at a time when autoreactivity is a normal feature, and high connectivity between lymphocytes plays an important role in repertoire development and establishment of the idiotype network. There are other possibilities, for example, CD5$^+$ B cells may act as antigen presenting cells for γδ T cells, γδ T cells may produce growth factors which augment CD5$^+$ B cell survival or growth. Alternatively, these subsets could be expanded in a nonspecific fashion by growth factors released from sites of inflammation.

Immunohistological analysis of RA synovial membrane has shown that the major population of lymphocytes is composed of T cells with the CD4 memory phenotype (CD4+CD45RO+) [53]. T lymphocytes with the CD8 phenotype are much less represented and are mainly found in the interaggregate area [32]. In addition to conventional T lymphocytes we observed an increase in γ/δ TCR T cells in RA joint tissue in about half the RA patients tested [3]. A similar increase has also been reported by another group [60] in RA synovial fluid. In both these studies γ/δ TCR T cells were detected using a pan-anti-δ chain antibody with an anti-γ antibody which detects the predominantly peripheral type of T cell (Vγ9-JγP-Cγ1). In a number of other unpublished studies, the phenotype of γ/δ TCR T cells in membrane was investigated. It was observed that there is a predominance of γ/δ TCR T cells which use the Vδ1 coupled to either Cδ1 or Cδ2 (Lydyard, personal communication), suggesting that a "thymic-like" situation may develop at the site of inflammation. The function of γ/δ TCR T cells remains speculative, although non-MHC restricted cytotoxicity [49] and reactivity against mycobacterial antigens [28] has been suggested. T lymphocyte reactivity to mycobacterial antigens has been described in cells isolated from RA synovial fluid [24], and double negative γ/δ[+] T cell clones reacting with mycobacteria have been isolated [25], raising the possibility of a specific involvement of heat-shock proteins and double negative γ/δ[+] T cells in the pathogenesis of RA.

α/β TCR[+] Cells

The large majority of T cells which are double-negative express the γ/δ TCR; however, a small proportion of cells express the conventional α/β TCR. These cells, first described in normal mouse thymocytes [14], are expanded in the thymus and periphery of autoimmune mice such as MRL/lpr [7]. In MRI/lpr mice, infection with IL-2 recombinant vaccinia virus led to a reduction in the number of double-negative cells and to amelioration of the disease with prolongation of life. It was concluded that the increase in double-negative T cells in MRL/lpr mice was the result of IL-2 deficiency resulting in maturation arrest of T cell differentiation and accumulation of immature T cells in the lymphoid organs of these mice [17].

Double-negative α/β T cells are found at very low levels ($<0.3\%$) in peripheral blood but are expanded in more than tenfold in the peripheral blood of patients with SLE [64]. The function of these cells in unknown but it has been speculated that they may arise from progenitors in the thymus which have escaped thymic deletion [30]. It is of interest therefore that double-negative α/β TCR T cells cloned from normal peripheral blood showed unusual growth requirements in proliferating in response to IL-3, a growth factor affecting chiefly progenitor cells.

It has been proposed that nonpolymorphic MHC class 1-like molecules such as the CD1 antigens may serve as ligands for double-negative T cells. Thus, it was of interest that 1 out of 13 double-negative T cell lines from the blood of a patient with SLE showed reactivity against CD1a[+] cells [58]. Also, T cell lines isolated from RA synovium which were 80%–90% γ/δ[+] double-negative TCR showed specific cytotoxicity for cells transfected with CD1c (Brenner, unpublished communication). This suggests that these molecules may serve as recognition ligands and/or presentation molecules for double-negative T cells and that such cells can be isolated from autoimmune diseases in which expansion of these subsets has been described.

It is unknown why double-negative T cells are expanded in SLE, but it is suggested that they may contribute to the pathogenesis of the disease as they have been found to induce the production of cationic auto anti-DNA antibodies. At this stage the "normal" function of either α/β or γ/δ double-negative T cells is unknown and their role in contributing to the pathogenesis of autoimmune disease remains speculative.

Since submission of this chapter, the ligand for CD5 has been identified and reported in: van de Velde H, von Hoegen I, Wei Luo, Parnes JR, Thielemans K (1991) The B cell surface protein CD72/Ly6-2 is the ligand for CD5. Nature 351:662–665.

References

1. Bergui L, Tesio L, Schena M, Riva M, Malavasi F, Schulz T, Marchision PC, Caligaris-Cappio F (1988) CD5 and CD21 molecules are a functional unit in the cell/substrate adhesion of B-chronic lymphocytic leukemia cells. Eur J Immunol 18:89–96
2. Boumsell L, Choppin H, Pham D, Raynall B, Lemerle J, Dausset J, Bernard A (1980) An antigen shared by a human T cell subset and B cell chronic lymphocytic leukemia cells. Distribution on normal and malignant lymphoid cells. J Exp Med 152:229–234
3. Brennan FM, Londei M, Jackson AM, Hercend T, Brenner MB, Maini RN, Feldmann M (1988) T cells expressing $\gamma\delta$ chain receptors in rheumatoid arthritis. J Autoimmunity 1:319–326
4. Brennan FM, Plater-Zyberk C, Feldmann M, Maini RN (1989) Coordinate expansion of 'feotal type' lymphocytes (TCR $\gamma\delta$ T+ and CD5+ B) in rheumatoid arthritis and primary Sjogren's syndrome. Clin Exp Immunol 77:175–178
5. Brenner MB, Strominger JL, Krangel MS (1988) The $\gamma\delta$ T cell receptor. Adv Immunol 34:133–192
6. Brown CMS, Plater-Zyberk C, Mageed RA, Jefferis R, Maini RN (1990) Analysis of immunoglobulins secreted by hybridomas derived from rheumatoid synovia. Clin Exp Immunol 80:366–372
7. Budd RC, Schreyer M, Miescher C, MacDonald HR (1987) T cell lineages in the thymus of lpr/lpr mice: evidence for parallel pathways of normal and abnormal T cell development. J Immunol 139:2200–2210
8. Burastero SE, Casali P (1989) Characterization of human CD5 (Leu-1)+B lymphocytes and the antibodies they produce. In: Del Guercio P, Cruse JM (eds) B lymphocytes: function and regulation. Contrib Microbiol Immunol, Karger, Basel 11:231–262
9. Cazenave PA, Martinez AC, Countinho A (1989) Differential L chain expression in the antibody response to phosphorylcholine of adult bone marrow or peritoneum-derived B lymphocytes. J Immunol 142:8–11
10. Cavender D, Haskard D, Yu CL, Igushi T, Miossec P, Oppenheim-Marks N, Ziff M (1987) Pathways to chronic inflammation in rheumatoid synovitis. Fed Proc 46:113–117
11. Dauphinee M, Yovar Z, Talal N (1988) B cells expressing CD5 are increased in Sjogren's syndrome. Arthritis Rheum 31:642–647
12. Erhardt CC, Mumford PA, Venables PJW, Maini RN (1989) Factors predicting a poor life prognosis in rheumatoid arthritis: an eight year prospective study. Ann Rheum Dis 48:7–13
13. Foster I, Rajewski K (1987) Expansion and functional activity of Ly-1+B cells upon transfer of peritoneal cells into allotype-congenic, newborn mice. Eur J Immunol 17:52–528
14. Fowlkes BJ, Kruisbeck AM, Ton-That H, Weston MA, Coligan JE, Schwartz RH, Pardoll DM (1988) A novel population of T-cell receptor $\alpha\beta$ bearing thymocytes which predominantly express a single Vb gene family. Nature 329:251–254

15. Freedman AS, Boyd AW, Bieber FR, Dayley J, Rosen K, Horowitz JC, Levy DN, Nadler LM (1987) Normal cellular counterparts of B cell chronic lymphocytic leukemia. Blood 70:418–427
16. Gadol N, Ault K (1986) Phenotypic and functional characterization of human Leu 1 (CD5) B cells. Immunol Rev 93:23–34
17. Gutierrez-Ramos JC, Andreu JL, Revilla Y, Vinuela E, Martinez-A C (1990) Recovery from autoimmunity of MRL/lpr mice after infection with an interleukin-2/vaccinia recombinant virus. Nature 346:271–274
18. Hale LP, Martin ME, McCollum DE, Nunley JA, Springer TA, Singer KH, Haynes BF (1989) Immunohistologic analysis of the distribution of the cell adhesion molecules within the inflammatory synovial microenvironment. Arthritis Rheum 32:22–30
19. Hara M, Atsushi K, Hirose T, Norioka K, Harigai M, Suzuki K, Tabata H, Kawakami M, Kawagoe M, Nakamura H (1988) Stimulatory effect of CD5 antibody on B cells from patients with rheumatoid arthritis. Clin Immunol Immunopathol 49:223–230
20. Hardy RR, Hayakawa K, Shimizu M, Yamasaki K, Kishimoto T (1987) Rheumatoid factor secretion from human Leu-1+B cells. Science 236:81–83
21. Hayakawa K, Hardy RR, Parks DR, Herzenberg LA (1983) The "Ly-1B" cell subpopulation in normal immunodefective and autoimmune mice. J Exp Med 157:202–218
22. Hayakawa K, Hardy RR, Herzenberg LA, Herzenberg LA (1985) Progenitors for Ly-1 B cells are distinct from progenitors for other B cells. J Exp Med 161:1554–1568
23. Herzenberg LA, Stall AM, Lalor PA, Sidman C, Moore WA, Parks DR (1986) The Ly-1 B cell lineage. Immunol Rev 93:81–102
24. Holoshitz J, Klamjma A, Drucker I, Lapidot Z, Yaretzky A, Van Eden W, Cohen IR (1986) T lymphocytes or rheumatoid arthritis patients show reactivity to a fraction of mycobacteria cross-reactive with cartilage. Lancet ii:305–309
25. Holoshitz J, Koning F, Je De Bruyn J, Strober S (1989) Isolation of CD4–CD8-mycobacteria-reactive T lymphocyte clones from rheumatoid arthritis synovial fluid. Nature 339:226–229
26. Humphries GC, Shen A, Kuziel WA, Capra JD, Blattner FR, Tucker PW (1988) A new human immunoglobulin VH family preferentially rearranged in immature B-cell tumors. Nature 331:446–449
27. Iwatani Y, Amino N, Kaneda T, Ichihara K, Tamaki H, Tachi J, Matsuzuka F, Fukata S, Kuma K, Miyai K (1989) Marked increase of CD5+B cells in hyperthyroid Graves' disease. Clin Exp Immunol 78:196–200
28. Janis EM, Kaufmann SHE, Schwartz RH, Pardoll DM (1989) Activation of $\gamma\delta$ T cells in the primary immune response to *Mycobacterium tuberculosis*. Science 244:713–716
29. Jones NH, Clabby ML, Dialynas DH, Huang HJ, Herzenberg LA, Strominger J (1986) Isolation of complementary DNA clones encoding the human lymphocyte glycoprotein T1/Leu-1. Nature 323:346–349
30. Kappler JW, Staerz U, White J, Marrack P (1988) Self tolerance eliminates T cells specific for Mls-modified products of the major histocompatibility complex. Nature 332:35–40
31. Kearney JF, Vakil M, Solvason N (1989) The role of idiotypic interactions and B-cell subsets in development of the B-cell repertoire. Cold Spring Harbor Symp Quant Biol LIV:23–207
32. Kennedy TD, Plater-Zyberk C, Partridge TA, Woodrow DF, Maini RN (1988) Morphometric comparison of synovium from patients with osteoarthritis and rheumatoid arthritis. J Clin Pathol 41:847–852
33. Kipps TJ, Vaughan JH (1987) Genetic influence on the levels of circulating CD5 B lymphocytes. J Immunol 139:1060–1064
34. Kipps TJ, Tomhave E, Chen PP, Carson D (1988) Autoantibody-associated kappa light chain variable region gene expressed in chronic lymphocytic leukemia with little or no somatic mutation. J Exp Med 167:840–852
35. Kipps TJ (1990) The CD5 B cell. Adv Immunol 47:117–185
36. Kipps TJ, Robbins BA, Carson DA (1990) Uniform high frequency expression of autoantibody-associated crossreactive idiotypes in the primary B cell follicles of human fetal spleen. J Exp Med 171:189–196

37. Kissonerghis AM, Maini RN, Feldmann M (1989) High rate of HLA class II mRNA synthesis in rheumatoid arthritis joints and its persistence in culture: down-regulation by recombinant interleukin 2. Scand J Immunol 29:73–82
38. Lanier LL, Ruitenberg J, Bolhuis RLH, Borst J, Phillips JH, Testi R (1988) Structural and serological heterogeneity of γδ T cell antigen receptor expression in thymus and peripheral blood. Eur J Immunol 18:1873–2112
39. Londei M, Savill C, Verhoef A, Brennan F, Leech ZA, Duance V, Maini RN, Feldmann M (1989) Persistence of collagen type II specific T cell clones in the synovial membrane of a patient with RA. Proc Natl Acad Sci 8:636–640
40. Maini RN, Plater-Zyberk C, Andrew E (1987) Autoimmunity in rheumatoid arthritis. An approach via the study of B lymphocytes. In: Zvaifler N, Saunders WB (eds) Pathogenesis of chronic inflammatory arthritis. Rheum Dis Clin North Am 13:319–337
41. Maini RN, Plater-Zyberk C (1988) The significance of CD5+B cells in rheumatic diseases. Scand J Rheumatology 76 (suppl):237–242
42. Marcos MA, de le Hera A, Pereira P, Marquez C, Toribio M, Coutinho A, Martinez C (1988) B cell participation in the recursive selection of T cell repertoires. Eur J Immunol 18:1015–1020
43. Martinez-A C, Bernabe R, de la Hera A, Pereira P, Cazenave P-A, Coutinho A (1985) Establishment of idiotypic helper T-cell repertoires early in life. Nature 317:721–723
44. Martinez C, Pereira P, de la Hera A, Bandeira A, Marquez C, Coutinho A (1986) The basis for major histocompatibility complex (MHC) and immunoglobulin gene control of helper T cell idiotopes. Eur J Immunol 16:417–422
45. Masmoudi H, Motas-Santos, Huetz F, Coutinho A, Cazenave P-A (1990) All T15 Id-positive antibodies (but not the majority of VH T15+ antibodies) are produced by peritoneal CD5+B lymphocytes. International Immunol 2:515–520
46. Mayer R, Logtenberg T, Strauchen J, Dimitriu-Bona A, Mayer L, Mechanic S, Chiorazzi N, Borche L, Dighiero G, Mannheimer-Lory A, Diamond B, Alt F, Bona C (1990) CD5 and immunoglobulin V gene expression in B-cell lymphomas and chronic lymphocytic leukemia. Blood 75:1518–1524
47. Mercolino TJ, Arnold LW, Hawkins LA, Haughton G (1988) Normal mouse peritoneum contains a large population of Ly-1+ (CD5) B cells that recognize phosphatidylcholine. Relationship to cells that secrete hemolytic antibody specific for autologous erythrocytes. J Exp Med 168:687–698
48. Mix E, Olsson T, Correale J, Baig S, Kostulas V, Olsson O, Link H (1990) B cells expressing CD5 are increased in cerebrospinal fluid of patients with multiple sclerosis. Clin Exp Immunol 79:21–27
49. Moingeon P, Ythier A, Goubin G, Faure F, Nowill A, Delmon L, Rainaud M, Forestier F, Daffos F, Bohuon C, Hercend T (1986) A unique T cell receptor complex expressed on human foetal lymphocytes displaying natural-killer like activity. Nature 323:638–640
50. Nicoletti F, Meroni PL, Barcellini W, Steinvag PO, di Mauro M, Lunetta M, Pagano M, Consoli U, Zanussi C (1990) Enhanced percentage of CD5+B lymphocytes in newly diagnosed IDDM patients. Immunol Lett 23:211–215
51. Nishimura Y, Bierer BE, Burakoff SJ (1988) Expression of CD5 regulates responsiveness to IL-1. J Immunol 141:3438–3444
52. Perlmutter RM, Kearney JF, Chang SP, Hood LE (1985) Developmentally controlled expression of immunoglobulin VH genes. Science 227:1597–1601
53. Pitzalis C, Kingsley G, Murphy J, Panayi G (1987) Abnormal distribution of the helper-inducer and suppressor-inducer T lymphocyte subsets in the rheumatoid joint. Clin Immunol Immunopathol 45:252–258
54. Plater-Zyberk C, Maini RN, Lam K, Kennedy TD, Janossy G (1985) A rheumatoid arthritis B cell subset express a phenotype similar to that in chronic lymphocytic leukemia. Arthritis Rheum 28:971–976
55. Plater-Zyberk C, Maini RN (1988) Phenotypic and functional features of CD5+B lymphocytes in rheumatid arthritis. Scand J Rheumatology 75 (suppl):76–83

56. Plater-Zyberk C, Brennan FM, Feldmann M, Maini RN (1989) 'Foetal-type' B and T lymphocytes in rheumatoid arthritis and primary Sjogren's syndrome. J Autoimmun 2 (suppl):233–241
57. Plater-Zyberk C, Brown CMS, Mageed RA, Jefferis R, Maini RN (1990) B cell hybridomas derived from rheumatoid synovium express CD5 antigen and cross-reactive idiotypes. to be published
58. Porcelli S, Brenner MB, Greenstein JL, Balk SP, Terhorst C, Bleicher PA (1989) Recognition of cluster antigens by human CD4–CD8- cytolytic T lymphocytes. Nature 341:447–450
59. Raulet DH (1989) The structure, function and molecular genetics of the γδ T cell receptor. Ann Rev Immunol 7:175–207
60. Reme T, Portier M, Frayssinoux F, Combe B, Miossec P, Favier F, Sany J (1990) T cell receptor expression and activation of synovial lymphocyte subsets in patients with rheumatoid arthritis. Phenotyping of multiple synovial sites. Arthritis Rheum 33:485–492
61. Sanz I, Casali P, Thomas JW, Notkins AL, Capra D (1989) Nucleotide sequences of eight human natural autoantibody VH regions reveal apparent restricted use of VH families. J Immunol 142:4054–4061
62. Schroeder HW Jr, Hillson JL, Perlmutter RM (1987) Early restriction of the human antibody repertoire. Science 238:791–793
63. Schroeder HW Jr, Wang JY (1990) Preferential utilization of conserved immunoglobulin heavy chain variable gene segments during fetal life. Proc Natl Acad Sci USA 87:614–6150
64. Shivakumar S, Tsokos GC, Datta SK (1989) T cell receptor αβ expressing double-negative (CD4-/CD8-) and CD4+ T helper cells in humans augment the production of pathogenic anti-DNA autoantibodies associated with lupus nephritis. J Immunol 143:103–112
65. Strominger JL (1989) The γδ T-cell receptor and class 1b MHC-related proteins: enigmatic molecules of immune recognition. Cell 57:875–898
66. Suranyi P, Szegedi G, Damjanovich S, Juhasz F, Stenszky V, Farid NR (1989) B lymphocytes in Hashimoto's thyroiditis. Immunol Lett 22:147–150
67. Taniguchi O, Miyajima H, Hirano T, Noguchi M, Ueda A, Hashimoto H, Hirose S, Okumura K (1987) The Leu-1 B cell subpopulation in patients with rheumatoid arthritis. J Clin Immunol 7:441–448
68. Tarkowski A, Klareskog L, Carlsten H, Herbets P, Koopman W (1989) Secretion of antibodies to type I and II collagen by synovial tissue cells in patients with rheumatoid arthritis. Arthritis Rheum 32:1087–1092
69. Vakil M, Kearney JF (1986) Functional characterization of monoclonal autoanti-idiotype antibodies from early B cell repertoire. Eur J Immunol 16:1159–1165
70. Waaler E (1945) On the occurrence of a factor in human serum activating the specific agglutination of sheep blood corpuscules. Acta Pathol Microbiol Scand 17:172–178
71. Yamada H, Shimizu H, Taniguchi O, Okumura K (1988) Leu-1 (CD5) B cell subpopulation in patients with various liver diseases, special reference to hepatitis B virus carrier and to changes caused by prednisolone therapy. Int Arch Allergy Appl Immunol 87:409–416
72. Youinou P, Mackenzie L, Katsikis P, Merdrignac DA, Isenberg DA, Tuallon N, Lamour A, Ie Goff P, Jouquan J, Drogou A, Muller B, Moutsopoulos HM, Lydyard PM (1990) The relationship between CD5 expressing B lymphocytes and serological abnormalities in rheumatoid arthritis patients and their relatives. Arthritis Rheum 33:339–348
73. Ziff M (1989) Role of endothelium in chronic inflammation. Springer Sem Immunopathol 11:199–214

The Genetics of Rheumatoid Factors (RF):
The V-gene Repertoire of RFs in Rheumatoid
Arthritis as Analyzed by Hybridoma Clones*

J. B. Natvig[1], I. Randen[1], K. Thompson[1], and Ø. Førre[2]

[1] Institute of Immunology and Rheumatology, Oslo, Norway and MRC Centre, Molecular Immunopathology Unit, and Department of Immunology, Institute of Animal Physiology and Genetics Research, Cambridge, United Kingdom
[2] Oslo Rheumatism Hospital, Oslo, Norway

Introduction

The rheumatoid factors have been investigated in three different phases. The first detection of rheumatid factors and the establishment of the relationship between rheumatoid factors and clinical symptoms of rheumatoid arthritis (RA) occurred 50 years ago [53]. The pioneering phase between 1940 and 1950 included the confirmation of Waaler's findings by Rose and collaborators [see 50]. This period brought an appreciation of the diagnostic significance of rheumatoid factors in RA, although it was clear that there is also a group of patients with seronegative rheumatoid arthritis [50].

In the second phase from 1950 to 1980, RFs were characterized immuno-chemically, primarily by Henry Kunkel and his associates, and were shown to be mostly of the IgM type in serum, but later also of the IgG type [55]. In addition, during this phase there were numerous studies that elucidated the pathogenetic mechanisms of rheumatoid arthritis in which RF was involved by analyzing immune complexes in joint fluid, joint tissues, and serum [28, 30, 31, 39, 55]. These studies led to the definite understanding that RF was important in the formation of immune complexes in rheumatoid arthritis and thus clearly could be pathogenetic. Particularly the IgG variant of RF was essensial because of the self-associating IgG RF complexes [33, 39]. In this relation detailed studies of the fine specificities of RFs in RA were performed [2, 20, 23, 26, 36, 42]. It was also realized that RF could be harmless in other conditions, as seen in normal subjects following vaccinations and infections [8, 12, 44, 54]. In fact, the harmless and possibly beneficial RF in healthy persons led some investigators to argue that the RF was not part of the pathogenesis of rheumatoid arthritis.

* This work was supported by grants from the Norma and Leon Hess Foundation for Research on Rheumatological Diseases, the Norwegian Women's Health Organization, the Grethe Harbitz Legacy, and the Norwegian Research Council for Science and the Humanities.

Smolen, Kalden, Maini (Eds.)
Rheumatoid Arthritis
© Springer-Verlag Berlin Heidelberg 1992

Finally, the third and newest phase of investigation into rheumatoid factors started in the late 1980s and is continuing into the 1990s. This phase represents the characterization of the genes, notably the variable genes encoding for RF [34, 35, 38, 40, 49, 52]. These studies are designed to answer the question of whether the genetic repertoire of RF in the different clinical and normal situations is the same and whether the RF genes are encoded directly in the germline or are the result of somatic mutations.

RFs appear in at least three different conditions. First, they are found in healthy individuals as a response to antigenic stimulation, for example after vaccination or infection [8, 12]. There is evidence that RFs were most likely preserved during evolution because of their advantageous role in protecting life, for example by increasing the lytic effect of weak anti-viral antibodies. Second, RF appears spontaneously in M-components, seen for example in Waldenström's macroglobulinemia and mixed cryoglobulinemia [6, 7, 24, 25]. Third, RFs are important autoantibodies in certain autoimmune diseases, particularly in RA [28, 30, 31, 33, 39, 50, 55], where they can form self-associating complexes locally in the synovial tissues and fluids and generate chronic inflammatory responses [33, 39, 55].

We will review the present situation of the genetics of rheumatoid factors in RA with particular reference to information recently obtained about the idiotypes and V-gene usage. In this way we will compare the V-gene usage and idiotypes in RF produced in RA with those of RFs produced in normal individuals and in malignancies. In this context we will try to answer the following questions: First, is the genetic background of the RF the same in the three different conditions? Second, what in particular characterizes the genetics of RFs involved in rheumatoid arthritis?

Methodological Considerations

Until very recently, nearly all studies of the structure of RF involved patients with Waldenströms macroglobulinemia and mixed cryoglobulinemia. They were done by isolating the M-component with RF activity and performing amino acid sequencing of the monoclonal RF [3, 6, 7, 24, 25]. A series of important discoveries concerning the idiotypes and V-genes of these M-components were thus made. Regarding the structure of RF in the polyclonal repertoire of RA patients, some early studies utilized V-gene markers and cross-idiotypes [18, 19]. However, new methods had to be used for further structural studies. The recent development of producing human monoclonal antibodies with the Epstein-Barr virus (EBV) and the hybridoma technology [48] have made it possible to study the structure and genetics of RF in both normal subjects and RA patients [5, 22, 40, 41, 45, 46, 49]. We chose to use synovial tissue or blood from patients with RA for such studies. The technical details of these studies have been published elsewhere [32, 34, 35, 40, 49]. The lymphocytes were isolated from the tissues [1], then transformed with EBV, and subsequently fused with a nonsecreting mouse myeloma cell line X63-Ag8. 653 in a ratio of 2:1, as described in detail earlier [40, 48, 49]. The RF activity was analyzed by Latex fixation and ELISA techniques, using either whole IgG or isolated IgG Fc fragments as antigen [40]. The determination of other autoantibodies was done mostly with ELISA or indirect immunofluorescence techniques. In our own studies we have also determined RF-related cross-idiotypes (CRI) [27, 49].

Finally, the RF-producing clones were subjected to isolation of total RNA, reverse transcription, and subsequent enhancement by the polymerase chain reaction, and then to sequencing of the specific variable heavy and variable light chain cDNA. The methods and results of these studies have also been described in detail elsewhere [38, 52].

We will now consider the RFs first in patients with Waldenström's macroglobulinemia and mixed cryoglobulinemia, then in normal subjects, and finally in patients with rheumatoid arthritis. RFs are certainly also seen in other pathological conditions such as Sjögren's syndrome and SLE in increased amounts, but not much is known about whether the RFs are intimately involved in the disease processes or just reflect a stimulation of the repertoire for RFs in these conditions. The RFs corresponding to the M-components in patients with Waldenström's macroglobulinemia and mixed cryoglobulinemia were earlier thought to elucidate the genetics of RF also in RA. Although they have some similarities, there are, however also dinstinct differences among these RF antibodies [9, 10, 19].

Rheumatoid Factors in Malignant Disorders

The RFs in malignant disorders were first characterized genetically by Kunkel et al. [24, 25], who described the cross-idiotypes (CRI) and light-chain variable subgroups. This was later extended by sequence studies by Capra et al. [6, 7] and by further idiotype studies by Carson et al. [9, 10]. From these studies several points appeared:

1. The RFs in M-components represent a restricted repertoire, particularly for light-chain determinants. These RFs utilize mainly the $V_\varkappa III$ subgroup and the $V_\varkappa III$b sub-subgroup carrying the WA idiotype (about 60%–80% of the M-component RFs). This idiotype was extensively studied by Kunkel et al. [6, 7, 24, 25], and later also by Carson et al. [9, 10], using a closely related idiotope 17.109. Another variant of RF M-components related to $V_\varkappa III$a light chains is the idiotype PO [24, 25]. A third idiotope, BLA, was characterized by Agnello et al. [3].
2. Two of the genes related to the rheumatoid factors of M-components and carrying the respective idiotopes 17.109 and 6B6.6 have been identified. The

Table 1. Comparison of RF antibodies in various conditions

	RF antibodies in		
	M-components	RA	Normal immunization
Antigen driven	−	+	+
T-cell dependent	−	+	+
Clonality	Monoclonal	Polyclonal	Polyclonal
Ig class	IgG or IgM	IgG and IgM	IgM
Character	Malignant	Benign, chronic, self-perpetuating	Benign, self-limiting

    corresponding germline genes are apparently the $V_x 325$ and the $V_x 328$ genes [9, 10].

3. When these idiotype systems were more carefully studied in RA, it became apparent that, although the related idiotypes were present in RA patients, they represented quite a small percentage of RF idiotypes seen in this condition [9, 19].

While helping to characterize the M-components with RF activities, these studies have only partially elucidated the structure and genes of RFs found in healthy individuals and in patients with RA. In fact, there is increasing evidence that the three main conditions in which RFs are seen are very different and mostly use different genes in their production of RFs (Table 1).

First, in patients with RA and normal individuals, RF production is antigen driven, is polyclonal, and might be T-cell dependent [32]. In patients with M-components with RF antibody activity the response is T-cell independent, not antigen driven, monoclonal, and may reflect a semimalignant or malignant disease.

Second, in RA, RF antibodies are largely produced locally in the synovial tissues, where they also exert their pathogenetic effects. In normal individuals and patients with M-component RFs, the RF antibodies are produced in ordinary lymphoid tissues and are not deposited in the joint tissues.

Third, in normal individuals virtually all RF antibodies are of the IgM type, while in M-components they may belong either to the IgM or to the IgG class. M-component RF antibodies of the IgG type, which are the most pathogenetic, circulate in immune complexes which are deposited in the kidneys. In RA, the RF antibodies are of both the IgM and the IgG class and are deposited in the joints, where they are mostly produced. The IgG-containing immune complexes seem to be more pathogenetic than IgM-containing complexes. IgM-RFs may escape more easily into the circulation than IgG-RFs and probably do not cause much harm locally in the diseased joint. They may even be protective.

Fourth, similarities and differrences in the structure of the variable regions of the different types of RF antibodies were identified by idiotypic reagents. Thus we and others have found cross-idiotypic groups between RFs from

RA patients, as were previously detected between RF M-components in other diseases. For example, cross-idiotypic patterns were observed between either the PO or WA idiotypic groups of the RF M-components and RF preparations from RA patients [19]. However, there were also differences indicating a more hetergenous picture of RFs in RA than in M-component RFs [19]. This fits well with the observation that the 17.109 idiotype represented only a minor portion of the RFs in a panel of RA sera [9].

Rheumatoid Factors in Normal Subjects

As indicated above, RFs in normal subjects appear to be different from RFs in M-components. Using the previously described technology for making human monoclonal antibodies after EBV transformation and subsequent cloning, Sanz et al. [41] have developed clones of RF-producing cells from normal individuals and have clarified their structure and genetic background. These studies have shown that RFs from normal individuals are in some ways distinct from RFs in M-components: First, they utilize a more divergent group of variable light-chain genes and they also use different families of heavy-chain variable genes. Thus the somewhat rarer subgroup $V_H IV$ is more frequently utilized in the production of RFs in normals compared with other types of RFs [37]. Second, RFs from normal individuals are virtually always IgM and not IgG. Most of them correspond to the newly described polyreactive IgM auto-antibodies. These polyreactive IgM-RFs probably have lower affinities for IgG than monoreactive RFs [I. Randen et al., unpublished observation, 41]. The polyreactive IgM-RFs are also likely to originate from CD5 B cells [41]. These autoantibodies show very broad cross-reactivity with a variety of autoantigens and foreign antigens [40, 41]. We believe that the broad reactivity of these RFs is also important for their selective advantage, for example, in promoting and enhancing the cytolytic effect of weak anti-viral and other anti-microbial antibodies.

Rheumatoid Factors in Rheumatoid Arthritis

Rheumatoid arthritis is an inflammatory disorder characterized by a genetic predisposition related to HLA DR4 (Dw4, Dw14, and Dw15) and DR1 antigen-presenting molecules [14, 17]. The disease processes result from an immune response due to interaction between these genetically determined antigen-presenting HLA class-II molecules on accessory cells and T helper cells [32]. This gives rise to a strong delayed-type hypersensitivity reaction and a T helper cell-induced B-cell proliferation [11] with immunoglobulin and RF production in the joints [15, 16, 32, 47, 51]. This may initiate a classical immune complex disease. The best approach to a detailed study of the structure of RF and other antibodies in RA is to make human B-cell hybridoma clones. We have focused on making hybridomas from autoantibody-producing B-cells derived from the synovial tissue of patients with RA.

Antibody Specificity of RF-producing Clones in Rheumatoid Arthritis

Among all the fusions with EBV-stimulated B lymphocytes made from three patients (TS, SJ, and KL), 20 clones developed from RF-producing hybridoma cell lines were selected for further study, as described in detail by Randen et al. [40]. The RF-producing clones were all of the IgM class; 13 were $\varkappa$ and seven were λ proteins. When these autoantibodies were tested for reactivity towards IgG and a series of other antigens, it turned out that 14 were monoreactive for IgG (Table 2). All of these 14 clones (12 $\varkappa$ and 2 λ) reacted with human IgG, and five of them also reacted with rabbit IgG. No reactivity was seen with other antigens tested for (Table 2). In contrast, antibodies from six clones were polyreactive (1 $\varkappa$ and 5 λ); they reacted more weakly with the IgG than the monoreactive antibodies did. In addition, they also reacted with a series of other antigens such as tetanus toxoid, human serum albumin (HSA), thyroglobulin, DNA, and cytoplasmic structures of fixed fibroblasts (Table 2). It thus appears that the RFs detected in the synovial tissues fell into two different groups, one group with monoreactive RFs reacting only with IgG and another group with polyreactive RFs reacting with IgG and several other antigens [40].

Table 2. Reaction patterns of RF-producing human hybridomas [40]

	Human IgG	Rabbit IgG	Tetanus toxin	HSA	Thyro-globulin	DNA	Staining of fixed cells
Monoreactive RF							
9 clones	++	−	−	−	−	−	−
5 clones	+++	+++	−	−	−	−	−
Polyreactive RF							
3 clones	+	+	++	+	+++	+++	+
1 clone	+	−	+	+	−	+	−
1 clone	+	−	++	+	+++	+++	+
1 clone	+	−	−	+	−	+++	+

HSA, Human serum albumin; −, optical density <0.1 when tested in and enzyme-linked immunosorbent assay; +, 0.1–0.4; ++, 0.5–0.8; +++, 0.8 and over

Table 3. Reactivities of monoclonal RF with human IgG subclasses; no relation to RF-related CRI and V_H or V_L subgroups

Clones	Reacting with rabbit IgG	Heavy chains		Light chains	
		VH subgroup	CRI	VL subgroup	CRI
Pan-specificity Reacts with all IgG subclasses:					
RF-TS1	−	I	G6	$\varkappa$IIIb	17.109
RF-SJ1	+	III	B6, D12	λ1	−
Classical Ga specificity Reacts with IgG1, IgG2 and IgG4:					
RF-TS2	+	III	−	$\varkappa$IIIa	−
RF-TS3	−	I	−	$\varkappa$II	−
RF-TS6	+	n.d.	−	n.d.	−
RF-SJ2	−	III	B6, D12	λ1	−
RF-SJ3	−	III	−	$\varkappa$IIIb	17.109
RF-SJ4	+	IV	−	$\varkappa$IIIb	17.109
RF-KL2	−	III	−	$\varkappa$I	−
RF-KL3	−	III	−	n.d.	−
RF-KL4	−	III	−	n.d.	−
New Ga-related specificity Reacts with IgG1, IgG2, IgG4 and G3m (st):					
RF-TS5	+	III	D12	n.d.	−
RF-KL1	−	III	−	$\varkappa$1	−
G3m (u) specificity Reacts with IgG3 of allotypes G3m (b) and G3m (g):					
RF-TS4	−	III	B6, D12	n.d.	−

n.d., Not done; −, clone is negaive for all idiotypes tested for, or negative for reactivitiy with rabbit IgG

The 14 monoreactive RFs were tested for specificity for fine determinants of IgG Fc fragments, using isolated myeloma proteins of the different IgG subclasses as antigens [40]. Two of the RF clones were panspecific (i. e., reacted with all IgG subclasses), nine showed a classical Ga specificity, two showed the new Ga-related specificity and one showed a Gm specificity, anti-Gm(u) (Table 3).

Expression of Heavy and Light Chain-associated Cross-idiotypes (CRI)

The 14 monoreactive RFs were then tested for heavy- and light-chain-associated CRI (Table 3). These studies are described in more detail by Thompson et al. [49]. Two findings were striking: First, the $V_\varkappa III$ subgroup and $V\varkappa IIIb$-related CRI 17.109 were expressed in only four and three, respectively, of the 14 monoreactive RF clones. None of the IgM RFs were positive for the $V_\varkappa IIIa$-related CRI 6B6.6. In addition, the heavy chain-related CRI G6, which is frequently seen in connection with the CRI 17.109 on light chains [21], was present in only one of the 12 IgM$\varkappa$-monoreactive RFs – a much rarer frequency of those CRIs than is seen in M-component RF [6]. In contrast, four RF clones were positive for one or both of the $V_H III$-related CRI B6 and D12. By reaction with staphylococcal protein A (SPA) and blotting techniques, six more of the RF clones turned out to be $V_H III$ – althogether 10 clones. Therefore, it appears that RF clones from synovial tissue of RA patients are somewhat different in their usage of variable light-chain subgroups and variable heavy-chain subgroups (mostly $V_H III$) than RFs from normal individuals (relatively frequently $V_H IV$) and RF M-components which have more restricted light and heavy chains (mostly $V\varkappa III$ and $V_H I$) [6–8, 24, 25, 27].

Second, we compared the expression of different fine specificities of RF from RA patients for IgG determinants and the usage of different heavy and light chain variable subgroups (see Table 3). No correlation was seen between these fine specificities of the RF autoantibodies and the heavy and light chain-related CRIs studied, or the usage of V_H and V_L subgroups.

Table 4. Usage of V_H and V_L subgroups as well as J_H and J_L segments

RF clones	Heavy chain	Light chain*
RF-TS-1	$V_H I,\ J_H 3$	$V_\varkappa IIIb,\ J_\varkappa I$
RF-TS-2	$V_H III, J_H 3$	$V_\varkappa IIIa,\ J_\varkappa V$
RF-TS-3	$V_H I,\ J_H 4$	$V_\varkappa II,\ J_\varkappa V$
RF-TS-4	$V_H III$	$V_\varkappa$
RF-TS-5	$V_H III$	$V_\varkappa$
RF-TS-6	n.d.	$V_\varkappa$
RF-SJ-1	$V_H III, J_H 6$	$V_\lambda I \quad J_\lambda II$
RF-SJ-2	$V_H III, J_H 6$	$V_\lambda I,\quad J_\lambda II$
RF-SJ-3	$V_H III$	$V_\varkappa IIIb$
RF-SJ-4	$V_H III$	$V_\varkappa IIIb$
RF-KL-1	$V_H III, J_H 4$	$V_\varkappa I,\quad J_\varkappa V$
RF-KL-2	$V_H III$	$V_\varkappa I$
RF-KL-3	$V_H III$	$V_\varkappa$
RF-KL-4	$V_H III$	$V_\varkappa$

* The proteins labeled $V_\varkappa$ belong to one of the $V\varkappa$ subgroups but have been shown clearly not to be $V_\varkappa III$.
n.d., Not done

Sequence Studies of RF-variable Heavy- and Light-Chain Segments

The details of the sequence studies are published elsewhere [37, 38, 52]. Usage of the V and J segments of the heavy and light chains in Tables 4 and 5 shows; First there is considerable heterogeneity in the usage not only of variable heavy and light chain segments but also of J segments. This extends the heterogeneity already indicated from the idiotype studies above. The D segments are also very diverse. Three of the D segments appear to have a germline counterpart, but the others are very different, both in their amino-acid sequence and in their length. Second, the sequence studies show that the actual gene segments utilized within a given V_H or V_L family is quite diverse. For example, among the RF clones using the $V_H III$ at least three different subfamilies are also utilized [38]. Third, most of these IgM RFs are identical or nearly identical to the germline. Most of them shows more than 99% homology with previosly identified germline genes. Some genes have, in addition, also been identified in the germline of the patients [38]. In contrast, other genes coding for the heavy chain of the RF are most likely somatically mutated [38].

The same pattern is found among the light-chain genes. Most of them are clearly germline related while others are most likely somatically mutated, as described in detail by Victor et al. [52].

Discussion

RFs appear in at least three distinct conditions. First, they are found in normal individuals as a response to antigenic stimulation, accomplished by vaccination or infectious agents [8, 12, 54]. The genes coding for these RFs were probably preserved during evolution because they are useful in increasing the lytic effect of weak anti-viral antibodies and in removing old and dead cells. Second, RF appears spontaneously in M-components, such as those seen in Waldenström's macroglobulinemia and mixed cryoglobulinemia [4, 6–9, 10, 13, 24, 25]. Third, RFs are important autoantibodies in certain autoimmune diseases such as RA, where they can form self-associating complexes locally in the synovial tissue and fluids and thus generate and perpetuate chronic inflammation [30, 31, 33, 35, 39, 55]. To further understand the pathogenetic mechanisms of RA we have cloned RFs from synovial B lymphocytes. There are some questions whether the EBV technique used selects for certain subtypes of B lymphocytes. However, at least two groups have recently presented work clearly indicating that no such selection is caused by the EBV transformation [21; L. MacKenzie and P. Lydyard, personal communication]. We therefore believe that the clones derived from our patients, two with RA (SJ and TS) and one with the polyarticular form of juvenile rheumatoid arthritis (KL), are representative for the polyclonal B-cell repertoires in the joints, although the total number of clones is limited.

Table 5. V_H and V_L segments of IgM RF*

Clone	V_H Family	Closest V_H gene	% Homology	V_L Family	Closest V_L gene	% Homology
Monoreactive RF from RA						
RF-TS1	V_HI	51P1	95	$\varkappa$IIIb	325	99.3
RF-TS3	V_HI	41.6	99.2	$\varkappa$II	A23	100
RF-TS2	V_HIII	1.9III	97.8	$\varkappa$IIIa	328	97
RF-TS5	V_HIII	222B	99.2	$\varkappa$I	Hk102	97.9
RF-KL1	V_HIII	VH26	96	$\varkappa$I	Vd	97.5
RF-SJ1	V_HIII	56P1	95.3	λI	FOG-B	93.0
RF-SJ2	V_HIII	56P1	99.4	λI	FOG-B	96.3
RF-SJ3	V_HIII	19III	99.4	$\varkappa$IIIb	325	98.7
RF-AN	V_HIII	?	–	λIII	ND[3]	ND
RF-SJ4	V_HIV	71.2	95.4	$\varkappa$IIIb	100	
Polyreactive RF from RA						
PR-TS1	V_HIII	3005	99.6	λI	FOG-B	98.3
PR-SJ2	V_HIII	1.9III	94.7	λII	Hum Ig VL21	91.0
PR-SJ1	V_HIV	71-4/MAR 1	99.6	λV	PAG1	83
PR-TS2	V_HIV	4.21	100	λIV	IGIV351	100

* Modified from ref. 37

Our findings show first of all that, in contrast to the RFs seen in M-components, the RFs in RA do not show a similar V-gene subgroup restriction for light chains. The light chains of the RFs in RA frequently utilize all the main $V_\varkappa$ subgroups, $V_\varkappa$I, $V_\varkappa$II, and $V_\varkappa$III. In addition, we have already identified V_λI, V_λII, V_λIII, V_λIV and V_λV RF clones [34, 37, 40, 49, 52]. This means that probably all the main $\varkappa$ and λ subgroups can be involved in RF production in RA. All the monoreactive IgM-RF clones studied except one utilize the frequent V_H groups V_HIII and V_HI (Table 5). This is in contrast to what is seen in polyreactive RFs, recently studied by Sanz et al. [41], which frequently utilize the rarer, V_HIV group. It is also apparent that the usage of heavy-chain variable subgroups in RFs related to RA is heterogeneous within a given V_H family. This is so both for V_HIII and for V_HI. The RFs from RA patients thus utilize different sub-subgroups within the main V_H families. At least three different subfamilies are represented among the RFs within the V_HIII group. The two V_HI proteins are also different in their V_HI composition. For example, only one of them carries the V_HI germline-related idiotope G6 [38, 49].

When we investigated the D segments it appeared that they also showed broad heterogeneity [38]. Three of the D segments appeared to have a germline origin, but the others were heterogeneous with respect to both sequence and length. In this way they presumably add much more diversity to the third diversity region CDR3 of the heavy chain. The J segments are also hetero-geneous, for both the heavy and the light chain. We also looked for certain amino acid residues that might be related to the RF antibody specificity. There was one conserved segment in the CDR1 region of the heavy chains, which is seen both in RFs and in some other autoantibodies of both the V_HI and V_HIII subgroups. This may indicate that this segment is preserved by gene conversion and is possibly related to the RF specificity. This is discussed in more detail by Pascual et al. [38]. In addition, we are now examining certain amino acids in the CDR 3 regions by means of site mutagenesis to evaluate whether they are related to the RF autoantibody specificity.

In conclusion, the RFs from the synovial tissues appear not to be restricted in their usage of V_H and V_L gene segments, nor in D- or J-segment utilization. Like the immune antibodies, RFs in RA utilize the frequent V_H gene families, mostly various subfamilies of V_HIII but also of V_HI. These findings indicate that the RF production is due to an antigenic drive. Continued search for an elusive antigen which might trigger and stimulate the T cells and promote the T cell help for RF autoantibody production might shed more light on the autoimmune process of rheumatoid pathology.

References

1. Ambrahamsen TG, Frøland SS, Natvig JB, Pahle J (1975) Elution and characterization of lymphocytes from rheumatoid inflammatory tissue. Scand J Immunol 4:823–830
2. Allen JC, Kunkel HG (1966) Hidden rheumatoid factors with specificity for native γ-globulins. Arthritis Rheum 9:758
3. Agnello V (1988) Rheumatoid factor cross-idiotypes. Springer Semin Immunopathol 10:203–214
4. Bona CA (1988) V genes encoding autoantibodies: molecular and phenotypic characteristics. Annu Rev Immunol 6:327–358
5. Brown CMS, Plater-Zyberk C, Mageed RA, Jefferis R, Maini RN (1990) Analysis of immunoglobulins by hybridomas derived from rheumatoid synovia. Clin Exp Immunol 80:366–372
6. Capra JD, Kehoe GM, Winchester RJ, Kunkel HJ (1971) Structure-function relationships among anti-γ globulin antibodies. Ann NY Acad Sci 190:371–381
7. Capra CD, Klapper DG (1976) Complete amino acid sequence of the variable regions domains of two human IgM anti-γ globulins (Lay/Pom) with shared idiotypic specificities. Scand J Immunol 5:677
8. Capra JD, Winchester RJ, Kunkel HG (1969) Cold reactive rheumatoid factors in infectious mononucleosis and other diseases. Arthritis Rheum 12:67
9. Carson DA, Chen PP, Kips TJ, Radouz V, Jirik F, Goldfien RD, Fox RI, Silverman GJ, Fong S (1987) Molecular basis for the cross-reactive idiotypes on human anti-IgG autoantibodies (rheumatoid factors). In: Autoimmunity and autoimmune disease. Ciba Foundation Symposium. Wiley, New York, pp 123–134
10. Carson DA, Chen PP, Fox RI, Kipps TJ, Jirik F, Goldfein RD, Silverman G, Radoux V, Fong S (1987) Rheumatoid factors and immune networks. Annu Rev Immunol 5:109–126
11. Chattopadhyay C, Chattopadhyay H, Natvig JB, Michaelsen TE, Mellbye OJ (1979) Lack of suppressor cell activity in rheumatoid synovial lymphocytes. Scand J Immunol 10:309
12. Coulie PG, Van Snik J (1985) Rheumatoid factor (RF) production during anamnestic immune response in the mouse. J Exp Med 161:88
13. Crowley JJ, Goldfein RD, Schrohenloher RE, Speigelberg HL, Silverman GJ, Mageed RA, Jefferis R, Koopman WJ, Carson DA, Fong S (1988) Incidence of three cross-reactive idiotypes on human rheumatoid factor paraproteins. J Immunol 140:3411
14. Dobloug JH, Førre Ø, Lea T, Solheim BG, Natvig JB (1980) HLA antigen and rheumatoid arthritis. Association between HLA-DRw4 positivity and IgM rheumatoid factor production. Arthritis Rheum 23:309–313

15. Egeland T, Lea T, Mellbye OJ, Pahle JA, Ottesen T, Natvig JB (1982) Quantitation of cells secreting immunoglobulins after elution from rheumatoid synovial tissue. Scand J Immunol 16:413
16. Egeland T, Lea T, Saari G, Mellbye OJ, Natvig JB (1982) Quantitation of cells secreting rheumatoid factor of IgG, IgA and IgM class after elution from rheumatoid synovial tissue. Arthritis Rheum 25:1445–1450
17. Førre Ø, Dobloug JH, Høyerall HM, Thorsby E (1983) HLA antigens in juvenile arthritis. Genetic basis for different subtypes. Arthritis Rheum 26:35–40
18. Førre Ø, Johnsen PM, Natvig JB (1977) A study of the variable heavy-chain (V_H) regions in human polyclonal IgM rheumatoid factors. Scand J Rheumatol 6:113–117
19. Førre Ø, Dobloug JH, Michaelsen TE, Natvig JB (1979) Evidence of similar idiotypic determinants on different rheumatoid factor populations. Scand J Immunol 9:281–189
20. Gaarder PA, Natvig JB (1979) Hidden rheumatoid factors reacting with a 'non-a' and other antigens of native autologous IgG. J Immunol 105:928
21. Guigou V, Cuisinier A-M, Tonnelle C, Moinier D, Fougereau M, Fumoux F (1990) Human immunoglobulin V_H and V_K repertoire revealed by in situ hybridization. Mol Immunol 27, 935–940
22. Haskard DO, Archer JR (1984) The production of human monoclonal antibodies from patients with rheumatoid arthritis by the EBV-hybridoma technique. J Immunol Methods 74:361
23. Jefferis R, Nik Jafaar MI, Steinitz M (1984) A monoclonal rheumatoid factor having specificity for a discontinuous epitope determined by His/Arg interchange at residue 435 of immunoglobulin G. Immunol Lett 7:191
24. Kunkel HG, Agnello V, Joslin FG, Winchester RJ, Capra JD (1973) Cross-idiotype specific among monoclonal IgM proteins with anti-gammaglobulin activity. J Exp Med 137:331–342
25. Kunkel HG, Winchester RJ, Joslin FG, Capra JD (1974) Similarities in the light chains of anti-gamma globulins showing cross-idiotypic specificities. J Exp Med 139:128–136
26. Loghem EV, Grobbelar BG (1971) A new genetic marker of human IgG3 immunoglobulins. Evolutionary dissociation of Gm allotypes. Vox Sang 21:405
27. Mageed RA, Dearlove M, Goodall DM, Jefferis R (1986) Immunogeneic and antigeneic epitopes of immunoglobulins. XVII. Monoclonal antibodies reactive with common and restricted idiotopes to the heavy chain of human rheumatoid factors. Rheumatol Int 6:179–183
28. Mannik M, Nardella FA, Sasso EH (1988) Rheumatoid factors in immune complexes of patients with rheumatooid arthritis. Springer Semin Immunopathol 10:215–230
29. Mellors RC, Heimer R, Corcos J, Korngold L (1959) Cellular origin of rheumatoid factor. J Exp med 110:875
30. Munthe E, Natvig JB (1971) Characterization of IgG complexes in eluates from rheumatoid tissues. Clin Exp Immunol 8:249–262
31. Munthe E, Natvig JB (1972) Complement-fixing intracellular complexes of IgG rheumatoid factor in rheumatoid plasma cells. Scand J Immunol 1:217
32. Natvig JB, Randen I, Thompson K, Førre Ø, Munthe E (1989) The B cell system in rheumatoid inflammation. New insights into the pathogenesis of rheumatoid arthritis using synovial B cell hybridoma clones. Springer Semin Immunopathol 11:301–313
33. Natvig JB, Munthe E (1975) Self-associating IgG rheumatoid factor represents a major response of plasma cells in rheumatoid inflammatory tissue. Ann NY Acad Sci 256:88–95
34. Natvig JB, Thompson KM, Randen I, Steinitz M, Taussig M, Beale D, Barker P, Sletten K, Waalen K, Førre Ø (1988) Partial amino acid sequence analysis and variable subgroup determination (V_H and V_L) of a monoclonal rheumatoid factor derived from a rheumatoid arthritis patient. Scand J Rheumatol 75:[Suppl] 127–132
35. Natvig JB, Førre Ø, Randen I, Steinitz M, Thompson K, Waalen K (1988) B lymphocyts, B cell clones and rheumatoid factor antibodies in rheumatoid inflammation. Scand J Rheumatol 76:[Suppl] 217–227
36. Normansell DE, Young CW (1974) The IgG sublclass specificity of anti-IgG immunoglobulin rheumatoid factors. Immunochemistry 12:187

37. Pascual V, Victor K, Randen I, Thompson K, Natvig J.B. and Capra J.D.: IgM rheumatoid factors in patients with rheumatoid arthritis derive from a diverse array of germline immunoglobulin genes and display little evidence of somatic variation. J Rheumatology, in press
38. Pascual V, Randen I, Thompson KM, Sioud M, Førre Ø, Natvig JB, Capra JD (1990) The complete nucleotide sequences of the heavy chain variable regions of six monospecific rheumatoid factors derived from EBV-transformed B cells isolated from the synovial tissue of patients with rheumatoid arthritis: further evidence that some autoantibodies are unmutated copies of germline genes. J Clin Invest 86, 1320–1328
39. Pope RM, Teller DC, Mannik M (1975) Intermediate complexes formed by self-association of IgG rheumatoid factors. Ann NY Acad Sci 256:82–87
40. Randen I, Thompson KM, Natvig JB, Førre Ä, Waalen K (1989) Human monoclonal rheumatoid factors derived from the polyclonal repertoire of rheumatoid synovial tissue: production and characterization. Clin Exp Immunol 78:13–18
41. Sanz I, Casali P, Thomas JW, Notkins AL, Capra JD (1989) Genetic basis of natural autoantibodies: organization, complexity and mechanisms of diversity of the human B cell repertoire. J Immunol 11:4054–4061
42. Schandfield MS, Fudenberg HH (1974) Gm- (Ray), a new allotypic marker on human IgG3. Vox Sang 26:133
43. Slaughter L, Carson DA, Jensen FC, Holbrook TL, Vaughan JH (1978) In vitro effects of Epstein-Barr virus on peripheral blood mononuclear cells from patients with rheumatoid arthritis and normal subjects. J Exp Med 148:1429
44. Stanley SLJR, Sischoff JK, Davie JM (1987) Antigen-induced rheumatoid factors. Protein and carbohydrate antigen induced diffeent rheumatoid factor responses. J Immunol 139:2936–2941
45. Steinitz M (1988) B cell clones in rheumatoid arthritis. Springer Semin Immunopathol 10:181
46. Steinitz M, Izak G, Cohen S, Ehrenfeld M, Flechner I (1980) Continuous production of monoclonal rheumatoid factor by EBV-transformed lymphocytes. Nature 287:443–445
47. Taylor-Upsahl NM, Abrahamsen TG, Natvig JB (1977) Rheumatoid factor plaque-forming cells in rheumatoid synovial tissue. Clin Exp Immunol 28:197–203
48. Thompson KM, Hough DK, Maddison PJ, Melamed MD, Hughes-Jones N (1986) The efficient production of stable, human monoclonal antibody-secreting hybridomas form EBV-transformed lymphocytes using the mouse myeloma X63-Ag8, 653 as a fusion partner. J Immunol Methods 94:7–12
49. Thompson KM, Randen I, Natvig JB, Mageed RA, Jefferis R, Carson DA, Tighe H, Førre Ø (1990) Human monoclonal rheumatoid factors derived from the polyclonal repertoire of rheumatoid synovial tissue: incidence of cross-reactive idiotopes and expressions of V_H and $V_\varkappa$ subgroups. Eur J Immunol 20:863–868
50. Tønder O (1962) Studies on the mechanism of the Waaler-Rose test with special regard to the reactant. Acta Univ Bergensis Ser Med 2:pp137
51. Vaughan JM, Chihara T, Moore TL, Robbins DL, Tanimoto K, Johnson JS, McMillan R (1976) Rheumatoid factor-producing cells detected by the direct hemolytic plaque assay. J Clin Invest 58:933
52. Victor KD, Randen I, Thompson KM, Førre Ø, Natvig JB, Fu SM, Capra JD (1991) Rheumatoid factors isolated from patients with autoimmune disorders are derived from germline distinct from those encoding the WA, PO and BLA cross-reactive idiotypes. J Clin Invest 87:1603–1613
53. Waaler E (1940) On the occurrence of a factor in human serum activating the specific agglutination of sheep blood corpuscles. Acta Pathol Microbiol Scand 17:177–88
54. Walsh MJ, Fong S, Vaughan JH, Varson DA (1983) Increased frequency of rheumatoid factor precursors in B lymphocytes after immunization of normal adults with tetanus toxoid. Clin Exp Immunol 51:299
55. Winchester RJ (1975) Characterization of IgG complexes in patients with rheumatoid arthritis. Ann NY Acad Sci 256:73–81

Neutrophil Polymorphonuclear Cell Function in Rheumatoid Arthritis

P. Youinou, A. Lamour, A. Dumay, and P. Le Goff

Laboratory of Immunology and Clinic of Rheumatology, Brest University Medical School Hospital, BP 824, F-29285 Brest Cedex, France

Introduction

Patients with rheumatoid arthritis (RA) suffer an excessive morbidity and mortality from pyogenic infections [1]. The neutrophil polymorphonuclear cell (PMN) system constitutes a crucial mechanism of defense due to its ability to recognize and ingest micro-organisms [2]. The question thus arises as to whether PMN function is modified in RA [3].

It has long been established that, although they are scarce within the pannus [4], such cells predominate in the synovial fluid (SF) during acute exacerbations of the disease [5]. Chemotaxis, phagocytosis, and degranulation are among major activities of PMN responding to a given stimulus. Convergent observations have shown that they are influential in the pathogenesis of RA [6]. Their activation generates lysosomal enzymes, mediators of inflammation, and derivatives from molecular oxygen at sites of inflammatory events [7]. All these products contribute to the disruption of cell membranes, and damage structural components of connective tissue such as collagen [8] or proteoglycans [9].

The above-mentioned lines of evidence have prompted a number of investigators to evaluate the functional comportment of PMN in RA. Their studies have yielded conflicting results, the interpretations of which are not wholly compatible with each other. A general consensus has not yet been reached, but it has become clear that the concept of PMN homogeneity is not valid [10], and that membrane receptors play a key role in the PMN competency [11]. It is also reasonable to suggest that part of this discrepancy may be due to differences in drug regimen [12]. There is controversy, however, concerning the effects of nonsteroidal anti-inflammatory drugs (NSAIDs) o PMN function [13]. Potential explanation will be discussed in this paper.

Smolen, Kalden, Maini (Eds.)
Rheumatoid Arthritis
© Springer-Verlag Berlin Heidelberg 1992

Activation of PMN in RA

Phenotypic Heterogeneity

PMN have been claimed to be heterogeneous according to several morphological parameters (Table 1). Analyses of PMN phenotype have consistently indicated that a fraction of these cells lack receptors for the Fc portion of IgG (FcR). Only 60%–80% of circulating PMN form rosettes with IgG-coated particles [14]. The rosette assay may, however, be influenced by a variety of trivial factors, while the advent of the monoclonal antibody (MAb) technology has allowed the extraordinary complexity of the FcR family to be substantiated [15]. At least three classes of FcR have been defined by a host of criteria: FcRI (CDw32), FcRII (CDw65), and FcRIII (CD16). PMN can bind to IgG-opsonized targets through FcRII and FcRIII [16], whereas the effector function so far ascribed to the latter is the release of granule proteins [17]. Additional FcR polymorphism has been identified on FcRIII, such as the neutrophil antigen system, by serological typing with alloantisera [18] or by using certain MAb [19].

Efficient phagocytosis also requires the participation of complement components. These bind to immune complexes and interact with specific receptors (CR) on PMN. Accordingly, the cells express receptors CR1 for C3b, CR3 for iC3b, and CR4 and for iC3b, C3dg, and C3d [20], but PMN are dissimilar in this respect. For example, the measurement of CR1 numbers in normal individuals has shown that PMN possess three distinct pools of CR1 [21].

Several MAb that recognize subpopulations of PMN have been raised since. A set of PMN-restricted surface antigens, termed granulocyte functional antigens 1 and 2, have been identified [22]. More recently, a PMN antigen belonging to the GpIb-IIIa complex has been shown to be a glycoprotein that serves as a receptor for fibrinogen and fibronectin [23].

Table 1. Some of the neutrophil polymorphonuclear cell membrane markers and their behavior in rheumatoid arthritis

Membrane markers	References	RA pattern	References
Fc-gamma receptor III	[15]	Diminution	[11, 71]
Neutrophil antigens (NA) 1 and 2	[18, 19]		
C3b receptor (CR1)	[21]	Augmentation	[29]
iC3b receptor (CR3)	[20]	Augmentation	[28, 30, 95]
iC3b/C3dg/C3d receptor (CR4)	[20]		
Granulocyte functional antigens (GFA) 1 and 2	[22]	Augmentation	[22]
GpIIb-IIIa complex	[23]	Diminution	[31]

The Effects of Activation

This heterogeneity does not reflect the existence of PMN subpopulations that proceed from distinct stem cells. Rather, it may represent maturation differences throughout a common cell lineage. For example, the proportion of PMN rosetting with sheep erythrocytes coated with IgG is enhanced upon activation with chemotactic agents [24]. Progressively, FcR would be shed by PMN [25]. Huizinga et al. have demonstrated that soluble FcRIII in human plasma originates from release by PMN [26], and cell-free FcRIII are indeed detectable in the serum of patients with RA [27].

Earlier studies have shown that exposure of PMN to chemotactic factors causes enhanced rosette formation with complement-coated sheep erythrocytes [28]. This phenomenon has been further analyzed by means of MAb and flow cytometry. The expression of CR1 [29] and CR3 [30] is markedly augmented following activation.

The density of GFA-1 and GFA-2 is also increased at inflammatory sites, i. e., in SF, whereas that of GpIIb-IIIa is diminished [31]. Thus, the phenotype of a PMN may well denote its functional status.

Functional Inferences

Klempner and Gallin have refined the rosette assay in order to separate the FcR-positive from the FcR-negative PMN [32]. They showed that, in addition to having different rosetting capabilities, these two categories of PMN differed functionally. The former were found to be superior in chemotaxis, phagocytosis, and bactericidal activity (BA). FcR expression was also required to distinquish PMN that produce an active form of lactoferrin capable of suppressing the synthesis of granulocyte-macrophage colony-stimulating activity by monocytes [33]. PMN with readily exposed FcR would thus be important in the regulation of myelopoiesis.

Other functional characteristics of certain PMN have been described. Resting PMN comprise a homogeneous density population [34], but a change in buoyancy results from interaction with chemotactic factors [35]. This could account for wide variations in the composition of cell preparations obtained by Ficoll-Hypaque (FH) gradient centrifugation, since the percentage of PMN at the interface is significantly higher in RA patients than in normal individuals [36]. Seligmann et al. have utilized the membrane potential-sensitive dye, 3-3′-dipentylocarbocyanine, to assess the heterogeneity of PMN upon activation [37]. Unstimulated PMN exhibited a unimodal distribution of fluorescence, suggesting that all the cells possessed the same resting membrane potential. In contrast, the chemoattractant N-formly-methionyl-leucyl-phenylalanine (f-Met-Leu-Phe) caused the PMN to assume a bimodal fluorescence distribution. It has been shown that the surface charge of PMN from patients with RA is lower than that of PMN from normal controls [38], and the cells of high surface charge are less adherent than those with a low surface charge [39]. As suggested by Brown et al. [40], an alteration in the electrophoretic distribution of PMN may represent changes that are related to the expression of functionally related membrane ionogenic groups.

The Consequences of Activation

Locomotion

The prerequisite for PMN diapedesis into the membrane and subsequent entry into the joint cavity is the margination of the cells to the synovial vessels. Several assay systems have been designed to estimate this PMN adhesive capacity [41]. Earlier studies have shown that rheumatoid PMN display adhesion greater than [42] or equal to [39] that of normal PMN. Other investigators pointed out that nylon fibers, previously used as an adhesion substrate, were a material of questionable biological application and thus preferred testing adhesion to porcine endothelial cell monolayers [43]. They came to the conclusion that the numbers of adhering cells were similar in RA patients and normal controls. Furthermore, the synovial PMN were less adherent than paired blood samples when autologous serum was present in the incubation medium, but more adherent when it was absent. The demonstration that most of the RA sera inhibited the adhesion of normal PMN is in agreement with a previous finding that the augmenting factor detected in plasma from patients with inflammation was not present in serum [44].

Types of motility include [3]: (a) random locomotion (occurring in the absence of any stimulus); (b) activated random locomotion, or chemokinesis (occurring when chemotactically active molecules are present in uniform concentration); and (c) directed locomotion, or chemotaxis (occurring when chemotactically active molecules are present in a concentration gradient).

PMN mobilization is determined by two general categories of methods: observations on the movement of individual cells and measurement of the migration of a cell population. For the latter, two techniques have been recommended. One is the Boyden chamber filter technique, first described in 1962 [45] and then simplified [46]. Locomotion is quantified by counting PMN which have crossed a predetermined interval from the cell source [47], or by determining the distance traveled by the PMN in leading front [48], i. e., the maximal migration in micrometers of at least two PMN in five random microscope fields. The other technique is a modified method of evaluating the PMN motility in agarose [49, 50]. The results may be expressed as absolute chemotaxis and/or chemotactic indices, which are calculated by subtracting the mean value for random migration from the mean value for direct migration, or by dividing the chemotactic distance by the chemokinetic distance. The differences between results obtained with the chamber and the agarose techniques may be due to increased random migration in agarose [51].

Table 2. Neutrophil polymorphonuclear cell locomotion in rheumatoid arthritis

Level of locomotion in RA [reference]	PMN isolation	Assay	Chemoattractant	Expression of the results
Reduced				
[52]	MC sedimentation	BC	Casein plus human serum	CI
[53]	Repeated centrif.	BC	Casein plus AB serum casein	Leading front plus CI
[54]	MC sedimentation	BC		Leading front plus CI
[55]	Plasmagel sedim. plus FH centrifugation	BC	f-Met-Leu-Phe	Leading front
Normal				
[39]	MC sedimentation plus FH centrifugation	BC	AB serum plus casein	Leading front
[56]	Dextran sedimentation	BC	Human c(zymosan)	Number of cells
[57]	Dextran sedimentation	BC	Human c (LPS)	Distance
[58]	Dextran sedimentation	Agarose	*E. coli* filtrate or AB serum	CI
[59]	Dextran sedimentation	Agarose	*E. coli* filtrate or human c (zymosan)	CI
Increased				
[60]	Dextran sedimentation	BC	casein	Counting of the cells
[61]	Dextran sedim. plus FH centrifugation	Agarose	Human c (zymosan)	CI
[62]	Dextran sedim. plus FH centrifugation	Agarose	Human c (zymosan)	CI
[63]	FH centrifugation	Agarose	f-Met-Leu-Phe	Leading front

PMN, Neutrophil polymorphonuclear cell; RA, rheumatoid arthritis; MC, methyl-cellulose; FH, Ficoll-Hypaque; BC, Boyden chamber; f-Met-Leu-Phe, *N*-formyl-methionyl-leucyl-phenylalamine; c, complement; LPS, lipopolysaccharides; CI, chemotactic indices

Studies of PMN chemotactic activity in RA have produced conflicting results (Table 2). Locomotion of peripheral blood (PB) has been found to be reduced [52–55], normal [39, 56–59], or exaggerated [60–63]. In addition to the interassay disparity [51], explanations for these discrepancies include technical differences in PMN isolation methods: dextran [56] or methyl-cellulose [52] sedimentation, repeated centrifugation [53], or sedimentation followed by centrifugation over FH [55]. It has been reported that these conditions modify the phenotype [29] and the function [36] of the cells. The nature of the chemoattractant is a source of further discrepancy: casein [60], human complement [56], *Escherichia coli* filtrate [58], and f-Met-Leu-Phe [55] have been applied together or separately. The diversity may also represent the different degrees of stimulus-directed cell processing in RA patients and the varying extent of disease activity. Finally, differences in drug regimens may account for part of the divergence. NSAIDs, such as diclofenac [59], ketoprofen [61], piroxicam [64], nabumetone, and indomethacin [65] affect chemotaxis, at least when this function is evaluated in vivo. This certainly holds true for slow-acting drugs, such as D-penicillamine [66], tiopronine [62], and gold compounds [67].

The results obtained in studies comparing the functional activity of SF cells with those from PB are as contrasted as the above findings. Here again, variable degrees of activation in vivo could render the PMN refractory to further stimulation in vitro.

Phagocytosis

No differences were found between PMN from RA patients and those from controls after 24 h, whereas serum-independent and serum-dependent phagocytosis by PMN from patients were increased compared with normal individuals [54]. In contrast, phagocytosis by normal PMN decreased equally and significantly in all SF from patients with RA, along with SF from patients with osteoarthritis and various other forms of arthritis [68].

Phagocytosis was further analyzed by Breedveld et al. They reported that circulating PMN from RA patients ingested *Staphylococcus aureus* opsonized with immunoglobulins and complement as effectively as did PMN from healthy donors [69]. This capacity was lower in patients than in controls when bacteria were incubated with sera lacking complement activity. However, in the presence of heat-inactivated SF, the ability of PMN from SF to phagocytos was greater than that of PMN from RA patients or donor PB [70]. The results of this test were correlated with FcR expression on the PMN membrane [71] and are in agreement with the finding of higher percentages of FcR-positive PMN in SF than in paired PB of RA patients [11].

Metabolic Functions

Phagocytosis and degranulation result in the formation of vacuoles and lead to a series of metabolic events, collectively termed the respiratory burst. Engulfment of particles is followed by an enhancement of oxygen consumption, hydrogen peroxide production, and hexose monophosphate shunt activity (comprehensively reviewed by Stossel [72]).

The nitroblue tetrazolium dye reduction test partially highlights the oxydoredution cascade. This effect had previously been found to be reduced in stimulated PMN from RA patients, without any correlation to the clinical and biological parameters [73], but the results have not been confirmed by other investigators [54]. PMN function can also be evaluated by the chemiluminescence (CL) assay [74]. Here, the response is amplified by luminol and accounts for the generation of oxygen radicals [75]. Opsonized zymosanstimulated CL appears to be depressed in untreated RA patients compared with normal individuals [76], particularly in patients with neutropenia in addition to RA [77]. In contrast, Gale et al. reported that the majority of paired sera and SF from RA patients produced a rapid CL response when incubated with control cells [78]. CL has been shown to be closely linked to bactericidal activity (BA). Once the bacteria are internalized, this would be normal within the PMN from RA patients [56, 69]. There is actually a wide variability of BA from one patient to another [12].

With regard to the inflammatory effects of PMN in RA, there is little dispute about the fact that increases occur in the synovial production of lactoferrin [79], elastase [64, 79], and leukotriene (LT) B4 [55, 80, 81]. Membrane phospholipase A2 activity has been shown to increase in RA [82], partly accounting for the augmented generation of LTB4 [83]. All these inflammatory mediators contribute to tissue destruction.

The Cause of Activation

Circulating Immune Complexes

Alteration in activity has been attributed to the prior ingestion of circulating immune complexes (CIC) by PMN. This is based on the following evidence: (a) immunoglobulin inclusions may represent internalized CIC [84]; (b) PMN were found to undergo similar changes when incubated with heat-aggregated IgG or with RA sera before assay [85]; and (c) ultrastructural changes seen in PMN from RA patients resemble those shown to occur in normal PMN which are phagocytosing heat-aggregated IgG or rheumatoid factor (RF)- containing complexes [86].

Serum, and particularly plasma, from RA patients reduces the adherence of PMN to cultured endothelium, and, according to Chasty et al., the inhibition of PMN is directly related to the level of CIC and is reproducible by heat-aggregated IgG [87]. Certain CIC may impede PMN adhesion to systemic vessel endothelium; thus, the number of cells available for attachment to synovial endothelial cells would be increased.

Kemp et al. noted that IgG aggregates inhibited only random migration of PMN, and suggested that the capacity of CIC to inhibit PMN migration contributes to the PMN accumulation at their formation sites [88]. Furthermore, Wikinson [89] and Goddard et al. [53] demonstrated that IgG aggregates may stimulate as well as impede PMN function, depending on the size, concentration, and immunochemical properties of the CIC and the presence or absence of RF. For example, the CL responses vary according to the CIC characteristics [90], and hexose monophosphate pathway activation is greater for insoluble than for soluble aggregates [85].

The possibility also exists that a decline in PMN function is related to folic acid (FA) deficiency. FA levels are indeed reduced in the serum of patients with RA [91], and we have previously reported that a lack of FA can diminish significantly the degree of bacterial engulfment and killing by PMN [92].

Nonsteroidal Anti-inflammatory Drugs

NSAIDs are believed to exert their action on PMN by preventing the peroxidative effect of arachidonic acid by cyclo-oxygenase and prostaglandin (PG) synthesis. However, the patterns of PMN functional inhibition vary from drug to drug [2, 13, 65], while there is no difference in the level of LTB4 production between the RA patients treated with NSAIDs and those not taking NSAIDs [81], suggesting that the anti-inflammatory effect of NSAIDs cannot be entirely explained by their inhibition of PG synthetase. This conclusion is supported by several observations, one of which is that significantly higher doses of NSAIDs are required to abate PMN than to restrict PG synthesis [93]. Thus, NSAIDs may directly affect PMN activation [13].

Felty's Syndrome

Since Felty first described the triad of RA, splenomegaly, and leukopenia [94], a variety of conflicting mechanisms have been suggested to play a role in chronic neutropenia.

Shortened survival of PMN has been demonstrated in some patients and is attributed to humoral factors. PMN-bound IgG has been reported more regularly than circulating anti-PMN autoantibodies, and the increased proportion of PMN carrying CR 3 [95] has been shown to contrast with the reduced number of FcR-expressing PMN [71] in the PB of patients with Felty's syndrome (FS). This abnormality can be mimicked by incubating normal PMN with aggregated IgG, due to the effect of CIC, which are larger in patients with FS than in those with regular RA [96].

However, the mechanism may be central, since circulating mononuclear cells from FS patients are capable of preventing normal marrow granulocyte colony growth [97]. This view is further supported by several lines of clinical evidence. The effectiveness of treatment with prednisone is due to its inhibition of suppressor T-cells, and the response to glucocorticoid therapy can be predicted with the agar PMN culture technique and cortisol dose responses in vitro [98].

Pathogenesis can be expected to differ from one patient to another. Humoral and cellular anomalies co-exist in a given patient [97], and the target of some circulating autoantibodies is demonstrable at the bone-marrow level [99]. Additional heterogeneity of central mechanisms responsible for neutropenia has been described [100]; e. g., depletion of bone-marrow suppressor T-cells, anti-precursor cell activity, and growth-factor deficiency have been shown to operate in a large number of patients with FS.

To conclude, it becomes increasingly evident that the role of PMN, with or without chronic leukopenia, is decisive in the pathogenesis of RA. An extensive literature has accumulated in this field. Nevertheless, more work is needed to better understand the mechanisms involved. Further investigations are justified by knowledge that NSAIDs, as well as second-line drugs, are active at the level of PMN.

Acknowledgements. The editorial assistance of Mrs. Simone Forest and Dr. Ian Humphery-Smith, and the technical expertise of Mrs. Annie Péron are appreciataed.

References

1. Prior P, Symmons DPM, Scott DL, Brown R, Hawkins CF (1984) Cause of death in rheumatoid arthritis. Br J Rheumatol 23:92–99
2. Metschnikoff E (1887) Sur la lutte des cellules de l'organisme contre l'invasion des microbes. Ann Inst Pasteur 1:321–336
3. Howe GB, Fordham JN (1981) Polymorphonuclear leucocytes: origins, functions and roles in rheumatic diseases. In: Carson-Dick W (ed) Immunological aspects of rheumatology. MTP Press, Lancaster, pp 149–170
4. Mohr W, Wessinghage D (1978) The relationship between polymorphonuclear granulocytes and cartilage destruction in rheumatoid arhritis. Z Rheumatol 37:81–86
5. Palmer DG (1968) Total leukocyte examination in pathologic synovial fluid. Am J Clin Pathol 49:812–813
6. Palmblad J (1984) The role of granulocytes in inflammation. Scand J Rheumatol 13:163–172
7. Weissmann G, Sehman C, Korchak HM, Smolen JE (1982) Neutrophils: release of mediators of inflammation, with special reference to rheumatoid arthritis. Ann NY Acad Sci 389:11–24
8. Lazarus GS, Daniels JR, Brown RS (1968) Degradation of collagen by a human granulocyte collagenolytic system. J Clin Invest 47:2622–2629
9. Janoff A, Blondin J (1970) Depletion of cartilage matrix by a neutral protease fraction of human leukocyte lysosomes. Proc Soc Exp Biol Med 135:302–306

10. Gallin JI (1984) Human neutrophil heterogeneity exists, but is it meaningful? Blood 63:977–983
11. Youinou P, Jouquan J, Muzellec Y, Le Goff P (1987) Polymorphonuclear cell Fc-gamma receptors in rheumatoid arthritis. In: Peeters H (ed) Protides of the biological fluids. Pergamon, Oxford, pp 251–254
12. Youinou P, Le Goff P (1987) Drug-induced impairment of polymorphonuclear cell bactericidal ability in rheumatoid arthritis. Ann Rheum Dis 46:46–50
13. Abramson SB, Weismann G (1989) The mechanisms of action of nonsteroidal anti-inflammatory drugs. Arthritis Rheum 32:1–9
14. Messner RP, Jelinek J (1970) Receptor for human gamma-globulins on human neutrophils. J Clin Invest 49:2165–2170
15. Unkeless JC (1989) Function and heterogeneity of human Fc receptors for immunoglobulin G. J Clin Invest 83:355–361
16. Huizinga TWJ, van Kemenade F, Koenderman L, Dolman KM, von dem Borne AEG Kr, Tetteroo PAT, Ross D (1989) The 40-kD Fc receptor (FcR II) on human neutrophils is essential for the IgG-induced respiratory burst and IgG-induced phagocytosis. J Immunol 142:2365–2369
17. Huizinga TWJ, Dolman KM, van der Linden NJ, Kleijer M, Nuijens JH, von dem Borne AEG Kr, Roos D (1990) PI-linked FcR III mediates exocytosis of neutrophil granule proteins, but does not mediate initiation of the respiratory burst. J Immunol 144:1432–1437
18. Werner G, von dem Brone AEG Kr, Bos MJE, Tromp JF, von der Plas-van Dalen CM, Visser FJ, Engelfriet CP, Tetteroo PAT (1985) Localization of the human NA1 alloantigen on neutrophils to Fc receptors. In: Reinherz EL, Haynes BF, Nadler LM, Bernstein ID (eds) Leucocyte typing II, vol 3. Springer, Berlin Heidelberg New York, pp 109–121
19. Tetteroo PAT, van der Schoot CE, Visser FJ, Bos MJE, von dem Borne AEG Jr (1987) Three different types of Fc-gamma receptors of human leukocytes defined by workshop antibodies: Fc-gamma R low of neutrophils, Fc-gamma R low of NK/K lymphocytes and Fc-gamma II. In: Mc Michael AJ (ed) Leucocyte typing III. Oxford University Press, Oxford, pp 702–706
20. Ross GD, Atkinson JP (1985) Complement receptor structure and function. Immunol Today 6:116–119
21. Fyfe A, Holme ER, Zoma A, Whaley K (1987) C3b receptor (CR1) expression on the polymorphonuclear leukocytes from patients with systemic lupus erythematosus. Clin Exp Immunol 67:300–308
22. Vadas MA, Lopez AF, Williamson DJ (1985) Selective enhancement of the expression of granulocyte functional antigen 1 and 2 on human neutrophils. Proc Natil Acad Sci USA 82:2503–2507
23. Burns GF, Cosgrove L, Triglia T (1986) The IIb–IIIa glycoprotein complex that mediates platelet aggregation is directly implicated in leukocyte adhesion. Cell 45:269–280
24. Kay AB, Walsh GM (1984) Chemotactic factor-induced enhancement of the binding of human immunoglobulin classes and subclasses to neutrophils and eosinophils. Clin Exp Immunol 57:729–734
25. Huizinga TWJ, van der Schoot CE, Jost C, Klaassen R, Kleijer M, van dem Borne AEG Jr, Roos D, Tetteroo PAT (1988) The Pi-linked receptor FcR III is released on stimulation of neutrophils. Nature 333:667–669
26. Huizinga TWJ, de Haas M, Kleijer M, Nuijens JH, Roos D, von dem Borne AEG Jr (1990) Soluble Fc-gamma receptor III in human plasma originates from release by neutrophils. J Clin Invest 86:416–423
27. Khayat D, Le Goff P, Soubrane C, Magadur G, Youinou P (1990) Fc-gamma receptor III shedding by polymorphonuclear cells in rheumatoid arthritis. Med Sci Res 18:893–894
28. Kay AB, Glass J, Salter D McG (1979) Leucoattractants enhance complement receptors on human phagocytic cells. Clin Exp Immunol 38:294–299

29. Fearon DT, Collins LA (1983) Increased expression of C3b receptors on polymorphonuclear leukocytes induced by chemotactic factors and by purification procedures. J Immunol 130:370–375
30. Berger M, O'Shea J, Cross AS, Folks TM, Chused TM, Brown EJ, Frank MM (1984) Human neutrophils increase expression of C3 bi as well as C3b receptors upon activation. J Clin Invest 74:1566–1571
31. Emery P, Lopez AF, Burns GF, Vadas MA (1988) Synovial fluid neutrophils of patients with rheumatoid arthritis have membrane antigen changes that reflect activation. Ann Rheum Dis 47:34–39
32. Klempner MS, Gallin JI (1978) Separation and functional characterization of human neutrophil subpopulations. Blood 51:659–669
33. Broxmeyer HE, Ralph P, Bognachi J, Kinkade PW, Desousa M (1980) A subpopulation of human polymorphonuclear neutrophils contains an active form of lactoferrin capable of binding to human monocytes and inhibiting production of granulocyte-macrophage colony-stimulating activity. J Immunol 125:90–909
34. Zeya HI, Keku E, De Chatelet LR, Cooper MR, Spurr CL (1978) Isolation of enzymatically homogeneous populations of human lymphocytes, monocytes and granulocytes by zonal centrifugation. Am J Pathol 90:33–45
35. Pember SO, Barnes KC, Brandt SJ, Kinkade JM Jr (1983) Density heterogeneity of neutrophilic polymorphonuclear leucocytes: gradient fractionation and relationship to chemotactic stimulation. Blood 61:1105–1115
36. Hacbarth E, Kajdacsy-Balla A (1986) Low-density neutrophils in patients with systemic lupus erythematosus, rheumatoid arthritis and acute rheumatic fever. Arthritis Rheum 29:1334–1342
37. Seligmann B, Chused TM, Gallin JI (1981) Human neutrophil heterogeneity identified using flow microfluorometry to monitor membrane potential. J Clin Invest 68:1125–1131
38. Brown KA, Collins AJ, Holborow EJ (1977) Cell electrophretic analysis of lymphocytes and polymorphonuclear cells from patients with rheumatid arthritis. Lancet 1:114–117
39. Howe GB, Fordham JN, Brown KA, Currey HLF (1981) Polymorphonuclear cell function in rheumatoid arthritis and in Felty's syndrome. Ann Rheum Dis 40:370–375
40. Brown KA, Perry JD, Black C, Dumonde DC (1988) Identification by cell electrophoresis of a subpopulation of polymorphonuclear cells which is increased in patients with rheumatoid arthritis and certain other rheumatological disorders. Ann Rheum Dis 47:353–358
41. Mac Gregor RR, Spagnuolo PJ, Lentrek AL (1974) Inhbition of granulocyte adherence by ethanol, prednisone and aspirin, measured with a new assay system. N Engl J Med 291:642–646
42. Lentrek AL, Schreiber AD, Mac Gregor RR (1976) The induction of augmented granulocyte adherence by inflammation: mediation by a plasma factor. J Clin Invest 57:1098–1103
43. Sheehan NJ, Brown KA, Perry JD, Chasty RC, Yates DAH, Dumonde DC (1987) Adherence of rheumatoid polymorphonuclear cells to cultured endothelial cell monolayers. Ann Rheum Dis 46:93–97
44. Mac Gregor RR (1976) The effect of anti-inflammatory agents and inflammation on granulocyte adherence: evidence for regulation by plasma factors. Am J Med 61:597–607
45. Boyden S (1962) Chemotactic effects of antibody and antigen on polymorphonuclear leucocytes. J Exp Med 115:453–466
46. Baum J, Mowat AG, Kirk JA (1977) A simplified method for the measurement of chemotaxis of polymorph leucocytes from human blood. J Lab Clin Med 77:501–509
47. Goetzl EJ, Austen FK (1972) A neutrophil-immobilizing factor derived from human leucocytes. I. Generation and partial characterization. J Exp Med 136:1564–1580
48. Zigmond SH, Hirsch JG (1973) Leukocyte locomotion and chemotaxis: new methods for evaluation and demonstration of a cell-derived chemotactic factor. J Exp Med 137:387–410

49. Nelson RD, Quie PG, Simmons RL (1975) Chemotaxis under agarose, a new and simple method for measuring chemotaxis and spontaneous migration of human polymorphonuclear leucocytes and monocytes. J Immunol 115:1650–1656
50. Chenoweth DE, Rowe JG, Hugli TE (1979) A modified method for chemotaxis under agarose. J Immunol Methods 25:337–353
51. Hindocha PJ, Hedges SB, Wood CBS (1985) Assessment of neutrophil chemotaxis and random migration in children and adults. Arch Allergy Appl Immunol 76:116–119
52. Mowat AG, Baum J (1971) Chemotaxis of polymorphonuclear leukocytes from patients with rheumatoid arthritis. J Clin Invest 50:2541–2549
53. Goddard DH, Kirk AP, Kirwan JR, Johnson GD, Holborow EJ (1984) Impaired polymorphonuclear leucocytes chemotaxis in rheumatoid arthritis. Ann Rheum Dis 43:151–156
54. Wandall JH (1985) Leucocyte function in patients with rheumatoid arthritis: quantitative in vivo leucocyte mobilization and in vitro functions of blood and exudate leucocytes. Ann Rheum Dis 44:694–700
55. Smith DM, Johnson JA, Turner RA (1989) Alterations in arachidonic acid metabolism and chemotactic response in polymorphonuclear leukocytes from patients with rheumatoid arthritis. Clin Exp Rheumatol 7:471–477
56. Walker JR, James DW, Smith MJH (1979) Directed migration of circulating polymorphonuclear leucocytes in patients with rheumatoid arthritis: a defect in the plasma. Ann Rheum Dis 38:215–218
57. Hanbon SM, Panayi GS, Laurent R (1980) Defective polymorphonuclear leucocyte chemotaxis in rheumatoid arthritis associated with a serum inhibitor. Ann Rheum Dis 39:68–74
58. Unden AM, Trang L, Venizelos N, Palmblad J (1983) Neutrophil functions and clinical performances after total fasting in patients with rheumatid arthritis. Ann Rheum Dis 42:45–51
59. Scheja A, Forsgren A, Marsal L, Wollheim F (1985) Inhibiton of in vivo leucocyte migration by NSAIDs. Clin Exp Rheumatol 3:53–58
60. Kemp AS, Brown S, Brooks PM, Neoh SH (1980) Migration of blood and synovial fluid neutrophils obtained from patients with rheumatoid arthritis. Clin Exp Immunol 39:2410–246
61. Baccino E, Harrewyn JM, Jouquan J, Swirsky H, Bressolette L, Mottier D, Youinou P (1987) Ketoprofen-induced reduction of polymorphonuclear cell activation in rheumatoid arthritis. Clin Exp Rheumatol 5:53–57
62. Lelong A, Delecoeuillerie G, Fauquert P, Le Goff P, Youinou P (1989) Tiopronine modifies polymorphonuclear cell functions in patients with rheumatoid arthritis. Int J Immunotherapy 5:123–127
63. Espersen GT, Ernst E, Vestergaard M, Pedersen JO, Grunnet M (1989) Changes in PMN leukocyte migration activity and complement C3d levels in RA patients with high disease activity during steroid treatment. Scand J Rheumatol 18:51–56
64. Montecucco C, Mazzone A, Pasotti D, Caporalli R, Longhi M, Casilli D, Ricedveiti G, Fratino P, Ruffilli MP (1989) Effect of piroxicam therapy on granulocyte function and granulocyte elastase concentration in peripheral blood and synovial fluid of rheumatoid arthritis patients. Inflammation 13:211–220
65. Ip M, Lomas DA, Shaw J, Burnett D, Stockley RA (1990) Effect of nonsteroidal anti-inflammatory drugs on neutrophil chemotaxis: an in vitro and in vivo study. Br J Rheumatol 29:363–367
66. Youinou P, Le Goff P, Lepoivre B, Mottier D (1984) D-penicillamine-induced impairment of plymorphonuclear leukocyte chemotaxis in rheumatoid arthritis. Med Sci Res 12:1062–1063
67. Elmgreen J, Ahnfelt-Ronne I, Nielsen OH (1989) Inhibition of human neutrophils by auranofin: chemotaxis and metabolism of arachidonate via the 5-lipoxygenase pathway. Ann Rheum Dis 48:134–138
68. Turner RA, Schumacher HR, Myers AR (1973) Phagocytic function of polymorphonuclear leukocytes in rheumatic diseases. J Clin Invest 52:1632–1635

69. Breedveld FC, van den Barselaar MT, Leijh PCJ, Cats A, van Furth R (1985) Phagocytosis and intracellular killing by polymorphonuclear cells from patients with rheumatoid arthritis and Felty's syndrome. Arthritis Rheum 28:395–404
70. Breedveld FC, Lafeber GJM, van den Barselaar MT, van Dissel JT, Leijh PCJ (1986) Phagocytosis and intracellular killing by polymorphonuclear cells from synovial fluid from patients with rheumatoid arthritis. Arthritis Rheum 29:166–173
71. Breedveld FC, Lafeber GJM, de Vries E, Leijh PCJ, Daha MR, Cats A (1984) Fc receptors on granulocytes from patients with rheumatoid arthritis and Felty's syndrome. Clin Exp Immunol 55:677–683
72. Stossel TP (1974) Phagocytosis. N Engl J Med 290:717–723, 774–780, 833–839
73. Corberand J, Amigues H, de Larrard B, Pradere J (1977) Neutrophil function in rheumatoid arthritis. Scand J Rheumatol 6:49–52
74. Wilson ME, Trush MA, van Kyke K, Kyle JM, Mullett MD, Neal WA (1978) Luminol-dependent chemiluminescence analysis of opsonophagocytic disfunctions. J Immunol Methods 23:315–326
75. De Chatelet LR, Long GD, Shirley PS, Bass DA, Thomas MJ, Henderson FW, Cohen MS (1982) Mechanism of the luminol-dependent chemiluminescence of human neutrophils. J Immunol 129:1589–1593
76. Piergiacomi G, Guiletti AA, Muti S, Silveri F, Cervini C (1988) Stimulated chemiluminescence of polymorphonuclear leukocytes in rheumatoid arthritis: in vivo enhancement by auranofin. Z Rheumatol 47:151–155
77. Davis P, Johnston C, Bertouch J, Starkebaum G (1987) Depressed superoxide radical generation by neutrophils from patients with rheumatoid arthritis and neutropenia: correlation with neutrophil reactive IgG. Ann Rheum Dis 46:51–54
78. Gale R, Bertouch J, Bradley J, Roberts-Thomson PJ (1983) Direct activation of neutrophil chemiluminescence by rheumatoid sera and synovial fluid. Ann Rheum Dis 42:158–162
79. Adeyemi EO, Campos LB, Loisou S, Walport MJ, Hodgson JH (1990) Plasma lactoferrin and neutrophil elastase in rheumatoiid arthritis and systemic lupus erythematosus. Br J Rheumatol 29:24
80. Moilanen E, Alanko J, Nissila M, Hamalainen M, Isomaki H, Vapaalalo H (1989) Eicosanoid production in rheumatoid arthritis. Agents Action 28:290–297
81. Belch JJ, O'Dowd A, Ansell D, Sturrock RD (1989) Leukotriene B4 production by peripheral blood neutrophils in rheumatoid arthritis. Scand J Rheumatol 18:213–219
82. Pruzanski W, Vadas P, Kim J, Jacobs H, Stefanski E (1988) Phospholipase A2 activity associated with synovial fluid cells. J Rheumatol 15:791–794
83. Bomalaski JS, Baker D, Resurreccion NV, Clark MA (1989) Rheumatoid arthritis synovial fluid phospholipase A3 activating protein stimulates human neutrophil degranulation and superoxide ion production. Agents Actions 27:425–427
84. Hurd ER, Lospalluto J, Ziff M (1970) Formation of leukocyte inclusions in normal polymorphonuclear cells incubated with synovial fluid. Arthritis Rheum 13:724–733
85. Treadway W, Collins RL, Turner RA, De Chatelet L (1979) Polymorphonuclear leucocyte secretory and metabolic response to immunoglobulin aggregates. J Rheumatol 6:636–644
86. McCarthy DA, Hollurn CM, Pell BK, Moore SR, Hirk AP, Perry JD (1986) Scanning electron microscopy of rheumatoid arthritis peripheral blood polymorphonuclear leucocytes. Ann Rheum Dis 45:899–910
87. Chasty RC, Brown KA, Sheehan NJ, Kirk AP, Perry JD, McCarthy D, Dumonde DC (1987) Rheumatoid blood decreases the adherence of polymorphonuclear cells to cultured endothelium. Ann Rheum Dis 46:98–103
88. Kemp AS, Roberts-Thomson P, Neoh SH, Brown S (1979) Inhibition of neutrophil migration by sera from patients with rheumatoid arthritis. Clin Exp Immunol 36:423–429
89. Wilkinson PC (1980) Effect of human IgG on locomotion of human neutrophils related to IgG binding to hydrophobic probe. Immunology 4:457–466

90. Gale R, Bertouch JV, Gordon JP, Bradley J, Roberts-Thomson PJ (1984) Neutrophil activation by immune complexes and the role of rheumatoid factor. Ann Rheum Dis 43:34–39
91. Gough KR, McCarthy C, Read AE, Mollin DL, Waters AH (1964) Folic acid deficiency in rheumatoid arthritis. Br Med J 1:212–214
92. Youinou P, Garré M, Ménez JF, Boles JM, Morin JF, Pennec Y, Miossec P, Morin PP, Le Menn G (1982) Folic acid deficiency and neutrophil disfunction. Am J Med 73:652–657
93. Atkinson DC, Collier HOJ (1980) Salicylates: molecular mechanism of therapeutic action. Adv Pharmacol Chemother 17:233–288
94. Felty AR (1924) Chronic arthritis in the adult associated with splenomegaly and leukopenia. Bull Johns Hopkins Hosp 35:16–20
95. Breedveld FC, Lafeber GJM, de Vries E, Daha MR, Cats A (1984) C3 receptors on granulocytes from patients with rheumatoid arthritis and Felty's syndrome. Clin Exp Immunol 57:557–563
96. Hurd ER, Chubick A, Jasin HE, Ziff M (1979) Increased Clq binding immune complexes in Felty's syndrome. Comparison with uncomplicated rheumatoid arthritis. Arthritis Rheum 22:697–702
97. Starkebaum G, Singer JW, Arend WP (1980) Humoral and cellular immune mechanisms of neutropenia in patients with Felty's syndrome. Clin Exp Immunol 39:307–314
98. Bagby JC Jr, Gabourel JD (1979) Neutropenia in three patients with rheumatic disorders. Suppression of granulopoiesis by cortisol-sensitive thymus-dependent lymphocytes. J Clin Invest 64:72–82
99. van der Veen JPW, Hack CE, Egelfriet CP, Pegels JG, van dem Borne AEG Jr (1986) Chronic idiopathic and secondary neutropenia: clinical and serological investigations. Br J Haematol 63:161–171
100. Abdou NI (1983) Heterogeneity of bone marrow-directed immune mechanisms in the pathogenesis of neutropenia of Felty's syndrome. Arthritis Rheum 26:947–953

Etiologic Factors –
Bacterial Antigens,
Autoantigens, Viruses

Heat-Shock Proteins and Mycobacterial Antigens

W. van Eden [1,2], C. J. P. Boog [1], E. J. M. Hogervorst [1],
M. H. M. Wauben [1], R. van der Zee [2], and J. D. A. van Embden [2]

[1] Department of Infectious Diseases & Immunology, Veterinary Faculty,
University of Utrecht, P. O. Box 80.165, 3508 TD Utrecht, The Netherlands
[2] Department of Bacteriology, National Institute of Public Health and
Environmental Hygiene, P. O. Box 1, 3720 BA Bilthoven, The Netherlands

Introduction

Most autoimmune diseases in humans are known to be associated with certain
HLA alleles. This means that genetic factors contribute to individual susceptibility and that at least some of these factors are encoded within or close to the
major histocompatibility complex (MHC). In the case of rheumatological
disorders, the association of HLA-B27 with ankylosing spondylitis is well-
known and impressive. Of less biological impact, but certainly very significant,
is the association of HLA-DR4 and HLA-DR1 with rheumatoid arthritis.
Furthermore, evidence has been put forward that the same DR4 allele
contributes to the development of arthritis in Lyme borreliosis [42].

In their attempts to explain the nature of such disease associations,
geneticists have argued that such associations are actually a consequence of the
evolutionary process that has generated the amazing degree of genetic
polymorphism of the MHC. It is generally assumed that in this evolutionary
process infectious diseases have been the major driving force for the development of polymorphism. On theoretical grounds, the phenomenon of antigenic
mimicry – the potential of microorganisms to develop structural similarities to
host antigens as a protective disguise – may be held particularly responsible
[28]. It is easy to understand that, for a microbe, the advantage of having
developed such similarities to a certain host is severely reduced as soon as the
next potential host has a different antigenic constitution. Thus, the teleological
reason for the existence of MHC polymorphism seems to be to provide effective
resistance against infections organisms. Autoimmune diseases are probably the
negative by-product of the same evolutionary process. Since selection is thought
to operate at the interface of successful mimicry and effective non-self
recognition, one may understand that coding for a good protective response
and for a tendency to respond to self may be two sides of the same coin. Genes
that ensured a strong and specific recognition of microbial antigens were
favored; the ability of the same selected genes, by coding for strong responses, to
overshoot their goal and lead to aberrant immune responses that destroy self-

Smolen, Kalden, Maini (Eds.)
Rheumatoid Arthritis
© Springer-Verlag Berlin Heidelberg 1992

tolerance was not adequately counterbalanced during the evolutionary process. In accordance with this is that the ensuing autoimmune disorders usually seem to peak only after the reproductive years. Furthermore, most autoimmune diseases have little effect on survival or fertility as such and the genetic associations are mostly seen with relatively frequently occurring HLA types. Rheumatoid arthritis (RA) may be a good example in this respect [22]. In rheumatological diseases the frequent involvement of microbial triggering has been suspected or proven in rheumatic fever, Lyme arthritis, and Reiter disease.

Theoretically, one would expect that the association between HLA and disease involved resistance rather than susceptibility. For statistical reasons associations with resistance are hard to investigate. Mycobacterial diseases have provided different possibilities for looking at the role of HLA polymorphism in disease, since these diseases are of a particularly diverse clinical nature. In some individuals, mycobacterial antigens are capable of inducing specific forms of immune suppression, e. g., lepromatous leprosy. In other individuals regulatory disbalance with subsequent (auto-)immune pathology, e. g., tuberculoid leprosy developes. HLA polymorphism has been found to contribute to a significant extent to such differences in clinical course [11]. Other in-depth studies have subsequently revealed the potential of various mycobacterial antigens to give direction to immune reponses in the context of certain MHC products [48].

In these respects mycobacterioses provide model diseases to study immune recognition and its pathological consequenses. Due to their versatile pathology, including forms with histopathological pictures resembling those in affected joints of RA patients, the possible relationship between mycobacterial diseases and RA has already been studied. Discussions on "rhumatisme tuberculeux" date back to before the advent of modern tuberculostatic drugs [4]. However, solid evidence regarding the role of mycobacteria in RA was never obtained and, together with the decrease in incidence of tuberculosis in the western world, the interest in a possible relationship between tuberculosis and RA gradually disappeared. It may be of some anecdotal interest to note that the introduction of gold therapy for treating rheumatoid disease, originally invented although without much success as a tuberculostatic therapy, was a direct spin-off of such an interest. Nonetheless, clinically no relationship between mycobacteriosis and chronic arthritic disease has been demonstrated. From the immunogeneticists point of view one would also not expect such a clinical relationship to exist. As discussed earlier, theoretically only those having a genetic predisposition to develop relative resistance to infectious problems would have a tendency to develop autoimmunity when exposed to microbial antigens. In keeping with such an argument may be the findings that were obtained when a group of individuals was skin-tested with a tuberculin of *M. tuberculosis* [30]. Individuals that exhibited a strong delayed-type hypersensitivity (DTH) and therefore T cell reactivity to this antigen were more frequently HLA-DR4 positive than the others. It was concluded from this that the HLA specificity which contributes to susceptibility to RA is a so-called immune response (Ir) gene coding for strong responsiveness to certain mycobacterial antigens. In addition, in vitro proliferative responses, for instance those elicited by an acetone precipitable fraction of *M. tuberculosis,* were found in lymphocytes obtained from donors carrying HLA-DR4 [32]. These relatively recent observations of the immunogenetic associations between the genetic predisposition to RA and responsiveness to mycobacteria, together with the newly emerging understanding of the pathogenic mechanisms that lead to arthritis after mycobacterial immunization in an experimental model of adjuvant arthritis, have stimulated a renewed interest in mycobacteria and human arthritis. That humans may develop arthritis when confronted with mycobacterial antigens has been known for some time, since repeated immune stimulations with BCG, used for cancer immunotherapy, frequently lead to complications such as a transient form of arthritis [46] (Steerenberg, personal communication). Artificial as the procedure of BCG immunotherapy is, it seems to be the direct human homologue of the experimental rat model of mycobacteria induced adjuvant arthritis.

Adjuvant Arthritis

Although adjuvant arthritis (AA) is not a natural disease, its study can extend our appreciation of the role of the host-parasite relationship in the induction of autoimmunity. In this model, the connections between mycobacterial antigens, host genes, and autoimmunity can be examined experimentally.

Three decades ago Pearson [34] described a subacute to chronic form of polyarthritis inducible in susceptible strains of rats by immunizing them against antigens of *M. tuberculosis.* AA has been considered to be a model of RA [35] because of its morphological features of synovitis, pannus formation, and erosion of cartilage and bone progressing to anyklosis, most prominently in the small joints of the extremities. The disease was found to be influenced by Ir genes linked to the MHC of the rat [3]. AA therefore provided an opportunity to explore experimentally the question of how the immune response to an environmental agent could trigger an immunological disease.

Although AA could be transmitted by inoculating rats with lymphocytes of affected donors [35, 6], some investigators questioned whether the disease was of autoimmune etiology since it was not clear whether arthritis could be produced in recipient rats by lymphocytes alone in the absence of mycobacterial antigens [38]. It was conceivable that mycobacterial antigens transferred into recipient rats seeded the joints and provided a target for an anti-mycobacterial immune response. Thus, the arthritis could be explained by inflammatory damage to the joint, which was an innocent bystander in the legitimate attack against mycobacterial antigens. Alternatively, it was conceivable that the joints were damaged by an autoimmune attack against an endogeneous, self-antigen. In this case, *M. tuberculosis* could have triggered the arthritis by expressing or modifying a self-antigen in the rat's connective tissues as a consequence of intracutaneous immunization. It was also possible that one of the antigens of

M. tuberculosis was structurally similar to a joint antigen and that immunization to this crossreactive epitope led to an attack against the self-antigen in the joints. As we shall describe here, this latter hypothesis turned out to be correct.

To distinguish between these alternative explanations of AA, we set out to isolate the lymphocytes that caused AA and then test their specificity. Although we were ignorant of the target antigen critical to arthritis, we reasoned that the disease-producing lymphocytes must have receptors capable of recognizing the target. Therefore, once isolated, these lymphocytes could be analyzed for their specificity. Holoshitz et al. [16] isolated a T cell line, A2, after in vivo immunization of susceptible Lewis rats with *M. tuberculosis* (Mt). The cells were cultured by repeated restimulations with Mt in vitro. The peculiar feature of this A2 cell line was that, upon inoculation into irradiated syngeneic Lewis rats, it caused arthritis. Furthermore, A2 inoculated nonirradiated rats were found to develop specific resistance against the induction of AA by Mt immunization. Apparently A2, with its specificity for mycobacterial antigens, was composed of T cells which also had a specificity for antigens of critical importance to the recognition or regulatory processes involved in AA. Subsequent subcloning of A2 gave rise to several clones, including clones A2b and A2c [17, 8]. Upon in vivo testing, A2b was found to be virulently arthritogenic, while A2c was protective. Thus, although both clones had a helper CD4 phenotype, their functional activities in vivo were clearly distinct. A2c not only induced specific resistance against AA, by inoculation before AA induction, but also caused rapid disease remission when administered into rats suffering from active AA. Cellular mixing experiments in vitro, using A2c primed lymph node cells, have indicated that, in contrast to A2b, A2c has the phenotype of a so-called suppressor inducer T cell [9]. Having isolated such monoclonal T cell reagents with functional activities in vivo disease, a search for the nature of the antigens critical to the arthritic processes was initiated. Although the original A2 cell line had been found to recognize, to some extent, collagen type II, the more virulent A2b clone did not [14]. However, when this clone was tested on various crude preparations enriched for cartilage proteoglycans, significant reactivity was seen [49]. Also, in synovial fluid of human origin and in supernatants of in vitro grown chicken chondrocytes a stimulatory activity was observed. Thus, in addition to an antigen present in mycobacteria, the T cells recognized an antigen associated with cartilage. Furthermore, following immunization of rats with mycobacteria in order to induce arthritis or following in vivo administration of A2b, DTH reactivity in the skin with specificity for proteoglycan containing preparations developed, especially with preparations enriched for core or link proteins of proteoglycans. Thus, A2b and A2c, although being monoclonal populations of T cells with single receptor specificities, were both capable of recognizing a cartilage associated antigen, despite the fact that they had been selected for their recognition of mycobacteria. The inevitable conclusion from this was that these clones were critical to arthritis because of their specificity either for one antigenic epitope shared between mycobacteria and proteoglycans or for two distinct epitopes that were structurally related and present in mycobacteria and proteoglycans [50, 52]. Both situations would be perfect examples of antigenic mimicry, this time identified at the level of the disease regulating agents themselves. The finding of such mimicry was the impetus for efforts to define the epitope in mycobacteria recognized by A2b and A2c. In collaboration with Thole and Van Embden of the Dutch National Institute of Public Health and Environmental Hygiene, a number of recombinant proteins of *M. bovis* BCG and *M. leprae,* expressed in *E. coli* [43], were screened for stimulatory activity on rat arthritis T cell clones. A remarkably strong reactivity was seen with a 65 kDa protein of *M. bovis* BCG [51]. Sequencing of the 65 kDa, gene revealed that its amino acid sequence was 100% identical to its *M. tuberculosis* homologue [44]. Thus, the mycobacterial antigen recognized by clones A2b and A2c and having a shared or mimicked epitope had been identified. In search for the mimicry epitope(s), fragments of the 65 kDa protein were obtained from deletion mutants of the gene or from deletion mutants after fusion with the beta-galactosidase gene. From the analysis of the fragments, the area between residues 170 and 234 in the molecule was found to be critical. Further analysis of peptides synthesized on the basis of sequences in the critical area showed that both A2b and A2c were specific for an epitope located at position 180–188. Comparing the sequence of 180–188 (TFGLQLELT in the one letter code) with known protein sequences in cartilage proteoglycans revealed a sequence homology, four out of nine identical, with a rat link protein sequence [51]. Whether this resemblance represents the mimicry we were looking for is uncertain, since A2b and A2c did not respond to this link protein nonapeptide. By further analysis the minimal size of the epitope was shown to be the 180–186 sequence [54].

Alternative possibilities, apart from a mimicry of the 65 kDa protein with a proteoglycan molecule, are, however, suggested by the very nature of the mycobacterial 65 kDa protein itself. It was already observed that antibodies raised against mycobacteria and recognizing the mycobacterial 65 kDa molecule frequently bound to many other bacterial organisms [45]. By western blotting it was observed that the cross-reactive antigen in the other bacterial organisms invariably was a 59–65 kDa antigen, which had been known already as the so-called common antigen of gram negatives. Based on the extensive sequence homologies of the mycobacterial 65 kDa antigen with a known heat-shock protein in *E. coli,* groEL, the mycobacterial 65 kDa antigen was considered to be a member of the 60 kDa heat-shock protein family [56]. This explained the cross-reactions of anti-mycobacterial 65 kDa antibodies with other bacterial organisms, since heat-shock proteins are exceptionally well-conserved not only throughout prokaryotic organisms, but also eukaryotes and even mammals. Therefore, one should take into account the possibility that the cartilage associated target molecule in AA is not proteoglycan itself, but a proteoglycan associated heat-shock protein of mammalian origin.

It can thus be concluded that exposure of rats to a conserved bacterial protein may result in the triggering of T cells exhibiting a specificity relationship with some cartilage associated antigen. Such T cells may be responsible both for inducing arthritis (A2b) and for down-regulation or control of such a disease process (A2c).

Heat-Shock Protein 65:
Molecular Definition and Immunogenicity

Heat-shock proteins are produced in cellular organisms after sudden rises in temperature. In addition many other stressful events elicit production of hsps; the term "stress proteins" has therefore also been used. Heat-shock proteins are particularly well-conserved molecules since they serve essential physiological functions. One of these is as housekeeping proteins or chaperonins [12, 33]. The chaperone function consists of their capacity to transient associate with other proteins to assist in folding, unfolding, translocation over intracellular membranes, and the assembly or disassembly of oligomeric protein complexes. The mycobacterial hsp65 belongs to the hsp60 family of hsps, together with the structurally related *E. coli* hsp groEL and plant Rubisco subunit-binding protein. Mammalian hsp65 has now been identified as a part of the proteinaceous machinery in mitochondrial matrix membranes that takes care of the (re)folding of proteins after translocation. It was termed an ATP-dependent "folding catalyst" [29]. How hsps exert such chaperonin activities is unknown. Recent crystallographic data have shown that, for a smaller, heat-shock inducible, periplasmatic *E. coli* protein, PapD, the secondary structure is related to immunoglobulins and that PapD has sequence homology with the human lymphocyte differentiation antigen CD5, a member of the supergene family of molecules [15]. It is expected that in the coming years much more will become known about the functional activities of hsps and that this will have implications for our understanding of various immunological processes. So far, however, most of the attention has been focused on the extreme degree of sequence conservation in hsps. For instance, hsp65 is identical in *M. bovis* BCG and *M. tuberculosis* [41]. These have roughly 95% identity with *M. leprae* hsp65. Sequence homologies with other bacterial species are also remarkably high. Alignment of such sequences in *Coxiella burnetii* [55], *Borrelia burgdorferi* (Hindersson, personal communication), *Saccharomyces cerevisiae* [39], *Ricinus communis* [61], *Triticum aestivum,* and in humans [19] indicated that, while some areas in the molecules are very conserved, some areas are particularly variable or non-conserved. The overall sequence homology between the bacterial and human hsp65 is about 65% when conserved substitutions are taken into account. The 180–186 epitope, recognized by the rat arthritis T cell clones, is located in a relatively nonconserved area. Compared to the human sequence only three out of seven residues were found to be identical [53]. Obviously, it makes sense that the rat responds to an epitope that differs from self. Preliminary data on the rat hsp65 180–186 sequence obtained with the polymerase chain reaction (PCR) (Van der Zee, unpublished data) revealed similarity, although not identity, to the human sequence. Thus, although hsp65, in analogy with hsp70, may have distinct isoforms, we have no evidence that A2b is arthritogenic due to recognition of the rat hsp65 itself. However, during the process of AA, there is a vigorous response to hsp65 as well as to a mutant mycobacterial hsp65 without the 180–186 epitope. Here we have arrived at one of the peculiar characteristics of hsp65, and that is its good immunogenicity. In patients with bacterial infections antibodies against hsp65 may easily dominate [21]. In tuberculosis and leprosy T cells reactive with hsp65 are also activated [60, 63]. The same is true for individuals after BCG vaccination [31]. In mice it was shown that after Mt immunization 10%–20% of all T cells respond by limiting dilution analysis [63]. Even in naive human individuals T cell reactivity to hsp65 can also be found against epitopes shared between the human and bacterial hsp65 [27, 25]. It is likely that repeated exposure to bacterial organisms has led to memory responses with specificity for the shared region in the hsp65 molecule. It is possible that such responses to the shared regions may add to resistance at an early stage of infection [21]. Could this be the evolutionary driving force for this dominant recognition? Facing the old dogma of "horror autotoxicus" one should expect responses to hsp65 to be down-regulated instead. The same paradox seems to occur for myelin basic protein, just one out of many electrostatically basic proteins in the CNS, which is also clearly a dominant self-antigen. Since the same dominance is seen to occur irrespective of animal species or MHC type, the explanation should be sought in preexisting idiotypic networks determining self-antigen dominance [10]. This level of selectivity in the immune system gives it the possibility to focus on certain antigens and so to guarantee efficient regulatory mechanisms to control disease. Fine regulation, within the framework of such preexisting networks, may then further depend on MHC controlled epitope selection. Lewis rats apparently run into trouble when they focus on the 180–186 epitope. Somehow, the recognition of this epitope seems to have pernicious consequences to the animal, which are likely to be caused by disregulation of the response to this critical hsp65.

Heat-Shock Protein 65 in Experimental Arthritis

As discussed, hsps are readily recognized by the immune system. This is also the case in AA. When rats are immunized with Mt strong responses to hsp65 are found in lymphocytes obtained from their draining lymph nodes. This has been seen not only in the case of Lewis rats, but also in BN and Fisher rats [62]. The latter is of interest since BN rats are intermediately susceptible and Fisher rats are resistant to AA. Thus, as mentioned above, such dominant recognition seems to occur irrespective of the genetic background of the animals. This is expected to be different for specific epitopes residing on such a molecule. Indeed, responses to the 180–188 arthritis epitope have been seen after Mt immunization in Lewis rats, but not in BN and Fisher rats.

That Fisher rats do not respond is intriguing since they have the same MHC haplotype as Lewis (RTI[1]). However, in an exceptional case of arthritis in Fisher rats, we have observed rigorous responses to the 180–188 synthetic peptide. So, although Fisher rats are capable of responding to 180–188, they can avoid doing this. These findings support the crucial significance of the 180–188 sequence in AA. How Fisher rats control their response to 180–188 is not clear at the moment. No evidence for a defect at the level of antigen presentation or for specific immunological suppression has been obtained [62].

Earlier findings in Fisher rats indicated that their resistance to AA is acquired, since germ-free bred Fisher rats were found to be susceptible. Colonizing such rats, with for instance *E. coli,* induced their resistance to AA [23]. From this, one could argue that exposure of Fisher rats to certain microbial antigens, for instance an *E. coli* hsp, makes them tolerant in such a way that resistance to AA ensues.

A similarly effective acquisition of tolerance seems to occur when susceptible rats are immunized at mature ages with hsp 65 itself. Immunization of Lewis rats in the skin with hsp 65 solubilized in incomplete Freund's adjuvant in the same manner as used to induce arthritis has never resulted in the development of arthritis [51]. However, hsp 65 immunized animals have shown a resistance to developing AA after being challenged with whole Mt [51, 7]. So, although it contains the critical 180–188 sequence, hsp 65 apparently induces a situation where potentially autoaggressive T cells are safely contained. The same has now been found in other models of experimental arthritis, such as in streptococcal cell wall (SCW) induced arthritis [47]; in nonmicrobially induced arthritis, such as pristane arthritis in mice (Thompson, personal communication) and, to a minor degree, also in collagen type II arthritis [7]. The latter findings are obviously suggestive of the fact that hsp 65 is associated with arthritis, irrespective of the inducing agent. It is attractive to assume that hsp 65 is related to a target antigen which is common to the joint inflammatory process. Be that as it may, hsp 65 is capable of inducing cell regulation effective in controlling disease. In in vitro proliferation experiments such regulation has been shown to operate, since priming in vivo with hsp 65 or restimulation in vitro has been found to reduce the 180–188 specific response obtained through immunizations with whole Mt or with the 180–188 peptide itself [62]. An example of cells capable of effecting such regulation is the newly obtained cell line M 1 [10] which is part of the "preemptive regulatory network" involved in resistance to development of AA. M 1 has now been found to recognize an epitope of hsp 65 that differs from the 180–188 epitope [10]. With the help of cloned T cells and well-defined antigens or epitopes understanding of such regulatory mechanisms is presently emerging. It is expected that the findings will aid in the development of specific forms of immunological intervention in arthritic disease. Prevention of experimental disease is already possible; treatment of existing disease seems more difficult. Administration of hsp 65 to arthritic animals usually leads to disease exacerbation, both in AA and in SCW induced arthritis [47]. Although such observations once more stress the critical role of the antigen in the disease, strategies to exploit the same antigen to mitigate existing disease still await development. It is the classical problem of inducing tolerance instead of immunity. Since the tools for tackling such a problem are now available in AA, we tend to be optimistic about the chances of success. What remains is of course the question how to extrapolate such findings to the human situation. The principles that we have learned from the AA model obviously influence our appreciation of the condition in humans. However, we have, at present, no solid indications that in humans a chronic condition such as RA also depends on certain well defined critical antigens or even epitopes. Nevertheless, facing the nagging blank spots in our understanding of the disease mechanisms in order to help patients, it is clear that we are obliged to explore fully any possibilities emerging from animal models. In this respect, hsps seem to be a category of antigens that deserve special attention.

Heat-Shock Proteins in Human Arthritis

As mentioned above, in humans, responses to microbial hsps are also seen following exposure to infectious organisms. Given the conserved nature of the hsps, both in microbes and their homologous endogenous counterparts in humans and rats, there is a realistic possibility that responses elicited by microbial hsp65 in the rat are of significance to human arthritis as well. Various groups have followed such reasoning and have reported data supportive of such a possibility. A most straightforward approach in these matters seemed to be the search for antibodies directed against hsps in patients. Anti-hsp antibodies have been found in sera obtained from patients with forms of reactive arthritis (Wauben et al. unpublished) and Lyme arthritis (Wauben et al. unpublished and Steere, personal communication). Certainly of more interest, however, is the finding that in RA patients [2] and in children with juvenile chronic arthritis raised levels of antibodies were found [58].

Further analysis indicated that such antibodies were more frequently positive with the mycobacterial hsp65 than with the *E. coli* groEL homologue. At the level of T cell responses positive findings have also been made. In this case, immunological reactivity appeared to confine itself to the site of action, namely the joint synovial compartments. T cells collected from affected joint synovial fluids were found to respond to mycobacterial antigens such as PPD [1], acetone precipitate of mycobacteria [17, 37], and hsp65 [40, 14, 37, 58]. These data clearly demonstrate that T cells with hsp65 specificity can be found to be present in affected joints. It is therefore of no surprise that some workers have been able to clone such cells from the synovial compartment [14, 18]; further analysis of such clones is eagerly awaited. It remains, however, difficult to judge the significance of such findings to our understanding of the disease. The "chicken and egg" type of question is difficult to answer: Is such reactivity specifically related to the initiation of the arthritic process? Or is it the specific result of responses directed at a target structure – possibly proteoglycan associated – that has a peculiar similarity with microbial hsp65?

Furthermore, apart from such questions, one may expect that a site of chronic inflammation a polyclonal activation of T cells may occur. It is possible that reactivity to hsps is thus the natural by-product of polyclonal activation of a repertoire that originally was molded by MHC molecules filled with self-protein epitopes. Given the readiness of the immune system to recognize hsp, one may suppose that this group of proteins especially dominates formation of the repertoire. Thus, although T cell responses to hsps are found at the sites of action in the joints, and such responses have been seen to supersede the responses to other recall antigens, one should be cautious in concluding from this that hsp65 is the critical antigen in human RA.

Probably of a more informative nature may be the recent finding of enhanced expression of endogenous hsp65 in inflamed synovium, as demonstrated by the reactivity of antibodies with specificity for mycobacterial hsp65. This has been seen in specimens taken from children suffering from juvenile chronic arthritis [59] and from adult RA patients [20, 13]. Control specimens obtained from nonsynovial inflammatory processes did not express hsp65 [20]. The latter would suggest that in inflamed joints not only are reactive T cells present, but also the relevant antigen itself. Further analysis of such hsp65 expression in the course of both actively and passively induced AA will possibly provide further insight into the pathogenic significance of hsp65 tissue expression.

In other rheumatological disorders evidence for the possible role of hsps is accumulating. In SLE raised titers against hsp70, hsp90, and ubiquitin (also an hsp) have been seen [57]. In scleroderma the hsp topoisomerase may be an important autoantigen. In ankylosing spondylitis antibodies have been found against hsp90 and, interestingly enough, also against a 63 kDa hsp present in heat-shocked *Drosophila* tissue culture cells [5]. Diagnostic use has already been made of the latter phenomenon [24]. Whether or not proof of a role for hsps in the etiology of rheumatological disorders will eventually be assured, further analysis of hsps in immune regulation will likely enough generate new approaches to diagnosis or, hopefully, even specific therapy.

References

1. Abrahamsen TG, Froland SS, Natvig JB (1978) In vitro stimulation of synovial fluid lymphocytes from rheumatoid arthritis and juvenile rheumatoid arthritis parents: dissociation between the response to antigens and polyclonal mitogens. Scan J Immunol 7:81–90
2. Bahr GM, Rook GAW, Al-Saffar M, Van Embden JDA, Stanford JL, Behbehani K (1989) An analysis of antibody levels to mycobacteria in relation to HLA type: evidence for non-HLA-linked high levels of antibody to the 65kD heat shock protein of *M. tuberculosis* in rheumatoid arthritis. Clin Exp Immunol 74:211–215
3. Batisto JR, Smith RN, Bechman K, Sternlight M, Welles WL (1982) Susceptibility to adjuvant arthritis in DA and F344 rats. A dominant trait controlled by an autosomal gene locus linked to the major histocompatibility complex. Arthritis Rheum 25:1194–1200
4. Brav EA, Hench PS (1934) Tuberculous rheumatism. J Bone Joint Surg 16:839–866
5. Bernstein RM (1989) Heat-shock proteins and arthritis. Brit J Rheum 28:369–373
6. Berry Y, Willoughby DA, Giroud JP (1973) Evidence for an endogenous antigen in the adjuvant arthritic rat. J Pathol 3:229–238

7. Billingham MEJ, Butler R, Colston MJ (1990) A mycobacterial 65-kD heat shock protein induces antigen-specific suppression of adjuvant arthritis, but is not itself arthritogenic. J Exp Med 171:339–344
8. Cohen IR, Holoshitz J, Van Eden W, Frenkel A (1985) Lines of T lymphocytes illuminate pathogenesis and affect therapy of experimental arthritis. Arthritis Rheum 28:841–845
9. Cohen IR (1986) Regulation of autoimmune disease: physiological and therapeutic. Immunol Rev 94:5–21
10. Cohen, IR (to be published) T cell vaccination and suppression of autoimmune disease. Prog Immunol 7:867–873
11. De Vries RPP, van Eden W, Ottenhoff THM (1987) HLA Class II immune response genes and products in leprosy. Prog Allergy 36:95–113
12. Ellis J (1987) Proteins as molecular chaperones. Cell 328:378–379
13. Evans D, Norton P, Ivanyi J (1990) Distribution in tissue sections of the human groEL stress-protein homologue. APMIS 98:437–441
14. Gaston JSH, Life PF, Bailey LC, Bacon PA (1989) In vitro responses to a 65 kilodalton mycobacterial protein by synovial T cells from inflammatory arthritis patients. J Immunol 143:2494–2500
15. Holmgren A, Branden C (1989) Crystal structure of chaperone protein PapD reveals an immunoglobulin fold. Nature 342:248–251
16. Holoshitz J, Naparstek V, Ben-Nun A, Cohen IR (1983) Lines of T lymphocytes induce or vaccinate against autoimmune arthritis. Science 219:56–58
17. Holoshitz J, Matitiau A, Cohen IR (1984) Arthritis induced in rats by clones of T lymphocytes responsiveness to mycobacteria but not to collagen type II. J Clin Invest 73:211–215
18. Holoshitz J, Koning F, Coligan JE, de Bruyn J, Strober S (1989) Isolation of CD4–CD8-mycobacteria reactive T lymphocyte clones from rheumatoid arthritis synovial fluid. Nature 339:226–229
19. Jindal S, Dudani AK, Harley CB, Singh B, Gupta RS (1989) Primary structure of a human mitochondrial protein homologous to bacterial and plant chaperonins and to 65 kD mycobacterial antigen. Mol Cell Biol 9:2279–2283
20. Karlsson-Parra A, Soderstrom K, Ferm M, Ivanyi J, Kiessling R, Klareskog L (1990) Presence of human 65kD heat shock protein (hsp) in inflamed joints and subcutaneous nodules of RA patients. Scand J Immunol 31:283–291
21. Kaufmann SHE (1990) Heat shock proteins and the immune response. Immunol Today 11:129–136
22. Klein J (1986) The natural history of the major histocompatibility complex. Wiley, New York, p 648–658
23. Kohashi O, Kohashi Y, Takahashi T, Ozawa A, Shigematsu N (1986) Suppressive effect of *E. coli* on adjuvant induced arthritis in germ-free rats. Arthrit Rheum 29:547–555
24. Lakomek H, Will H, Zech M, Krüskemper HL (1984) A new serologic marker in ankylosing spondylitis. Arth Rheum 27:961–967
25. Lamb JR, Bal V, Mendez-Samperio P, Mehlert A, So A, Rothbard J, Jindal S, Young RA, Young DB (1989) Stress proteins may provide a link between the immune response to infection and autoimmunity. Int Immunol 1:191–196
27. Munk ME, Schoel B, Modrow S, Karr RW, Young RA, Kaufmann SHE (1989) T lymphocytes from healthy individuals with specificity to self epitopes shared by the mycobacterial and human 65 kDa heat shock protein. J Immunol 143:2844–2849
28. Nagy ZA, Lehmann PV, Falcioni F, Muller S, Adorini L (1989) Why peptides? Their possible role in the evolution of MHC restricted T-cell recognition. Immunol Today 10:132–138
29. Ostermann J, Horwich AL, Neupert W, Hartl FU (1989) Protein folding in mitochondria requires complex formation with hsp60 and ATP hydrolysis. Nature 341:125–130
30. Ottenhoff THM, Torres P, De Las Aguas JT, Fernandez R, Van Eden W, De Vries RRP, Stanford JL (1986) Evidence for an HLA-DR4 associated immune response gene for *Mycobacterium tuberculosis:* a clue to the pathogenesis of rheumatoid arthritis. Lancet ii:310–312

31. Ottenhoff THM, Birhane Kale AB, Van Embden JDA, Thole JER, Kiessling R (1988) The recombinant 65kD heat-shock protein of M. bovis BCG is a target molecule for CD4 cytotoxic T lymphocytes that lyse human monocytes. J Exp Med 168:1947–1952
32. Palacios-Boix AA, Estrad GI, Colston MJ, Panayi GS (1988) HLA-DR4 restricted lymphocyte proliferation to a *Mycobacterium tuberculosis* extract in rheumatoid arthritis and healthy subjects. J Immunol 140:2–13
33. Pelham HRB (1989) Heat shock and the sorting of luminal ER proteins. EMBO J 8:3171–3176
34. Pearson CM (1956) Development of arthritis, periarthritis and periostitis in rats given adjuvant. Proc Soc Exp Biol Med 91:95–101
35. Pearson CM, Wood FD (1964) Studies of polyarthritis and other lesions induced in rats by injection of mycobacterial adjuvant: I. General clinical and pathologic characteristics and some modifying factors. Arthritis Rheum 2:440–459
36. Piercy DWT (1971) Synovitis induced by killed *Erysipelothrix rhusiopathiae*. J Comp Path 81:557–562
37. Pope RM, Pahlavani MA, LaCour E, Sambol S, Desai BV (1989) Antigenic specificity of rheumatoid synovial fluid lymphocytes. Arthritis Rheum 32:1371–1380
38. Quagliata F, Phillips-Quagliata JM (1972) Competence of thoracic duct cells to the transfer of adjuvant disease and delayed hypersensitivity. Evidence that mycobacterial components are required for successful transfer of the disease. Cell Immunol 3:78–87
39. Reading DS, Hallberg RL, Myers AM (1989) Characterization of the yeast HSP60 gene coding for a mitochondrial assembly factor. Nature 337:655–659
40. Res PCM, Schaar CG, Breedveld FC, Van Eden W, Van Embden JDA, Cohen IR, De Vries RRP (1988) Synovial fluid T cell reactivity against the 65 kD heat-shock protein of mycobacteria in early onset of chronic arthritis. Lancet ii:478–482
41. Shinnick TM, Vodkin MH, Williams JC (1988) The *Mycobacterium tuberculosis* 65 kD antigen is a heat-shock protein which corresponds to common antigen and to the *Escherichia coli* GroEL protein. Infect Immun 56:446–451
42. Steere AC, Malawista SE, Suydman DR, Shope RE, Andiman WA, Ross MR, Steele FM (1977) Lyme arthritis: an epidemic of oligoarticular arthritis in children and adults in three Connecticut communities. Arthritis Rheum 20:7–17
43. Thole JER, Dauwerse HG, Das PK, Groothuis DG, Schouls LM, Van Embden JDA (1985) Cloning of the *Mycobacterium bovis* BCG DNA and expression of antigens in *Escherichia coli*. Infect Immun 50:800–806
44. Thole JER, Keulen WJ, Kolk AHJ, Groothuis DG, Berwald LG, Tiesjema RH, Van Embden JDA (1987) Characterization, sequence determination, and immunogenicity of a 64kD protein of M. bovis BCG expressed in E. coli K12. Infect Immun 55:1466–1475
45. Thole JER, Hindersson P, De Bruyn J, Cremers F, Van der Zee J, De Cock H, Tommassen J, Van Eden W, Van Embden JDA (1988) Antigenic relatedness of a strongly immunogenic 65kD mycobacterial protein antigen with a similarly sized ubiquitous bacterial common antigen. Microbiol Pathog 4:71–83
46. Torisu M, Miyahara T, Shinohara N, Ohsato K, Sonozaki H (1978) A new side effect of BCG immunotherapy: BCG-induced arthritis in man. Cancer Immunol Immunother 5:77–83
47. Van den Broek MF, Van Bruggen MCJ, Hogervorst EJM, Van Eden W, Van der Zee R, Van der Berg WB (1989) Protection against streptococcal cell wall induced arthritis by pretreatment with the mycobacterial 65kD heat-shock protein. J Exp Med 170:449–466
48. Van Eden W, de Vries RRP (1984) HLA and leprosy: a re-evaluation. Lep Rev 55:89–104
49. Van Eden W, Holoshitz J, Nevo Z, Frenkel A, Klajman A, Cohen IR (1985) Arthritis induced by a T lymphocyte clone that responds to *Mycobacterium tuberculosis* and to cartilage proteoglycans. Proc Nat Acad Sci USA 82:5064–5067
50. Van Eden W, Holoshitz J, Cohen IR (1987) Antigenic mimicry between mycobacteria and cartilage proteoglycans: the model of adjuvant arthritis. In: Cruse TM (ed) Concepts Immunopathol, 4th edn. Karger, Basel, pp 144–170

51. Van Eden W, Thole JER, van der Zee R, Noordzij A, van Embden JDA, Hensen EJ, Cohen IR (1988) Cloning of the mycobacterial epitope recognized by T lymphocytes in adjuvant arthritis. Nature 331:171–173

52. Van Eden W, Hogervorst EJM, Hensen EJ, Van der Zee R, Van Embden JDA, Cohen IR (1989) A cartilage mimicking T cell epitope on a 65 kD mycobacterial heat-shock protein: adjuvant arthritis as a model for human rheumatoid arthritis. In: Oldstone MB (ed) cross-reactivity between microbes and host proteins as a cause of autoimmunity. Curr Top Microbiol Immunol 145:27–43 Springer, Heidelberg New York

53. Van Eden W, Boog CJP, Hogervorst EJM, Wauben MH, van der Zee R, van Embden JDA (1991) A mycobacterial heat-shock protein T cells in experimental arthritis: possibilities for immunotherapy. In: Kresina T (ed) Monoclonal antibodies and immunotherapy of rheumatoid arthritis. Marcel Dekker, New York, pp 253–268

54. Van der Zee R, Van Eden W, Meloen RH, Noordzij A, Van Embden JDA (1989) Efficient mapping and characterization of a T cell epitope by the simultaneous synthesis of multiple peptides. Eur J Immunol 19:43–47

55. Vodkin MH, Williams JC (1988) A heat shock operon in *Coxiella burnetii* produces a major antigen homologous to a protein in both mycobacteria and *Escherichia coli*. J Bacteriol 170:1227–34

56. Young DB, Ivanyi J, Cox JH, Lamb JR (1987) The 65 kDa antigen of mycobacteria – a common bacterial protein? Immunol Today 8:215–219

57. Winfield JB (1990) Stress proteins, arthritis, and autoimmunity. Arthritis Rheum 32:1497–1504

58. Danieli MG, Markovitz D, Gabrielli A, Corvetta A, Giorgi PL, van der Zee R, van Embden JDA, Danieli G, Cohen IR (1991) Juvenile Rheumatoid Arthritis patients manifest immune reactivity to the mycobacterial 65 kd heat shock protein, to its 180–188 peptide and to a partially homologous peptide of the proteoglycan link protein. J Clin Invest (submitted)

59. De Graeff-Meeder ER, van der Zee R, Rijkers GT, Schuurman HJ, Bijlsma JWJ, Kuis W, Zegers BJM, van Eden W (1991) Recognition of human 60 kD heat shock protein by mononuclear cells from patients with juvenile chronic arthritis. Lancet 337:1368–1372

60. Emmrich F, Thole J, van Embden J, Kaufmann SHE (1986) A recombinant 64 kilodalton protein of Mycobacterium bovis Bacillus Calmette-Guerin specificially stimulates human T4 clones reactive to mycobacterial antigens. J Exp Med 163:1024–1029

61. Hemmingsen SM, Woolford C, van der Vies SM, Tilly K, Dennis DT, Georgopoulos CP, Hendrix RW, Ellis RJ (1988) Homologous plant and bacterial proteins chaperone oligomeric protein assembly. Nature 333:330–334

62. Hogervorst EJM, Boog CJP, Wagenaar JPA, Wauben MHM, van der Zee R, van Eden W (1991) T cell reactivity to an epitope of the mycobacterial 65-kDa heat shock protein (hsp 65) corresponds with arthritis susceptibility in rats and is regulated by hsp 65 specific cellular responses. Eur J Immunol 21:1289–1296

63. Kaufmann SHE, Väth U, Thole JER, van Embden JDA, Emmrich F (1987) Enumeration of T cells reactive with Mycobacterium tuberculosis organisms and specific for the recombinant mycobacterial 64 kilodalton protein. Eur J Immunol 17:351–357

Type-II Collagen
in the Pathogenesis of Rheumatoid Arthritis*

R. Holmdahl

Department of Medical and Physiological Chemistry, Box 575 Uppsala University, S-75123 Uppsala, Sweden

Remarks on Genetics and Pathogenesis of Rheumatoid Arthritis

Rheumatoid arthritis (RA) is now generally regarded as an autoimmune disease with relapsing or progressive occurrence of arthritis affecting preferentially peripheral joints. In spite of the fact that it is a severe and crippling disease affecting a large population, very little is known of its etiology and pathogenesis, although many of its seconday manifestations have been well described. Fortunately, basic research has made considerable progress which now make it possible (a) to evolve the structural requirements for one critical event of importance in RA, the trimolecular interaction between an autoantigenic peptide on major histocompatibility complex (MHC) class-II molecule and the T-cell receptor, and (b) to rapidly increase our knowledge of the basic rules for self- and non-self-discrimination by the immune system. Analysis of the MHC class-II genes which confer a high risk of developing RA suggests that many, perhaps a majority of patients suffering from the syndrome classified as RA according to the criteria of the Arthritis Rheumatism Association actually suffer from a single disease entity with a pathologic response to a particular autoantigen. Considering the preferential involvement of peripheral joints in RA, it is likely that this particular antigen is a molecule specifically located in joint tissues. In this chapter the descriptive findings of autoimmune reactions to cartilage-specific type-II collagen (CII) in RA are reviewed and the general requirements for recognition of these molecules by the immune system are discussed. The possible pathologic relevance is evaluated in light of recent findings in experimental models in which arthritis is induced with cartilage-specific molecules.

* This work was supported by the Swedish Medical Research Council, the Craaford Foundation, the King Gustav V 80-years Foundation, the Nanna Swartz Foundation, and National League against Rheumatism.

Smolen, Kalden, Maini (Eds.)
Rheumatoid Arthritis
© Springer-Verlag Berlin Heidelberg 1992

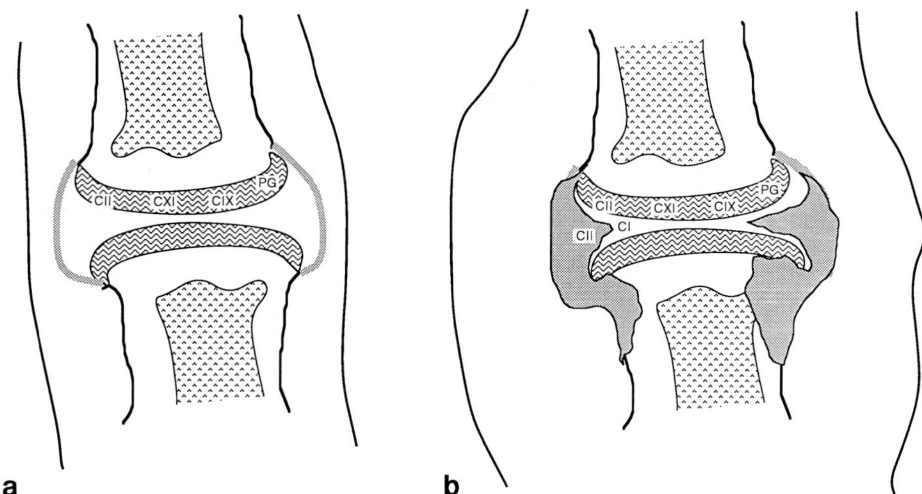

Fig. 1 a, b. Location of different matrix components in **(a)** a normal and **(b)** a rheumatoid joint. The cartilage contains type-II collagen (*CII*), type-IX collagen (*CIX*), type-XI collagen (*CXI*) and chondroitin sulphate proteoglycans (PC) as well as other proteins of cartilage-nonspecific location. During the erosion of joints by the pannus tissue, collagen molecules can be detected in synovial cells (*CII*) [142, 143] and in synovial fluid (mainly *CI,* probably also *CII*) [75, 76]

Joint Cartilage, Synvial Tissue and the Immune System

The joint is composed of several different types of connective tissue as depicted in Fig. 1. Known joint-specific molecules are localized to the articular cartilage. Joint cartilage is composed of a meshwork of CII fibers with connecting CIX molecules and cartilage-specific chondroitin sulphate proteoglycans. The proteoglycan core protein is anchored to hyaluronan with a special region (the hook region) at the end of the molecule, and the binding is stabilized by the link protein. The structure functions as a water-containing elastic sponge and harbors a considerable amount of fluid under resting conditions. Intermittent pressure on the cartilage facilitates diffusion transport of nutrients, which is necessary since the cartilaginous tissue lacks vascularization. The synovial membrane is continuous with the periosteum and forms the joint capsule. The lining layer of the synovial membrane facing the joint space consists of cells with several functions: to produce hyaluronate, and to scavenge "garbage material" in the synovia, such as breakdown products from cartilage; it thereby also picks up antigens which are possibly presented to the immune system. The cells of the synovial membrane are fibroblasts, macrophages, and dendritic cells. The synovium is most likely a part of the reticuloendothelial system, which specifically absorbs systemically spread opsonized particles such as bacteria and bacteria cell walls.

A basic, unresolved question concerning the autoimmune response to joint molecules is whether the cartilage tissue might be immunoprivileged. Although cartilage is not vascularized, we suggest that it is available to immune system. CII is expressed early in fetal development and is extensively metabolized during this period [1, 2]. Furthermore, cartilage channels containing blood vessels have been shown to penetrate cartilage matrix for a long period, up to adolescence in mammals [3]. The synovial membrane is a richly vascularized tissue and is drained by lympoid vessels. It is likely, although it has not been directly demonstrated, that synovial cells of bone marrow origin [4], e. g., macrophages and dendritic cells, pick up cartilage antigens which will be processed to peptides and bound to class-II molecules. Subsequently, the synovial dendritic cells might migrate to draining lymph nodes, as has been shown for dendritic cells in the epidermis [5, 6]. Hence, autoantigenic peptides from CII and other cartilage-specific molecules may be accessible also in the lymph nodes, where they can be presented to lymphocytes. Moreover, in spite of the nonvascularized nature of cartilage, it can be shown that CII is exposed to antibody binding *in vivo*. This has been demonstrated by induction of arthritis via injection of polyclonal antiserum [7–9] and of syngeneic monoclonal autoantibodies specific for different epitopes on the CII molecule into experimental animals [10, 11]. Thus, it is likely that CII molecules, as well as other cartilage-specific molecules, are accessible to the immune system during ontogeny and in adult life. In conclusion, it can be anticipated that CII is a self-protein recognized by the peripheral immune system. Whether CII molecules or CII peptides are available in the thymus and bone marrow during lymphocyte maturation is not clear, however. From these considerations it follows that CII must be regarded as a true self-protein without "non-self" properties, as can be postulated for self-proteins localized at immunoprivileged sites.

Immunogenetics of RA

It has been known for a long time that the susceptibility for developing RA is weakly associated with certain HLA specificities, particularly HLA-DR4 and DR1 [12]. This linkage was more exactly defined recently, and thereby made stronger, by sequencing a series of DR4 and DR1 subtypes [13]. Thus, a strong correlation has been found with the HLA-Dw4 and Dw14 subtypes of DR4, and sequence information reveals that critical residues of importance for RA susceptibility are located at positions 69, 70, 71, and 74 on the DRB chain [14, 15]. Since the three-dimensional structure of the class-II molecule has been calculated from crystallographic data on a class-I molecule [16], the exact positions of these sites can be anticipated. From such comparisons it is clear that the critical sites are located in the alpha-helix of the DRB chain and therefore may be involved in both the peptide binding and the interaction with the T-cell receptor. One of the potentially important conclusions from this observed linkage between the certain MHC class-II haplotypes and RA is that it may be only one self-peptide, or more likely a set of related self-peptides, that is critically recognized in the majority of RA patients. It should be stressed, however, that the critical structures on class-II molecules are far from being fully characterized and that there may also be important contributions from DQ alleles to RA susceptibility [17].

The Rheumatoid Inflammatory Attack on the Joints

Several observations indicate that local T-cell activation against as yet unknown antigens occurs in the synovial tissue in RA, which may be of importance for the perpetuation of the inflammation. Evidence that T cells in the synovial tissue are activated to a larger extent than T cells in the synovial fluid or in peripheral blood has been provided from observations of increased expression of class-II molecules and IL-2 receptors on synovial T cells from patients with active RA [18, 19]. Immunohistochemical studies have demonstrated a multitude of MHC class-II-expressing cells with potential antigen-presenting function in the rheumatoid synovial tissue [20, 21]. Thus, a cellular basis for local class-II-restricted T-cell activation exists. In the rheumatoid joint, chondrocytes in the cartilage, and macrophages, fibroblasts, B lymphocytes and endothelial cells in the pannus tissue are activated by a multitude of cytokines, some of them derived from activated T cells, such as gamma-interferon [22–25].

RA is also characterized by activation of autoreactive B cells, and immune complexes precipitating in the joints are believed to be important factors contributing to the pathogenesis [26]. A hallmark of RA is the production of rheumatoid factor. This is an autoimmune reaction toward autologous IgG, which has been shown to be dependent on activated T helper cells [27, 28]. Antibodies against other autoantigens, such as CII, have also been demonstrated (see below). It is likely that gamma-interferon and other T-cell-derived interleukins, as well as immune complexes formed by the locally produced immunoglobulins and autoantigens, contribute to the activation of synovial macrophages and fibroblasts in the synovial tissue and to the accumulation of granulocytes in the synovial fluid.

A challenging question for the study of RA concerns the specificity of the immune reactions which initiate and perpetuate the autoimmune pathology. These reactions are most likely dependent on both activated autoreactive T cells and certain autoreactive B cells. Thus, immunespecific lymphocytes are of importance for both delayed hypersensitivity and immune complex mediated pathogenetic mechanisms. It is now pertinent to determine the specificity of such activated lymphocytes infiltrating the synovial tissue during rheumatoid disease. It is also possible that the critical interactions of autoreactive T cells and B cells are localized to the lymph nodes draining the actively affected joints, although only a limited number of studies have been performed on such lymph nodes in RA. Isolation of lymphocytes with critical specificities may prove to be a complicated task, however. First, the activated lymphocytes in the joints are not monoclonal but rather polyclonal or possibly oligoclonal [29] in origin and, as judged from experimental autoimmune models, very few of them can be postulated to have direct importance for the initiation and perpetuation of the disease [30]. Second, it will be difficult to prove the pathogenicity of a given isolated lymphocyte. Third, we have limited basic knowledge on how autoreactive T cells and B cells are regulated in vivo. For instance, the presence per se of autoreactive lymphocytes may not be the pathologic event but rather a failure to regulate such physiologically occurring cells. For an understanding of the basic mechanisms leading to autoimmune arthritis we think that experimental models of RA are useful, even though the specific molecular interactions in these models cannot be directly applied to human diseases.

Animal Models for Rheumatoid Arthritis

One approach to studying the development of autoimmune arthritis has been to induce disease by immunization with joint-specific macromolecules in experimental animals. To date, CII [31] and CXI (which has one of its alpha-chains in common with CII) [32] have been shown to induce rheumatoid-like diseases in rodents, and cartilage-specific proteoglycan has been shown to induce an ankylosing spondylitis-like disease in mice [33]. The most widely used model, collagen-induced arthritis (CIA), can be induced in several species, such as mice [34], rats [31], and monkeys [35], after intradermal immunization with CII.

Immunogenetics of CIA
Only certain inbred rat and mouse strains are susceptible for CIA, suggesting a genetic linkage of CII responsiveness. Susceptibility for CIA is inherited polygenically but with a major contributing gene within MHC. Development of arthritis after immunization with heterologous [36–39] or autologous CII [39] is restricted to mouse strains of $H-2^q$ related or $H-2^r$ haplotypes, while $H-2^p$ confers resistance. By using mouse strains recombinant at the MHC region it has been shown that CIA susceptibility is associated with genes in the class-II region [36, 37]. The relevant class-II molecules A^q and A^p differ only by four amino acids, which then can be defined as the critical residues determining responsiveness to CIA [40]. Recent sequence data also suggest that the $I-A^r$ molecule shares important structures with the $I-A^q$ molecule [41]. Not only do the $H-2^q$ and $H-2^r$ haplotypes share the susceptibility for development of CIA; they also mount a specific autoimmune response after immunization with autologous mouse CII [39, 42]. Thus, in CIA there is evidence for involvement of specific structures on I-A class-II molecules, which are of critical importance for presentation of CII to autoreactive T cells. Structural analysis of the site determining the responsiveness to CIA in mice and of the site in the DRB chain linked with RA shows that the critical residues might interact with both the antigenic peptide and the T-cell receptor.

Pathogenesis of CIA
Irrespective of the species source of CII, a severe erosive arthritis develops that has many histopathologic similarities with RA [43–45]. In the heterologous CII-induced diseases a relatively stronger anti-CII autoantibody response develops, and this disease seems to be more self-limited in its course, possibly

because of downregulation by anti-CII antibodies [46, 47]. On the other hand, immunization with autologous CII leads to a chronic and progressive arthritic disease, which may be self-perpetuating, in both rats and mice [42, 47, 48].

Of considerable relevance for the understanding of RA is the finding that the immune response after immunization with autologous CII differs dramatically compared with the immune response after immunization with heterologous CII. First, T cells reactive with autologous CII can be isolated from spleens of normal, not immunized, DBA/1 (H-2^q) mice, but only when stimulated with high antigen doses [49]. Second, autoantibodies to CII develop after immunization with autologous CII, but at variable and often low levels [39, 42]. It is conceivable that a large fraction of the anti-CII autoantibodies produced are absorbed by cartilage.

Some properties of the immune response after immunization with heterologous CII may also be of importance for an understanding of RA. Thus a strong anti-CII antibody response develops early after immunization with rat CII in H-2^q high-responder mice which is almost totally cross-reactive to mouse CII [50, 51]. Approximately one third of the antibody-producing B cells in a lymph node primed 9 days earlier produce anti-CII autoantibodies. These are mainly of the IgG type and are encoded by many different V genes. Most of the anti-CII autoantibodies react exclusively with epitopes present on the native triple helix and are specific for CII with no cross-reactions to CI. One interpretation of these findings is that anti-CII-reactive B cells are not deleted from the repertoire but occur naturally before immunization, and that these B cells have already been primed to be ready for a secondary immune response. The physiological role of such naturally occurring autoreactive and primed B cells is presently unknown. As they may be antigen-presenting cells for autoreactive T cells, this is a very important issue to investigate for the understanding of CIA and most likely also for RA.

As to the effector mechanisms, the triggering of an anti-CII immune response and CIA are T-cell dependent [52–54], leading to enhancement of both macrophage-mediated erosive destruction of the joints [55–58] and antibody or immune complex-mediated development of edematous synovitis [7, 8, 59, 60]. Thus, apart from the CII immunization, which precipitates a chronic arthritic disease in genetically susceptible animals, the CIA model has many major similarities to RA and a few major differences [43–45]. This may reflect that both are dependent on the critical recognition of a joint-specific antigen, altough most certainly different antigenic peptides are recognized in the different diseases.

Observed Autoimmune Reactions to CII in RA

The possibility of the involvement of autoimmunity to collagen was first suggested by Steffen and co-workers [61]. In a series of studies, these authors demonstrated the occurrence of antibodies toward collagen in serum and collagen-anti-collagen immune complexes in the synovial fluid of RA patients [61–62]. Subsequent studies using passive hemagglutinin methods revealed a high frequency (more than 50%) of serum from RA patients to have positive titers to denatured collagens [63, 64]. Thus, these earlier studies showed that RA patients possess hyperreactivity toward collagens. However, most of these investigations were performed with type-I collagen (CI), and the results showed that the reactivity was directed mainly toward collagen alpha-chain and not to quaternary epitopes on the triple helix. However, since the RA attack is directed mainly against joints, joint-specific proteins have attracted increasing interest as possible targets for the autoimmune attack, especially after David Trentham's finding in 1977 that cartilage-specific CII induces a rheumatoid-like arthritic disease (CIA) in rats [31].

Immune Reactivities to Collagen Alpha Chains

The early studies by Steffen et al. have been confirmed by a number of more recent reports showing that RA serum often contains positive titers against denatured collagen alpha-chains [65–66]. The measured serum antibodies are generally not type specific and seem to be directed to common collagen alpha-chain structures which presumably are dependent on the Gly-X-Y kind of repetitive units. It is likely that antibodies with relatively low affinity for such structures may be determined due to the repetitive occurrence of the epitope. Earlier animal studies suggested that B cells producing antibodies to repetitive (Pro-Gly-Pro)^n polypeptides were T-cell independent [67]. In contrast, the immune response to native collagens, e. g., against quaternary epitopes, is T-cell dependent, associated with specific MHC haplotypes and often, but not always, type specific [36–40, 68–72]. Furthermore, immunization of mice with native CI (nCI), as well as with other collagen types except native CII (nCII), induces an antibody response which is usually species specific, and in particular, does not cross-react with homologous collagen [68–71]. In man there is some direct experience with bovine CI immunization due to the widespread use of Zyderm collagen implants [73]. Patients developed antibody responses to bovine CI which did not cross-react with CI from other species. The response was not entirely type specific and cross-reacted with other investigated collagens such as CII and CIII [73].

High serum and synovial fluid titers to collagen alpha-chains are not specific for RA, but are seen also in a number of other inflammatory disorders [74]. This finding is expected, since collagens are the most abundant proteins in the body and are present at all inflammatory sites. In rheumatoid inflammation, collagens are present also in the synovial fluid during active arthritis [75, 76]. This collagen is mainly CI, and there is evidence that the collagen forms immune complexes with anti-collagen IgG in the synovial fluid and synovial membrane [62, 77]. It is likely that exposed collagens at inflamatory sites trigger the production of anti-collagen antibodies. Accordingly, the levels of anti-denatured CII (dCII) antibodies, presumably directed to denatured collagen alpha-chains, irrespective of collagen type, have been found to be higher in synovial fluid than in serum [65, 78] and correlated to disease activity [79].

B-Cell Responses to Native CII (nCII)

Similar to the immune response toward certain other native collagens, for example CI, CIII, and CV, the immune response to CII is inducible in animal strains expressing certain immune response genes. However, in contrast to the immune response to systemically occurring collagens, the antibodies to nCII strongly cross-react with the homologous counterpart [50, 51, 68–71], which means that the B cells producing autoantibodies to CII are not deleted in a manner which has been demonstrated to occur for certain other autoreactive B cells using transgenic mice and bonemarrow chimeras [80, 81].

In man, both frequency and titers of antibodies to nCII detected in RA patients have varied between different studies, depending mainly on differences in sensitivity of the methods used [82]. In addition, there are some methodologic pitfalls which may influence the assay results [82–85]. Nevertheless, it is clear from a number of studies that some patients with RA have an elevated antibody response specifically directed to nCII [65, 66, 74, 82, 84, 86–93]. Such an anti-CII immune response is elevated in RA and in relapsing polychondritis (RP) [93] and juvenile RA (JRA) [84] but generally not in other arthritides or in normal controls. One of the most discriminatory assays used is immunofluorescence on articular cartilage, used by Greenbury and Skingle [86], who investigated a large number of sera from RA patients and normal controls. Positive reactivity was restricted to RA sera, although among these only 3% bound cartilage. These sera were all specific for nCII and did not cross-react with denatured collagens or other types of native collagens. Sera from patients with RP, an autoimmune systemic chondritis disease, show a higher frequency (30%–60%) of cartilage-specific antibodies using the same assay [94]. In a series of papers [66, 82, 92, 94–99], Clague and co-workers have described the anti-CII antibody responses in RA patients and found that the various methods (hemagglutination, RIA, and immunofluorescence) correlated well with each other but had different levels of discrimination [82]. Using these methods, they and others have found that the frequency of RA sera with specific reactivity to nCII varied between 3% and 15% [65, 82, 84–92]. A few RA patients develop relatively high serum titers of anti-nCII antibodies [65]. Assessment of these studies is complicated by the fact that the production of anti-CII antibodies fluctuates during the course of disease [79, 90, 92]. The levels have been suggested to be maximal during the first acute onset of disease [89] but not to precede the onset [100]. Also, the production of anti nCII antibodies most likely occurs preferentially in the RA synovia, since the relative titers are higher in the synovial fluid than in serum [96], although there is no correlation between the severity of arthritis and the occurrence of anti nCII antibody titers [89, 101]. However, the value of frequency data on specific antibody content in serum and synovial fluid is questionable, since it is likely that autoantibodies directed to nCII are bound to cartilage surfaces in vivo. In fact, one recent study by Tarkowski [102], using the ELISPOT technique to enumerate the frequency of B cells producing anti-CII antibodies in situ, suggests that the majority of investigated RA patients have B cells secreting IgG antibodies to nCII in the synovial tissue, while no reactions were determined in the sera of the same patients. Although this study confirms earlier reports of local anti-nCII antibody production in situ [65, 78, 103], the occurrence of anti-nCII-reactive B cells at other locations, e. g., in lymphoid organs, is not excluded.

A Pathogenic Role for Anti-CII Antibodies?

Presumably, autoantibodies reactive with CII are present and also produced in the rheumatoid joint, but do they play a pathogenic role? Experiments in animal models point toward such an arthritogenic role of autoantibodies or immune complexes. Thus an arthritic disease, although transient and lacking the erosive component, is inducible with passive transfer of anti-nCII antibody-containing serum [7–9, 59, 60]. In fact, also human anti–nCII serum has been shown to transfer arthritic disease to mice [104]. However, transfer with monoclonal anti-CII antibodies induced only very mild signs of synovitis [105, 106], despite efficient binding to cartilage in vivo [10, 11]. Therefore, we have suggested that anti-CII antibodies may become more active by inducing formation of immune complexes precipitate in the joints and may participate in triggering a local immune complex mediated inflammatory reaction [44, 45]. Data on the specificity of the anti-CII antibody response support this hypothesis. Thus monoclonal anti-CII antibodies and anti-CII anti-idiotypic antibodies which cross-react with syngenic IgG-Fc, thus being rheumatoid factors, have been described [107, 108]. Another monoclonal anti-CII antibody cross-reacts with type-I collagen and the collagenous part of $C1^q$, and seems to inhibit activation of $C1^q$ [105, 109]. If such an inhibition of $C1^q$ activation occurs in vivo, it is likely that this will prevent dissolution of immune complexes in situ. These cross-reactive antibodies are not of the multispecific, IgM type with low avidity reactions to autoantigens, as described by many investigators [51, 110, 111]. The existence of dual specific antibodies connected with the anti-CII antibody response would allow local precipitation of immune complexes of anti-collagen antibodies, rheumatoid factors, and collagen. As a matter of fact, the occurrence of anti-CII-CII immune complexes in human rheumatoid joints has been described by several investigators. Jasin [112] analyzed immune complexes, composed of both anti-CII antibodies and rheumatoid factors, trapped in the articular cartilage. Clague and Moore [96] analyzed immune complexes isolated from synovial fluid and found that the anti-CII activity increased after collagenase treatment. To conclude, it seems likely that immune complexes with CII, anti-CII, and rheumatoid factors do play a role in arthritic inflammation. However, this does not explain the cause entirely, since immune complex-mediated reactions may be one of many aspects of the secondary phenomenon of the inflammatory response in the joints. The critical question is whether there are any specific events that trigger the observed anti-CII reactions in the joints, events which might be correlated to the genetic immune response restrictions of the disease.

T-Cell Reactivities to CII

Cellular reactivities were first measured with various lymphokine-based assays. In a leukocyte inhibitory factor (LIF) assay, Trentham and co-workers found that the peripheral blood leukocytes (PBL) from RA and psoriasis arthritis (PA) patients were specifically stimulated by nCII and nCIII but not nCI, nCIV, nCV, or denatured collagens of all types [113]. In contrast, employing a macrophage inhibitory factor (MIF) assay, Stuart et al. found significant stimulation with denatured collagens in PBL from patients suffering from various arthritides, although stimulation with native collagens showed a relatively specific correlation with RA [114]. Contrasting results have also been obtained with the LIF assay. Thus, Solinger et al. found stimulation with denatured collagens and with Pro-Gly synthetic polypeptides also in PBL from normal individuals and no correlation with RA [115], while others have reported an enhanced anti-collagen response in RA [116–119]. Reports measuring the antigen specificity of PBLs using assays measuring DNA synthesis after antigen challenge in vitro by [^{3}H]thymidine incorporation have given somewhat more convincing evidence that a more or less type-specific anti-CII activity is elevated in RA [21, 113, 114, 11, 119].

It is not surprising that no clear evidence has so far been provided for the possible involvement of cell reactivities with any particular autoantigens involved in the pathogenesis of RA. Even in the CIA model in mice it is difficult to detect and characterize the autoreactive T cells involved in the critical interactions leading to arthritis development. Clearly, T cells reactive with autologous CII are in a different functional state from T cells reactive with heterologous CII after immunization. Since such cells are not deleted in thymus or in the periphery, and autologous CII most likely is available, they must have reacted with CII in vivo without giving rise to arthritis under habitual conditions. There is at present no way of adequately measuring a potential arthritogenic activity of these anti-CII-reactive T cells in mice susceptible for CIA or in human beings suffering from RA. Other complications may stem from the fact that CII peptides can be present in the antigen-presenting cells and thereby raise background values of stimulation in vitro. However, it was recently shown that anti-CII reactive T cells are present in rheumatoid synovia [120]. From a patient with high anti-nCII antibody reactivity in serum, T-cell clones were established from the rheumatoid synovia, and 12% of the T-cell clones reacted with CII. These T-cell reactivities were persistent; a similar series of clones was isolated 3 years later from the joints of the same patient. The isolated T cells were oligoclonal since they had receptors with different V elements, they were class-II restricted since they expressed CD4, and they had potential effector functions since they secreted various interleukins such as gamma-interferon, TNFα, and TNFβ after stimulation with CII. Although this study was limited to one patient, it clearly shows that anti-CII-reactive T cells are present in situ, although we do not know about their frequency, potential pathogenic function, or regulation.

Genetic Associations of the Anti-CII Response
A more direct approach to understanding whether anti-CII reactivities in RA play a critical role is to investigate their association with immune response genes. Not surprisingly, very divergent results have been reported, partly

dependent on the assays used and the collagen specificities investigated. Solinger presented evidence that the PBL response to collagen alpha-chains using an LIF assay was associated with HLA-DR4 [115]. This was not confirmed by other investigators using the same assay [117, 118, 121]. However, the serum antibody reactivity to denatured CII was correlated with HLA-DR4 in another study [122]. Also, investigations of the reactivities to nCII show divergent results. In one study the serum antibody reactivity to nCII correlated with HLA-DR4 [101], but in another study it correlated with DR3 and DR7 and not with DR4 [97]. Since it is not likely that the assays used mirror the actual anti-CII response in the disease, as has been discussed above, the picture might become clearer when assays specifically designed to measure antigen-induced activities of autoreactive T and B cells are employed.

Is CII Immunity of Etiologic Importance in RA?

Based on the above-described data, it is reasonable to suggest that autoreactive T cells and B cells specific for CII are present in the peripheral immune system in both man and experimental animals, such as rat and mouse strains susceptible for CIA. It is possible that T cells specific also for other cartilage components occur naturally, and at least for proteoglycans some evidence had been reported of increased immune response in patients with ankylosing spondylitis, but not in RA [123]. From the accumulated work on anti-CII immunity, it can be concluded that this is more or less confined to RA, RP [94], and possibly JRA [84] diseases. If we suppose that CII is the crucial autoantigen in RA, we are provided with two possibilities. The first is that the occurrence of anti-CII reactive T and B cells is genetically restricted, by V gene germline repertoire or MHC restrictions, to individuals with a high risk of developing RA. The second is that all individuals have these autoreactive lymphocytes which may play some sort of physiological role, but that disregulation of these cells may lead to RA. These possibilities may be combined. It is apparent that autoreactive T cells must be present in individuals susceptible for RA but without disease and that they are not doing any harm, since T cells are not known to somatically mutate their receptors. Hence, these cells must be under strict regulatory control and/ or be anergic, and are thereby prevented from triggering arthritis. The critical phenomenon may therefore not be the presence of autoreactive lymphocytes per se but rather the regulatory cells controlling their activity.

Evidence that CII May Specifically Affect
the Antigen-presenting Cell Function

At least three different cell types with potential antigen-presenting functions, e. g., expressing class-II molecules, may be of importance in rheumatoid disease. First, there are dendritic cells in the lymph nodes (interdigitating cells), which constitutively express class-II molecules and are believed to pick up antigen in body tissue and transport antigenic peptides to the lymph node where the activation of T cells occurs [6]. The synovial tissue harbours dendritic cells, expressing class-II molecules which may have this function [124]. Second, macrophages can be induced to express class-II molecules after activation. Such activated and class-II-expressing macrophages occur in the rheumatoid pannus [125]. Third, B cells express class-II molecules and may function as efficient antigen-presenting cells after activation due to enhanced class-II expression and also because their Ig receptors are able to pick up specific antigen and present them to T cells reactive with the same protein [126].

To get a clue as to why normally occurring CII-reactive lymphocytes are activated in a way leading to induction of arthritis, it is important to ask whether antigen-presenting cell function might be disturbed. In this context, some potentially important observations should be mentioned. It is possible that macrophages and dendritic cells may be activated by some nonspecific stimuli in the joints and thereby become able to deliver a second signal believed to be crucial for an efficient activation of T cells [127]. Such nonspecific stimuli might be bacterial cell wall components which are known to persist in synovial tissue for a long time. This might be an explanation for the finding that patients infected with *Mycobacterium leprae* develop anti-nCII antibody responses [74], or for the finding that some rats injected with mycobacteria cell wall fragments to induce adjuvant arthritis also develop anti-CII immunity [128–130]. CII may also have a direct role in the stimulation of macrophages. Human monocytes can be activated with CII, but not with other types of collagen, to secrete IL-1α and IL-1β [131]. In addition, the regions on the CII molecule with these macrophage-activating properties was located om the CB11 and CB9 cyanogen bromide peptides. It would be useful to investigate whether this treatment changes the capacity of macrophages to activate autoreactive T cells.

There is also another intriguing, but again rather speculative, possibility. From animal studies it is clear that B cells reactive with autologous CII are not deleted, but rather seem to be present in the functional repertoire. From studies of the antigen-presenting functions of B cells it is known that activated B cells are efficient antigen-presenting cells and can deliver second signals to an interacting T cell [6, 126, 127]. Thus, it is conceivable that in rheumatoid disease the first event is that CII-reactive B cells are stimulated, for example by mimicry of CII with a bacterial antigen or mimicry with a self-antigen of importance in cell regulation; the last possibility was actually first proposed by Kunkel as a mechanism for the production of rheumatoid factors [132]. The latter possibility might be exemplified by the finding that CII immunity seems to be connected with a rheumatoid factor response [107, 108, 133]. Monoclonal anti-CII antibodies and anti-CII anti-idiotypic antibodies with dual function as rheumatoid factors have been isolated, and it is possible that when such rheumatoid factor-producing B-cells are activated they can also activate autoreactive CII-specific T cells.

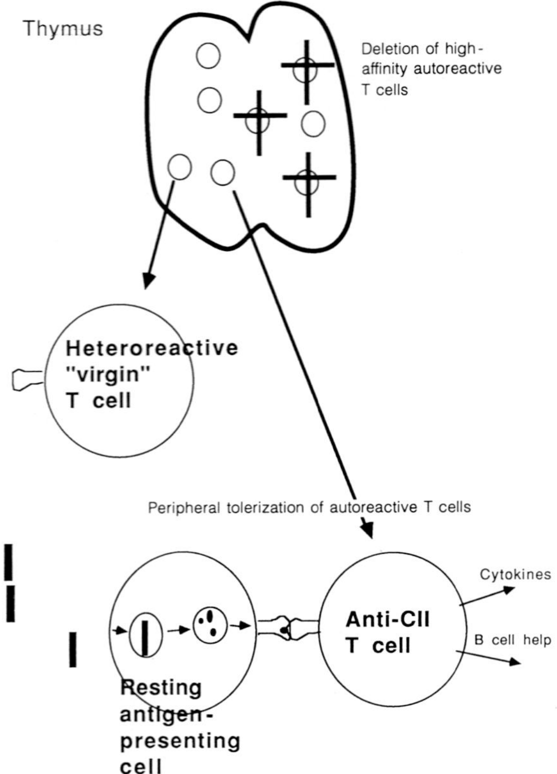

Fig. 2. Hypothetical illustration of the physiological maturation of T cells and its relevance for self-non-self-discrimination. In the thymus negative selection of self-reactive thymocytes occurs [144]. Some autoreactive thymocytes do escape negative selection by mechanisms – which are not yet completely understood [145 146]. All newly exported T cells, regarded as virgin, if stimulated by resting antigen-presenting cells, will give only a "first signal" mediated by the T-cell receptor, which will lead to tolerization of the T cells. Such tolerization will render the T cell anergic in response to the autoantigen, perhaps by an impaired proliferative capacity but retainment of some effector functions. Heteroactive T cells will be fully stimulated by their specific foreign antigen, which will presumably be presented in the context of a "second signal" by an activated antigen-presenting cell and eventually proliferate and develop into competent effector cells and memory cells. If not stimulated they will die

T-Cell Clonality and the Regulatory Control of Autoreactive T Cells

An interesting possibility for activation of autoreactive T cells in vivo has been highlighted recently by the studies of "superantigens" [134]. These "superantigens" bind to certain V-elements of the T-cell receptor and to nonpolymorphic regions of class-II antigens. The families of staphylococcal enterotoxins are examples of such antigens in the mouse [134], there are other examples, such as the *Mycoplasma arthritidis* mitogen (MAM) [135, 136]. MAM activates T cells expressing Vβ8 and Vβ6 V genes [136] and also induces arthritis after intravenous injection [137]. This finding might be of importance for CIA in

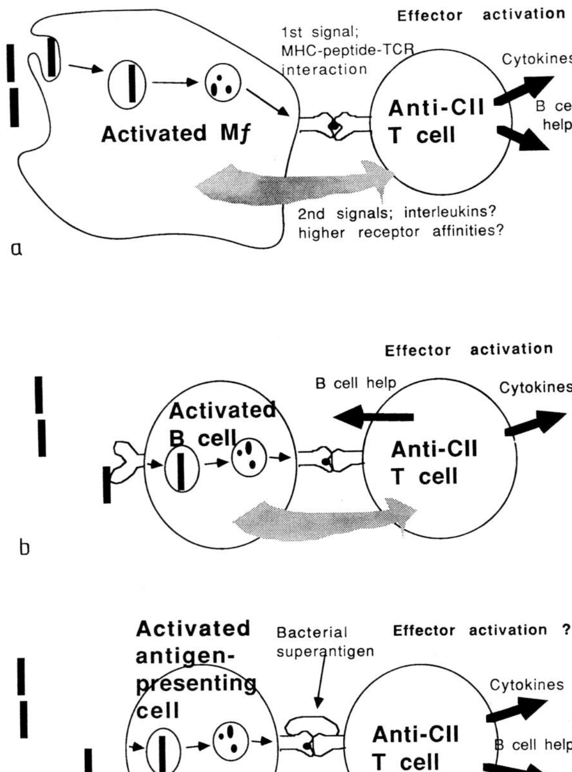

Fig. 3a–c. Some hypothetical possibilities for triggering of autoreactive T cells in vivo. **a** An antigen-presenting cell, which may be a macrophage MA or another cell expressing class-II molecules. This antigen-presenting cell must be activated, by some inflammatory or infectious stimuli, to be able to provide the second signal necessary to induce full stimulation of the interacting T cell. **b** An antigen-specific B cell, which may develop into an efficient antigen-presenting cell after stimulation with the appropriate antigen. **c** Stimulation of the antigen-presenting cell – T cell interaction by a superantigen, which may cross-link class-II molecules with certian V elements on the T-cell receptor. This will activate polyclonally activated T cells, including autoreactive T cells. Many superantigens described so far originate from bacteria; it is therefore possible to imagine that a simultaneous infection also will activate the antigen-presenting cells to provide a necessary second signal to the T cell

mice in which activation of Vβ8- or Vβ6-expressing T cells has been postulated to be critical for development of disease [138], although this hypothesis is debatable [139, 140]. However, no clear-cut association with a particular pathogen in RA has been demonstrated.

On the other hand, in experimental allergic encephalomyelitis (EAE), induced with basic protein peptide 1–10 in mice, it has been demonstrated that the pathogenic, myelin-basic protein-reactive T cells express only T-cell receptors with a certain V-element (Vβ8.2) [141]. It is therefore at lest theoretically possible that recognition of a specific arthritogenic epitope on CII is mediated only by T cells with certain V elements. However, we predict that it will be almost impossible to find such a monoclonal population of T cells in rheumatoid joints since the overwhelming majority must be "passenger" T cells of no relevance for the maintenance of disease.

To avoid getting further into areas which are only dimly illuminated, I have not discussed the challenging possibility of active regulatory cells. In order to sum up several very hypothetical mechanisms whereby autoreactive T cells – here CII-reactive T cells – might be activated into becoming competent effector cells of pathologic importance, I present physiologic interactions in Fig. 2 and the possible pathologic interactions in Fig. 3.

Acknowledgements. Im am very grateful to Kristofer Rubin, Barbara Bröker, Mikael Andersson, and Tom Goldschmidt for their critical reading of the manuscript.

References

1. Von Der Mark H, Von Der Mark K, Gay S (1976) Study of differential collagen synthesis during development of the chick embryo by immunofluorescence. I. Preparation of collagen type I and type II specific antibodies and their application to early stages of the chick embryo. Dev Biol 48:237–249
2. Thorogood P, Bee J, Von Der Mark K (1986) Transient expression of collagen type II at epitheliomesenchymal interfaces during morphogenesis of cartilaginous neurocranium. Dev Biol 116:497–509
3. Denecke R, Trautwein G, Kaup FJ (1986) The role of cartilage canals in the pathogenesis of experimentally induced polyarthritis. Rheumatol Int 6:239–243
4. Klareskog L, Forsum U, Wigzell H (1982) Murine synovial intima contains I-A-, I-E/C-positive bone marrow-derived cells. Scand J Immunol 15:509–514
5. Inaba K, Steinman R (1983) Dendritic cells are critical accessory cells for thymus-dependent antibody responses in mouse and in man. Proc Natl Acad Sci USA 80:6041–6045
6. Metlay JP, Puré E, Steinman RM (1989) Control of the immune response at the level of antigen-presenting cells: a comparison of the function of dendritic cells and B lymphocytes. Adv Immunol 47:45–116
7. Stuart JM, Cremer MA, Townes AS, Kang AH (1982) Type-II-collagen-induced arthritis in rats. Passive transfer with serum and evidence that IgG anti-collagen antibodies can cause arthritis. J Exp Med 155:1–16
8. Stuart JM, Dixon FJ (1983) Serum transfer of collagen-induced arthritis in mice. J Exp Med 158:378–392
9. Stuart JM, Tomoda K, Yoo TJ, Townes AS, Kang AH (1983) Serum transfer of collagen-induced arthritis. II. Identification and localization of autoantibody to type II collagen in donor and recipient rats. Arthritis Rheum 26:1237–1244
10. Jonsson R, Karlsson AL, Holmdahl R (1989) Demonstration of immune-reactive sites on cartilage after in vivo administration of biotinylated anti-type II collagen antibodies. J Histochem Cytochem 37:265–268

11. Holmdahl R, Mo J, Jonsson R, Karlström K, Scheynius A (1991) Multiple epitopes on cartilage type II collagen are accesible for antibody binding in vivo. Autoimmunity (in press)
12. Stastny P (1978) Association of the B-cell alloantigen DRw4 with rheumatoid arthritis. N Engl J Med (1978) 298:869–871
13. Gregersen PK, Shen M, Song Q, Merryman P, Dagar S, Seki T, Maccari J, Goldberg D, Murphy H, Schwenzer J, Wang CY, Winchester RJ, Nepom GT, Silver J (1986) Molecular diversity of HLA-DR4 haplotypes. Proc Natil Acad Sci USA 83:2642–2646
14. Gregersen PK, Silver J, Wincester RJ (1987) The shared epitope hypothesis. An approach to understanding the molecular genetics of susceptibility to rheumatoid arthritis. Arthritis Rheum 30:1205–1213
15. Nepom GT, Byers P, Seyfried C, Healey LA, Wilske KR, Stage D, Nepom BS (1989) HLA genes associated with rheumatoid arthritis. Identification of susceptibility alleles using specific oligonucleotide probes. Arthritis Rheum 32:15–21
16. Brown JH, Jardetzky T, Saper MA, Samraoui B, Bjorkman PJ, Wiley DC (1988) A hypothetical model of the foreign antigen-binding site of class-II histocompatibility molecules. Nature 332:845–850
17. Howell WM, Evans PR, Wilson PJ, Cawley MID, Smith JL (1989) HLA class-II DR, DQ, and DP restriction fragment length polymorphisms in rheumatoid arthritis. Ann Rheum Dis 48:295–301
18. Burmester GR, Yu DTY, Irani AM, Kunkel HG, Winchester RJ (1981) Ia+ T cells in synovial fluid and tissue of patients with rheumatoid arthritis. Arthritis Rheum 24:1370–1376
19. Burmester GR, Jahn B, Gramatzki M, Zacher J, Kalden JR (1984) Activated T cells in vitro and in vivo: divergence in expression of Tac and Ia antigens in the nonblastoid small T cells of inflammation and normal T cells activated in vitro. J Immunol 133:1230–1234
20. Janossy G, Panai G, Duke O, Bofill M, Poulter LW, Goldstein G (1981) Rheumatoid arthritis: a disease of T lymphocyte/macrophage immunoregulation. Lancet 2:839–843
21. Klareskog L, Forsum U, Scheynius A, Kabelitz D, Wigzell H (1982) Evidence in support of a self-perpetuating HLA-DR dependent delayed-type hypersensitivity reaction in rheumatid arthritis. Proc Natl Acad Sci USA 79:3632–3636
22. Scher MG, Beller DI, Unanue ER (1980) Demonstration of a soluble mediator that induces exudates rich in Ia-positive macrophages. J Exp Med 152:1684–1698
23 Mosmann TR, Coffman RL (1989) TH1 and TH2 cells: different patterns of lymphokine secretion lead to different functional properties. Annu Rev Immunol 7:145–173
24. Husby G, Williams RC (1985) Immunohistochemical studies of interleukin-2 and gamma-interferon in rheumatoid arthritis. Arthritis Rheum 28:174–181
25. Buchan G, Barrett K, Fujita T, Taniguchi T, Maini R, Feldmann M (1988) Detection of activated T cell products in the rheumatoid joint using cDNA probes to interleukin-2 (IL-2),IL-2 receptor and IFN-gamma. Clin Exp Immunol 71:295–301
26. Zvaifler NJ (1973) The immunopathology of joint inflammation in rheumatoid arthritis. Adv Immunol 16:265–336
27. Carson DA, Chen PP, Fox RI, Kipps TJ, Jirik F, Goldfien RD, Silverman G, Radoux V, Fong S (1987) Rheumatoid factor and immune networks. Annu Rev Immunol 5:109–126
28. Nemazee DA (1985) Immune complexes can trigger specific T-cell-dependent, autoanti-IgG antibody production in mice. J Exp Med 161:242–256
29. Stamenkovic I, Stegano M, Wright KA, Krane SM, Amento EP, Colvin RB, Duquesnoy RJ, Kurnick JT (1988) Clonal dominance among T-lymphocyte infiltrates in arthritis. Proc Natl Acad Sci USA 85:1179–1183
30. Schluesener HJ, Wekerle H (1985) Autoaggressive T lymphocyte lines recognizing the encephalitogenic region of myelin basic protein: in vitro selection from unprimed T lymphocyte populations. J Immunol 135:3128–3133
31. Trentham DE, Townes AS, Kang AH (1977) Autoimmunity to type II collagen: an experimental model of arthritis. J Exp Med 146:857–868

32. Morgan K, Evans HB, Firth SA, Smith MN, Ayad S, Weiss JB, Holt PJL (1983) 1-alpha, 2-alpha, 3-alpha collagen is arthritogenic. Ann Rheum Dis 42:680–683
33. Glant TT, Mikecz K, Arzoumanian A, Poole AR (1987) Proteoglycan-induced arthritis in Balb/c mice. Arthritis Rheum 30:201–212
34. Courtenay JS, Dallman MJ, Dayan AD, Martin A, Mosedal B (1980) Immunization against heterologous type II collagen induces arthritis in mice. Nature 283:666–667
35. Yoo TJ, Kim SY, Stuart JM, Floyd RA, Olson GA, Cremer MA, Kang AH (1988) Induction of arthritis in monkeys by immunization with type II collagen. J Exp Med 168:777–782
36. Wooley PH, Luthra HS, Stuart JM, David CS (1981) Type II collagen induced arthritis in mice. I. Major histocompatibility complex (I-region) linkage and antibody correlates. J Exp Med 154:688–700
37. Wooley PH, Luthra HS, Griffiths MM, Stuart JM, Huse A, David CS (1985) Type II collagen induced arthritis in mice. IV. Variations in immunogenetic regulation provide evidence for multiple arthritogenic epitopes on the collagen molecule. J Immunol 135:2443–2451
38. Holmdahl R, Klareskog L, Andersson M, Hansen C (1986) High antibody response to autologous type II collagen is restricted to H-2q. Immunogenetics 24:84–89
39. Holmdahl R, Jansson L, Andersson M, Larsson E (1988) Immunogenetics of type II collagen autoimmunity and susceptibility to collagen arthritis. Immunology 65:305–310
40. Holmdahl R, Karlsson M, Andersson ME, Rask L, Andersson L (1989) Localization of a critical restriction site on the I-A-beta chain which determines susceptibility to collagen-induced arthritis. Proc Natl Acad Sci USA 86:9475–9479
41. Gustafsson K, KarlssonM, Andersson L, Holmdahl R (1990) Structures on the I-A molecule which predisposes for susceptibiity to collagen-induced arthritis and for type II collagen autoimmune response. Eur J Immunol 20:2127–2131
42. Holmdahl R, Jansson L, Larsson E, Rubin K, Klareskog L (1986) Homologous type II collagen induces chronic and progressive arthritis in mice. Arthritis Rheum 29:106–113
43. Trentham DE (1982) Collagen arthritis as a relevant model for rheumatoid arthritis. Evidence pro and con. Arthritis Rheum 25:911–916
44. Holmdahl R (1988) Collagen-induced arthritis , Int Rev Immunol Vol 4 Harwood, New York
45. Holmdahl R, Andersson ME, Goldschmidt TJ, Gustafsson K, Jansson L, Mo J (1990) Type II collagen autoimmunity in animals and provocations leading to arthritis. Immunol Rev 118:193–232
46. Kresina TF, Moskowitz RW (1985) Adoptive transfer of suppression of arthritis in the mouse model of collagen-induced arthritis. J Clin Invest 75:1990–1998
47. Englert M, McReynolds RA, Landes MJ, Oronsky AL, Kerwar SS (1985) Pretreatment of rats with anticollagen IgG renders them resistant to active type II collagen arthritis. Cell Immunol 90:258–266
48. Larsson P, Kleinau S, Holmdahl R, Klareskog L (1990) Autologous collagen-II-inducd arthritis in rats. Demonstration of clinically distinct forms of arthritis in two strains of rats. Arthritis Rheum (in press)
49. Andersson M, Holmdahl R (1990) Analysis of type II collagen-reactive T cells in the mouse. I. Different regulation of autoreactie versus non-autoreactive anti-C II T cells in the DBA/1 mouse. Eur J Immunol 20:1061–1066
50. Holmdahl R, Andersson M, Tarkowski A (1987) Origin of the autoreactive anti-type II collagen response. I. Frequency of specific and multispecific B cells in primed murine lymph nodes. Immunology 61:369–374
51. Holmdahl R, Bailey C, Enander I, Mayer R, Klareskog L, Moran T, Bona C (1989) Origin of the autoreactive anti-type II collagen response. II. Specificities, isotypes and usage of V gene families of anti-type II collagen autoantibodies. J Immunol 142:1881–1886
52. Klareskog L, Holmdahl R, Larsson E, Wigzell H (1983) Role of lymphocytes in collagen-II-induced arthritis in rats. Clin Exp Immunol 51:117–125

53. Brahn E, Trentham DE (1984) Effect of antithymocyte serum on collagen arthritis in rats: evidence that T cells are involved in its pathogenesis. Cell Immunol 86:421–428
54. Ranges GE, Sriram S, Cooper SM (985) Prevention of type II collagen-induced arthritis by in vivo treatment with anti-L3T4. J Exp Med 162:1105–1110
55. Holmdahl R, Jonsson R, Larsson P, Klareskog L (1988) Early appearance of activated CD4 positive T lymphocytes and Ia-expressing cells in joints of DBA/1 mice immunized with type II collagen. Lab Invest 58:53–60
56. Holmdahl R, Tarkowski A, Jonsson R (1991) Involvement of macrophages and dendritic cells in synovial inflammation of collagen-induced arthritis in DBA/1 mice and spontaneous arthritis in MRL/lpr mice. Autoimmunity (in press)
57. Mauritz NJ, Holmdahl R, Jonsson R, Van Der Meide P, Scheynius A, Klareskog L (1988) Treatment with interferon-gamma triggers onset of collagen arthritis in mice. Arthritis Rheum 31:1297–1304
58. Caulfield JP, Hein A, Dynesius-Trentham R, Trentham DE (1982) Morphological demonstration of two stages in the development of type II collagen-induced arthritis. Lab Invest 46:321–343
59. Kerwar SS, Englert ME, McReynolds RA, Landes MJ, Lloyd JM, Oronsky AL, Wilson FJ (1983) Type II collagen-induced arthritis. Studies with purified anticollagen immunoglobulin. Arthritis Rheum 26:1120–1131
60. Holmdahl R, Jansson L, Larsson A, Jonsson R (1990) Arthritis in DBA/1 mice induced with passively transferred type II collagen immune serum. Immunohistopathology and serum levels of anti-type II collagen autoantibodies. Scand J Immunol 31:147–157
61. Steffen C, Ludwig H, Knapp W (1974) Collagen-anticollagen immune complexes in rheumatoid arthritis synovial fluid cells. Z Immuni Aaetsforsch 147:229–235
62. Menzel J, Steffen C (1982) Demonstration of C1q – binding to collagen-anticollagen immune complexes in synovial fluids of RA patients. Z Rheumatol 41:47–49
63. Michaeli D, Fudenberg HH (1974) The incidence and antigenic specificity of antibodies against denatured human collagen in rheumatoid arthritis. Clin Immunol Immunopathol 2:153–159
64. Andriopoulos NA, Mestecky J, Miller EJ, Bradley EL (1976) Antibodies to native and denatured collagens in sera of patients with rheumatoid arthritis. Arthritis Rheum 19:613–617
65. Stuart JM, Huffstutter EH, Townes AS, Kang AH (1983) Incidence and specificity of antibodies to types I, II, III, IV, and V collagen in rheumatoid arthritis and other rheumatoid diseases as measured by ^{125}I-radioimmunoassay. Arthritis Rheum 26:832–840
66. Morgan K, Clague RB, Collins I, Ayad S, Phinn SD, Holt PJL (1987) Incidence of antibodies to native and denatured cartilage collagens (type II, IX, and XI) and to type I collagen in rheumatoid arthritis. Ann Rheum Dis 46:902–907
67. Fuchs S, Mozes E, Maoz A, Sela M (1974) Thymus independence of a collagen-like synthetic polypeptide and of collagen, and the need for thymus and bone marrow-cell cooperation in the immune response to gelatin. J Exp Med 139:148–158
68. Nowack H, Hahn E, Timpl R (1975) Specificity of the antibody response in inbred mice to bovine type I and type II collagen. Immunol 29:621–628
69. Hahn E, Nowack H, Götze D, Timpl R (1975) H-2 linked genetic control of antibody response to soluble calfskin collagen in mice. Eur J Immunol 5:288–291
70. Hahn E, Timpl R, Miller EJ (1974) The production of specific antibodies to native collagens with the chain compositions, [alpha1(I))]3, [alpha1(II)3], and [alpha1(I)-2alpha2. J Immunol 113:421–423
71. Kemp JD, Madri JA (1981) The immune response to human type II and type V (AB2) collagen: antigenic determinants and genetic control in mice. Eur J Immunol 11:90–94
72. Beard HK, Ueda M, Faulk WP, Glynn LE (1978) Cell-mediated and humoral immunity to chick type II collagen and its cyanogen bromide peptides in guinea pigs. Immunology 34:323–334
73. Ellingsworth LR, DeLustro F, Brennan JE, Sawamura S, McPherson J (1986) The human immune response to reconstituted bovine collagen. J Immmunol 136:877–882

74. Choi EKK, Gatenby PA, McGill NW, Bateman JF, Cole WG, York JR (1988) Autoantibodies to type II collagen: occurrence in rheumatoid arthritis, other arthritides, autoimmune connective tissue diseases, and chronic inflammatory syndromes. Ann Rheum Dis 47:313–322
75. Cheung HS, Ryan LM, Kozin F, McCarty DJ (1980) Identification of collagen subtypes in synovial fluid sediments from arthritic patients. Am J Med 68:73–79
76. Kitridou R, McCarty DJ, Prockop DJ, Hummeler K (1969) Identification of collagen in synovial fluid. Arthritis Rheum 12:580–588
77. Wozniczko-Orlowska G, Milgrom F (1982) Collagen-anti-collagen complexes in rheumatoid arthritis sera. Int Arch Allergy Appl Immunol 68:28–34
78. Rowley MJ, Williamson DJ, Mackay IR (1987) Evidence for local synthesis of antibodies to denatured collagen in the synovium in rheumatoid arthritis. Arthritis Rheum 30:1420–1425
79. Stockman A, Rowley MJ, Emery P, Muirden KD (1989) Activity of rheumatoid arthritis and levels of collagen antibodies: a prospective study. Rheumatol Int 8:239–243
80. Goodnow CC, Crosbie J, Jorgensen H, Brink RA, Basten A (1989) Induction of self-tolerance in mature peripheral B lymphocytes. Nature 342:385–391
81. Nemazee D, Buerki K (1989) Clonal deletion of autoreactive B lymphocytes in bonemarrow chimeras. Proc Natl Acad Sci USA 86:8039–8043
82. Clague RB, Firth SA, Holt PJL, Skingle J, Greenbury CL, Webley M (1983) Serum antibodies to type II collagen in rheumatoid arthritis: comparison of 6 immunological methods and clinical features. Ann Rheum Dis 42:537–544
83. Alomari WRS, Archer JR, Brocklehurst R, Currey HLF (1983) Binding of immunoglobulins and immune complexes to cartilage-derived extracts. Clin Exp Immunol 54:716–722
84. Rosenberg AM, Hunt WC, Petty RE (1984) Antibodies to native and denatured type II collagen in children with rheumatic diseases. J Rheumatol 11:425–431
85. Kirk AP, O'Hara BP, Mageed RAK, McMahon MS, McCarthy D, Menashi S, Archer JR, Currey HLF. Pepsinogen – an immunoglobulin-binding artefact in collagen preparations. Clin Exp Immunol 65:671–678
86. Greenbury CL, Skingle J (1979) Anti-cartilage antibody. J Clin Pathol 32:826–831
87. Beard HK, Ryvar R, Skingle J, Greenbury CL (1980) Anti-collagen antibodies in sera from rheumatoid arthritis patients. J Clin Pathol 33:1077–1081
88. Dyer PA, Clague RB, Klouda PT, Firth S, Harris R, Holt PJL (1982) HLA antigens in patients with rheumatoid arthritis and antibodies to native type II collagen. Tissue Antigens 20:394–396
89. Gioud M, Meghlaoui A, Costa O, Monier JC (1982) Antibodies to native type I and type II collagens detected by an enzyme-linked immunosorbent assay (ELISA) in rheumatoid arthritis and systemic lupus erythematosus. Coll Relat Res 2:557–564
90. Pereira RS, Black CM, Duance VC, Jones VE, Jacoby RK, Welsh KI (1985) Disappearing collagen antibodies in rheumatoid arthritis. Lancet 2:501–502
91. Watson WC, Cremer MA, Wooley PH, Townes AS (1986) Assessment of the potential pathogenicity of type II collagen autoantibodies in patients with rheumatoid arthritis. Evidence of restricted IgG3 subclass expression and activation of complement C5 to C5a. Arthritis Rheum 29:1316–1321
92. Morgan K, Clague RB, Collins I, Ayad S, Phinn SD, Holt PJL (1989) A longitudinal study of anticollagen antibodies in patients with rheumatoid arthritis. Arthritis Rheum 32:139–145
93. Foidart JM, ABe S, Martin GR, Zizic TM, Barnett EV, Lawley TJ, Katz SI (1978) Antibodies to type II collagen in relapsing polychondritis. N Engl J Med 299:1203–1207
94. Clague RB, Shaw MJ, Holt PJL (1980) Incidence of serum antibodies to native type I and type II collagens in patients with inflammatory arthritis. Ann Rheum Dis 39:201–206
95. Morgan K, Buckee C, Collins I, Ayad S, Clague RB, Holt PJL (1988) Antibodies to type II and type XI collagens: evidence for the formation of antigen-specific as well as

cross-reacting antibodies in patients with rheumatoid arthritis. Ann Rheum Dis 47:1008–1013
96. Clague RB, Morre LJ (1984) IgG and IgM antibody to native type II collagen in rheumatoid arthritis serum and synovial fluid. Arthritis Rheum 27:1370–1377
97. Klimiuk PS, Clague RB, Grennan DM, Dyer PA, Smeaton I, Harris R (1985) Autoimmunity to native type II collagen – a distinct genetic subset of rheumatoid arthritis. J Rheumatol 12:865–870
98. Sanders PA, Grennan DM, Klimiuk PS, Clague RB, de Lange CG, Collins I, Dyer PA (1987) Gm allotypes and HLA in rheumatoid arthritis patients with circulating antibodies to native type II collagen. Ann Rheum Dis 46:391–394
99. Collins I, Morgan K, Clague RB, Brenchley PEC, Holt PJL (1988) IgG subclass distribution of anti-native type II collagen and anti-denatured type II collagen antibodies in patients with rheumatoid arthritis. J Rheumatol 15:770–774
100. Möttönen T, Hannonen P, Oka M, Rautiainen J, Jokinen I, Arvilommi H, Palosuo T, Aho K (1988) Antibodies against native type II collagen do not precede the clinical onset of rheumatoid arthritis. Arthritis Rheum 31:776–779
101. Banerjee S, Luthra HS, Moore SB, O'Fallon WM (1988) Serum IgG anti-native type II collagen antibodies in rheumatoid arthritis: association with HLA DR4 and lack of clinical correlation. Clin Exp Rheumatol 6:373–380
102. Tarkowski A, Klareskog L, Carlsten H, Herberts P, Koopman WJ (1989) Secretion of antibodies to types I and II collagen by synovial tissue cells in patients with rheumatoid arthritis. Arthritis Rheum 32:1087–1092
103. Klareskog L, Holmdahl R, Rubin K (1987) Binding of collagen type II to rheumatoid synovial cells. Scand J Immunol 24:705–714
104. Wooley PH, Luthra HS, Huse AR, Stuart JM, David CS (1984) Passive transfer of arthritis to mice by injection of human anti-type II collagne antibody. Mayo Clin Proc 59:737–743
105. Wooley PH, Luthra HS, Krco CJ, Stuart JM, David CS (1984) Type II collagen induced arthritis in mice. II. Passive transfer and suppression by intravenous injection of anti-type II collagen antibody of free native type II collagen. Arthritis Rheum 27:1010–1017
106. Holmdahl R, Rubin K, Klareskog L, Larsson E, Wigzell H (1986) Characterization of the antibody response in mice with type II collagen-induced arthritis, using monoclonal anti-type II collagen antibodies. Arthritis Rheum 29:400–410
107. Holmdahl R, Tarkowski A, Nordling C, Rubin K, Klareskog L (1987) Connection between autoimmunity to cartilage type II collagen and rheumatoid factor production. Monogr Allergy 22:71–80
108. Holmdahl R, Nordling C, Rubin K, Tarkowski A, Klareskog L (1986) Generation of monoclonal rheumatoid factors after immunization with collagen II –anti-collagen II immune complexes. Scand J Immunol 24:197–203
109. Heinz HP, Rubin K, Laurell AB, Loos M (1989) Common epitopes in C1q and collagen type II. Mol Immunol 26:163–169
110. Rolink AG, Radaszkiewicz T, Melchers F (1987) The autoantigen-binding B-cell repertoires of normal and of chronically graft- versus host- diseased mice. J Exp Med 165:1675–1687
111. Portnoi D, Freitas A, Holmberg D, Bandeira A, Coutinho A (1986) Immunocompetent autoreactive B lymphocytes are activated cycling cells in normal mice. J Exp Med 164:25–35
112. Jasin HE (1985) Autoantibody specificities of immune complexes sequestered in articular cartilage of patients with rheumatoid arthritis and osteoarthritis. Arthritis Rheum 28:241–248
113. Trentham DE, Dynesius RA, Rocklin RE, David JR (1978) Cellular sensitivity to collagen in rheumatoid arthritis. N Engl J Med 299:327–332
114. Stuart JM, Postlethwaite AE, Townes AS, Kang AH (1980) Cell-mediated immunity to collagen and collagen alpha-chains in rheumatoid arthritis and other rheumatic diseases. Am J Med 69:13–18

115. Solinger AM, Bhatnagar R, Stobo JD (1981) Cellular, molecular, and genetic characteristics of T cell reactivity to collagen in man. Proc Natl Acad Sci USA 78:3877–3881
116. Trentham DE, Kammer GM, McCune WJ, David JR (1981) Autoimmunity to collagen. A shared feature of psoriatic and rheumatoid arthritis. Arthritis Rheum 24:1363–1369
117. Kammer GM, Trentham DE (1984) HLA-DR4 is not a requisite for autoimmunity to collagen in rheumatoid arthritis. Arthritis Rheum 27:489–494
118. Vullo CM, Pesoa SA, Onetti CM, Riera CM (1987) Rheumatoid arthritis and its association with HLA-DR antigens. I. Cell-mediated immune response against connective tissue antigens. J Rheumatol 14:221–225
119. Golds EE, Stephen IBM, Esdaile JM, Strawczynski Strawczynski, Poole AR (1983) Lymphocyte transformation to connective tissue antigens in adult and juvenile rheumatoid arthritis, osteoarthritis, ankylosing spondylitis, systemic lupus erythematosus, and a non-arthritic control population. Cell Immunol 82:196–209
120. Londei M, Savill CM, Verhoef A, Brennan F, Leech ZA, Duance V, Maini RN, Feldmann M (1989) Persistence of collagen type-II-specific T-cell clones in the synovial membrane of a patient with rheumatoid arthritis. Proc Natl Acad Sci USA 86:636–640
121. Ström H, Al-Balaghi S, Möller E (1984) No demonstrable association between HLA DR4 and in vitro collagen reactivity as determined by the production of leukocyte inhibition factor. Tissue Antigens 24:174–183
122. Rowley M, Tait B, Mackay IR, Cunningham T, Phillips B (1986) Collagen antibodies in rheumatoid arthritis. Significance of antibodies to denatured collagen and their association with HLA-DR4. Arthritis Rheum 29:174–184
123. Mikecz K, Glant TT, Baron M, Poole AR (1988) Isolation of proteoglycan-specific T lymphocytes from patients with ankylosing spondylitis. Cell Immunol 112:55–63A
124. Poulter LW, Duke O, Hobbs S, Janossy G, Panayi G (1982) Histochemical discrimination of HLA-DR-positive cell populations in the normal and arthritic synovial lining. Clin Exp Immunol 48:381–388
125. Klareskog L, Holmdahl R, Rubin K, Victorin Å (1985) Different populations of rheumatoid adherent cells mediate activation versus suppression of T lymphocyte proliferation. Arthritis Rheum 28:863–872
126. Janeway CA, Ron Y, Katz ME (1987) The B cell is the initiating antigen-presenting cell in peripheral lymph nodes. J Immunol 138:1051–1055
127. Schwartz R (1989) Acquisition of immunological self-tolerance. Cell 57:1073–1081
128. Trentham DE, McCune JW, Susman P, David JR (1980) Autoimmunity to collagen in adjuvant arthritis of rats. J Clin Invest 66:1109–1117
129. Trentham DE, Dynesius-Trentham RA (1983) Attenuation of an adjuvant arthritis by type II collagen. J Immunol 130:2689–2692
130. Petty RE, Johnston W, McCormick AQ, Hunt DWC, Rootman J, Rollins DF (1989) Uveitis and arthritis induced by adjuvant: clinical, immunologic and histologic characteristics. J Rheumatol 16:499–505
131. Goto M, Yoshinoya S, Miyamoto T, Sasano M, Okamoto M, Nishioka K, Terato K, Nagai Y (1988) Stimulation of interleukin-1-alpha and interleukin-1-beta release from human monocytes by cyanogen bromide peptides of type II collagen. Arthritis Rheum 31:1508–1514
132. Kunken HG, Posnett DN, Pernis B (1983) Anti-immunoglobulins and their idiotypes: are they part of the immune network? Ann N Y Acad Sci 418:324–329
133. Wolf B, Bashey RI, Newton CD, Jimenez SA (1986) Development of rheumatoid factors and anti-F(ab)2 antibodies in guinea pigs immunized with type II collagen. Int Arch Allergy Appl Immunol 80:214–220
134. White J, Herman A, Pullen AM, Kubo R, Kappler JW, Marrack P (1989) The V beta-specific superantigen staphylococcal enterotoxin B: stimulation of mature T cells and clonal deletion in neonatal mice. Cell 56:27–35
135. Cole BC, David CS, Lynch DH, Kartchner DR (1990) The use of transfected fibroblast and transgenic mice establishes that stimulation of T cells by the *Mycoplasma arthritidis* mitogen is mediated by E-alpha. J Immunol 144:420–424

136. Cole BC, Kartchner DR, Wells DJ (1990) Stimulation of mouse lymphocytes by a mitogen derived from *Mycoplasma arthritidis* (MAM). VIII. Selective activation of T cells expressing V-beta T cell receptors from various strains of mice by the "superantigen" MAM. J Immunol 144:425–431
137. Cole BC, Ward JR, Jones RS, Cahill JF (1971) Chronic proliferative arthritis of mice induced by *Mycoplasma arthritidis*. I. Induction of disease and histopathologic characteristics. Infect Immun 4:344–355
138. Banerjee S, Haqqi TM, Luthra HS, Stuart JM, David CS (1988) Possible role of V-beta T-cell receptor genes in susceptibility to collagen-induced arthritis in mice. J Exp Med 167:832–839
139. Fujita M, Mishima M, Iwabuchi K, Katsume C, Gotohda T, Ogasawara K, Mizuno Y, Good RA, Onoe K (1989) A study of type II collagen-induced arthritis in allogeneic bone marrow chimaeras. Immunology 66:422–427
140. Goldschmidt T, Holmdahl R, Klareskog L (1988) Depletion of murine T cells by in vivo monoclonal antibody treatment is enhanced by adding an autologous anti-rat kappa chain antibody. J Immunol Methods 111:219–226
141. Acha-Orbea H, Mitchell DJ, Timmerman L, Wraith DC, Tausch GS, Waldor MK, Zamvil SS, McDevitt HO, Steinman L (1988) Limited heterogeneity of T-cell receptors from lymphocytes mediating autoimmune encephalomyelitis allows specific intervention. Cell 54:263–273
142. Klareskog L, Johnell O, Hulth A, Holmdahl R, Rubin K (1986) Reactivity of monoclonal anti-type II collagen antibodies with cartilage and synovial tissue in rheumatoid arthritis and osteoarthritis. Arthritis Rheum 29:730–738
143. Moreland LW, Stewart T, Gay R, Huang GQ, McGee N, Gay S (1989) Immunohistological demonstration of type-II collagen in synovial fluid phagocytes of osteoarthritis and rheumatoid arthritis patients. Arthritis Rheum 32:1458–1464
144. Kappler JW, Staerz U, White J, Marrac PC (1988) Self-tolerance eliminates T cells specific for Mls-modified products of the major histocompatibility comlex. Nature 332:35–40
145. Rammensee HG, Kroschewski R, Frangoulis B (1989) Clonal anergy induced in mature Vbeta 6 T lymphocytes on immunizing Mls-1 b mice with Mls-1 a-expressing cells. Nature 339:541–544
146. McDonald HR (1989) T-cell repertoire selection during development. Curr Opinion Immunol 2:199–203

Streptococcal Cell Wall Antigens and Rheumatoid Arthritis

L. J. Crofford and R. L. Wilder

Arthritis and Rheumatism Branch, National Institute of Arthritis and Musculoskeletal and Skin Diseases, National Institutes of Health, Building 10, Room 9N240, Bethesda, Maryland 20892, USA

Introduction

Although detailed mechanistic questions still remain, Group A streptococci are the established causative agents of rheumatic fever and poststreptococcal reactive arthritis [4, 14, 18]. The possibility exists that streptococcal or related bacterial antigens are the etiologic agents in some cases of adult or juvenile forms of rheumatoid arthritis. Indeed, a large body of data in support of this hypothesis demonstrates that cell walls from selected types of streptococci and other bacteria are potent inducers of experimental rheumatoid arthritis-like disease in certain strains of rats [11, 58, 59, 60, 62, 64]. Additional data link streptococcal cell wall proteins and related bacterial substances to rheumatoid factor production [9, 32, 42, 58]. Accordingly, this review will summarize some of the more recent information on these issues.

Streptococcal Cell Wall Arthritis in Rats

A single aqueous intraperitoneal injection of group A streptococcal cell wall fragments (SCW; specifically, the peptidoglycan-group-specific polysaccharide) into a susceptible rat induces a highly reproducible model of proliferative and erosive synovitis that resembles juvenile and adult rheumatoid arthritis (RA) [11, 58–61]. This animal model has provided important insights into potential etiologic mechanisms, pathogenesis, and therapy of inflammatory arthritis in humans.

Smolen, Kalden, Maini (Eds.)
Rheumatoid Arthritis
© Springer-Verlag Berlin Heidelberg 1992

Clinical and Histological Features

Injection of SCW into susceptible female inbred rats, such as Lewis rats, induces acute arthritis within 24 h. This rapid onset, clinically apparent disease is characterized by swelling and erythema. The wrists and ankles are most frequently involved, but other peripheral joints may be affected. The axial skeleton is spared, as is typical of RA in humans. The acute arthritis reaches maximum severity in about 3 days and then decreases, but is followed by an exacerbation of joint swelling, 14–28 days after cell wall injection, that persists for months. This later chronic phase exhibits a waxing and waning course and eventually results in deformity and functional impairment of the most severely affected joints [20, 64, 65, 67].

Other clinical manifestations of SCW arthritis include splenomegaly and a chronic microcytic anemia with decreased red cell survival. Serum iron and transferrin levels are depressed, but stainable iron in the liver, spleen, and mesenteric lymph nodes increases above normal [41]. In other words, this anemia is quite similar to the anemia of chronic disease that is a characteristic feature of most patients with long-standing RA. In addition, immunologic testing characteristically reveals defective cell mediated immunity which is very similar to the immunodeficiency commonly noted in patients with RA, particularly those with severe disease [35, 39, 69]. This will be further discussed below.

On histologic examination of the joints, the earliest changes during the development of the acute phase disease include swollen synovial microvascular endothelial cells consistent with cell activation/injury. Blood vessel lumens are frequently obliterated by platelet and fibrin thrombi. A perivascular mononuclear and polymorphonuclear cell infiltrate appears concomitantly that is most prominent around histologically abnormal blood vessels [20, 64, 67]. These endothelial cells are usually intensely positive when immunostained for markers of activation, e. g., class II antigen expression develops rapidly and persists [64]. Interstitial edema is also a prominent feature of the acute inflammatory process. Mild synovial lining cell layer thickening develops concomitantly with the appearance of fibrin and polymorphonuclear phagocytic cell-rich exudate in the joint cavity. Pronounced hyperplasia of subchondral bone marrow cells also develops early with an increased ratio of myeloid to erythoid cell precursors [8, 19, 40, 67].

The chronic phase of arthritis that is superimposed on the early developing but persistent microvascular activation/injury is characterized by pronounced thickening of the synovial lining with villus formation and diffuse and nodular lymphocytic infiltration consisting predominantly of the CD4+ T cell subset [2]. Exuberant proliferation of synovial stromal fibroblast-like cells and blood vessels (angiogenesis) is also a characteristic feature of this phase of disease [2, 8, 40, 68]. This highly proliferative inflammatory tissue is "tumor-like" in that it invasively destroys juxtaposed cartilage and bone. Cartilage loss is also evident at sites not immediately adjacent to the invasive synovium. Loss of bone also develops as an apparent result of increased osteoclastic activity in the periarticular subchondral bone. Thus, joint destruction appears to proceed by three separate but related pathways: (1) proliferative and invasive synovial resorption of marginal bone and cartilage of the joint, (2) increased degradation of cartilage matrix by chondrocytes themselves, and (3) increased osteoclastic activity in the subchondral bone. The ultimate result is fibrous ankylosis of the severely involved joints [8, 20, 64, 65, 67, 68].

Other histopathologic changes may include hepatic and splenic granuloma formation, leukocytosis, thymic atrophy, and occasional, mild, transient anterior uveitis. The inflammatory changes in other organs tend to parallel the severity of inflammation of the joints [2, 56, 57, 65].

Radiologic examination during the rapid onset, acute phase reveals soft tissue swelling and periarticular osteoporosis. As the chronic arthritis is superimposed on the microvascular activation/injury of the acute phase, radiologically apparent joint space narrowing and marginal erosions begin to appear. New bone formation is not apparent unless secondary degenerative disease develops [10, 20].

The major clinical differences between SCW arthritis in the Lewis female rat and human RA are: (a) the rapid progression and telescoped course of disease in the rat as compared with the long natural history in human disease; (b) low titer rheumatoid factor (RF) in the rat as opposed to high titer RF, with 80% incidence in human RA and absence of anti-collagen antibodies in the rat; (c) the development of hepatic granulomas in some inbred strains of rats; and (d) the lack of rheumatoid nodules in the rat model [58, 61]. While the clinical features of SCW induced arthritis in the Lewis rat do not exactly mimic all the clinical features of human RA, it provides a well-characterized reproducible model of erosive and proliferative synovitis that has advanced our understanding of potential pathogenic mechanisms in humans.

Inflammatory Stimulus

As noted above, the arthritogenic SCW are comprised of a complex heteropolymer containing peptidoglycan and a group-specific carbohydrate side chain. The rhamnose-rich side chain appears to protect the peptidoglycan from in vivo cleavage by lysozyme [44]. Resistance to degradation allows these proinflammatory agents to persist in vivo for weeks to months, i.e., small fragments ($<5\times10^6$ kDa) induce rapid onset transient disease, while large fragments ($>500\times10^6$ kDa) induce slow onset persistent disease [58, 61]. The carbohydrate moieties may act as an antigen [16]. It should be noted that the smallest biologically active subunit of the bacterial peptidoglycan is muramyl dipeptide. Muramyl dipeptides are adjuvant active substances with multiple proinflammatory properties, including a capacity to directly activate macrophages, endothelial cells, and B cells. SCW directly stimulates cell activation

[35, 58]. SCW also induces mast cell degranulation and localized edema when injected intravenously [12].

Following systemic injection of SCW into Lewis female rats, the fragments localize to endothelial and phagocytic inflammatory cells in the synovium, subchondral bone marrow, liver, and spleen [2, 3, 64]. These events are accompanied by activation of the complement cascade during the early evolution of the disease and persistent endothelial cell and macrophage activation throughout the course of the disease. Activated cells markedly amplify the intensity of joint destruction, in part by enhancing the release of cytokines and other proinflammatory substances in the joint [24, 38, 43, 64, 67].

Efforts to delineate specific antigenic epitopes in SCW have not been conclusive, but T cell lines reactive with SCW have been generated. Of importance, these T cell lines are capable of inducing arthritis in naive recipient Lewis rats, i. e., Lewis rats that have never been injected with SCW. These data suggest that antigenic epitopes present on the SCW are also expressed by host tissues, i. e., molecular mimicry. As discussed further below, one group of workers has suggested that 65 kDa heat shock proteins may be antigenically involved in the molecular mimicry [52], but this hypothesis is controversial since heat shock proteins are not a necessary component of arthritogenic cell walls and T cell lines that transfer disease have not shown reactivity with the 65 kDa heat shock protein [16]. This subject is still under active investigation.

Because of the cross-reactivity between the M protein of streptococci and cardiac and skeletal myosin and tropomyosin as well as renal glomeruli, M protein has been implicated in the development of autoimmune diseases such as rheumatic fever and poststreptococcal acute glomerulonephritis [15]. However, recent work has shown that SCW from both M+ and M− strains of Group A streptococci induce both acute and chronic arthritis, and there is no difference in the diseases [15]. The authors concluded that M protein is not critical in the pathogenesis of SCW arthritis in Lewis rats.

Genetics

Inbred strains of rats vary tremendously in their susceptibility to SCW arthritis, from 100% incidence with severe disease to no observable arthritis [1, 61, 66]. The Lewis female rat is the most susceptible to the injection of SCW. This rat strain is also susceptible to a wide array of other inflammatory autoimmune diseases including collagen arthritis [23], experimental autoimmune encephalomyelitis (EAE) [55], experimental autoimmune myasthenia gravis [5, 70], experimental autoimmune orchitis [49], experimental autoimmune oophoritis [13], experimental autoimmune hepatitis [29], experimental autoimmune uveitis [17], and experimental diabetes mellitus [71]. This strain is also highly susceptible to various infectious diseases, including Lyme arthritis [31], arthritis in response to *Erysipelothrix rhusiopathiae* [37], and encephalomyelitis in response to infectious agents [28, 50, 72]. Moreover, cell walls from various other bacteria can induce arthritis in these inbred rats [11, 26, 27, 45]. By contrast, Fischer female rats, a histocompatible inbred strain, are relatively resistant to chronic arthritis and many, if not most, of these other diseases [22, 63, 65, 66]. This strain has been studied extensively along with the Lewis strain in an attempt to understand the genetic mechanisms underlying susceptibility to inflammatory autoimmune disease [47, 48, 51, 54, 64]. For example, SCW rapidly up-regulate class II major histocompatibility antigen expression on synovial endothelial cells in both euthymic and athymic Lewis rats. This up-regulation is not observed in euthymic or athymic Fisher rats [64], although the cell walls localize and persist similarly in the joints of these rat strains [3, 63, 64].

Follow-up studies based on these observations have focused on activation of the hypothalamic-pituitary-adrenal (HPA) axis and the production of corticosteroids in these two strains. When HPA axis responses to SCW and other inflammatory mediators were compared, striking differences were documented. Compared to Fischer rats, Lewis female rats have a profound defect in their ability to increase the transcription of hypothalamic corticotropin releasing hormone (CRH) and enkephalin, to increase the level of pituitary adrenocorticotrophic hormone (ACTH), and to increase the level of plasma corticosterone in response to SCW and other inflammatory stimuli [47, 48]. Lewis rats also have smaller adrenal glands and larger thymuses, both of which may be a consequence of chronic understimulation by the HPA axis and mild chronic hyposecretion of corticosterone [48]. The glucocorticoid receptor antagonist RU 486 was administered with SCW to Fischer 344/N rats, and caused them to develop marked, often fatal inflammatory disease in a dose-dependent fashion [48]. Physiologic replacement doses of glucocorticoids as low as 1 µg/day, either split dose or single intraperitoneal injection, for 72 h at the time of SCW administration markedly diminished the severity of the arthritis in Lewis rats [48]. Similar effects of physiological corticosteroids and RU 486 have also been reported for experimental allergic encephalomyelitis in Lewis rats [6]. The data suggest that blunted HPA axis responsiveness and corticosteroid production in Lewis rats may be a critical factor in the susceptibility of this inbred strain to a wide array of autoimmune inflammatory and infectious diseases, while resistance to similar diseases in Fischer rats may be mediated by the robust counter-regulatory activity of the HPA axis and corticosteroids. Although similar defects have not, as yet, been identified in humans with RA, the data in the rat suggest that inadequate cortisol production, or, possibly, inadequate cortisol effects, may predispose to auto-immune diseases such as RA.

Other types of variation have been described in these rats. For example, it has been reported that there is a difference in the ability of T cells to respond to bacterial antigens and cross-react with cartilage components. Lewis rats mount a measurable, but weak, T cell proliferative response to SCW after immunization with SCW or arthritis induction, but Fischer animals do not [51, 54]. It has also been reported that the development of tolerance to bacterial antigens could be inhibited in Fischer rats, thereby making them susceptible to arthritis by maintaining them as germ-free animals [54].

The mechanisms underlying all of these phenotypic differences remain uncertain [47, 48, 51, 53, 54, 64], but it is conceivable that many of them may have the same molecular biological basis. More detailed examination of Lewis and Fischer rats and other inbred rat strains should clarify these questions and may provide new insights into the genetic factors that influence the development of inflammatory joint disease in humans.

Sex hormones also play a major role in the development of SCW arthritis [1, 66]. Male Lewis rats are much less susceptible to the development of severe chronic arthritic disease [1], but castration or treatment with estradiol renders them susceptible to the development of arthritis comparable to females [1]. These data may provide insights into the predominant expression of RA in females, i. e., the 4:1 female to male ratio. Moreover, these observations are interesting in light of recent observations demonstrating subnormal levels of testosterone in male patients with RA [46].

Immune Response

The acute phase of SCW arthritis is similar in euthymic, athymic, and cyclosporin A treated Lewis rats, indicating that it is thymic independent. However, the chronic phase is dependent on T cells, as shown by the finding that athymic and cyclosporin A treated Lewis rats do not develop the severe proliferative and erosive chronic arthritis [38, 64, 67]. Instead, the T cell immunodeficient rats exhibit a chronic low-grade, non-erosive inflammatory process. Reconstitution of athymic rats with T cells permits development of the severe chronic proliferative and erosive disease [38]. SCW distribution and persistence is similar in the euthymic and athymic rats [2, 64].

As noted above, the importance of T cells in the development of chronic arthritis has been intensively studied. T cell lines derived from SCW-induced arthritic rats can produce disease in naive recipients [16]. The 65 kDa heat shock protein may be an important antigen because of possible immunologic cross-reactivity between SCW antigens, the 65 kDa heat shock protein, and joint proteins. Disagreement exists, however, in the literature on this point. One group failed to find T cell proliferation in the presence of the 65 kDa antigen derived from *Mycobacterium tuberculosis,* although these T cells did proliferate in response to SCW and other antigens derived from *M. tuberculosis.* These cells were able to passively transfer disease [16]. Another group prevented the development of SCW arthritis by pretreatment of animals with the 65 kDa heat shock protein [52]. The protection against SCW arthritis was passively transferable by splenic T cells to a naive recipient [52]. SCW arthritis produced by intra-articular injection of cell wall fragments can be reactivated by IV injection of the same antigen and by other bacterial antigens.

Removal of T cells by monoclonal antibodies prevented the reactivation of disease [53].

One mechanism by which CD4+ T cells are directed to localize in the synovium was suggested by the study of the up-regulation of class II major histocompatibility complex (MHC) antigens (Ia antigens) expressed on the endothelial cells of the post-capillary venules that take up the SCW fragments [64]. Up-regulation develops early and persists throughout the chronic phase of arthritis [64]. Class II MHC antigens are part of the molecular complex on antigen-presenting cells recognized by CD4+ T cells. Thus, up-regulated expression in the joint suggests that "antigen presentation" is part of the developmental physiology of the joint disease. Athymic and cyclosporin A treated animals only transiently express class II MHC antigens during the rapid onset phases of the disease [64]. Therefore, expession of Ia antigens on endothelial cells and various other inflammatory cells during the acute response to the inflammatory stimulus may play a role in recruitment of T cells to the inflammatory site and enhancement of the intensity of the inflammatory process. T cells, in turn, enhance and sustain the exrpression of Ia antigen in the synovium. In other words, Ia expression is a molecular marker of severity in this model disease [64]. Similar observations have been made in RA.

There are other changes in the immune system which are manifested by both the rat model and in human RA. These include anergy, defective production of the lymphocyte cytokine interleukin-2 (IL-2), and diminished splenic mononuclear cell proliferation in response to mitogenic stimuli [35, 39, 65]. These changes parallel the development of arthritis. Interestingly, these abnormalities are reversed, both in the rat model and in humans with RA, by treatment with cyclosporin A, suggesting that the immune abnormalities reflect disease severity [69].

Molecular Mechanisms of Tissue Destruction

As noted, inflammatory arthritis in the SCW model is characterized by marked hypertrophy of synovium with proliferation of stromal fibroblast-like cells and new blood vessels and invasive destruction of juxtaposed cartilage and bone. New blood vessels and fibroblast-like cells predominate at the sites of cartilage resorption and bony erosion. Lesser numbers of macrophages are also present; osteoclasts are the dominant bone resorbing cell in the subchondral bone. Morphologically, the fibroblast-like cells at the margins of these erosions are spindle-shaped and have minimal condensed chromatin and an extensive endoplasmic reticulum which is characteristic of metabolically active cells. Due to the invasive behavior of the synovial tissue, the analogy has been made to tumor-like behavior. Synovial tissues from SCW arthritis and human RA synovium form short-lived nodules when implanted in nude, athymic mice. This phenotype, typically exhibited by transformed cells, is *not* inherent in the synovial cells, but depends on the inflammatory milieu in which these cells grow. In vitro, synovial fibroblasts from inflammatory joints behave like transformed cells when stimulated with certain growth factors (discussed below), i. e., rapid growth in monolayer culture, absence of contact inhibition, formation of foci, and anchorage-independent growth in soft agarose [24, 68]. All of these characteristics have been associated with the transformed phenotype. This abnormal phenotype is evident only in fresh explants and early passage cells and is progressively lost with in vitro passage of the cells [24]. Immunohistochemical studies have shown that the proliferative synovia in SCW arthritis and human RA produce high levels of c-*myc* and c-*fos,* nuclear proto-oncogenes that are highly expressed in activated or proliferating cells [7, 8, 40]. These cells also produce relatively high levels of vimentin, a microfilament that is prominent in immature and transformed mesenchymal cells [68].

Invasive tissue, whether in development or in carcinogenesis, must be able to degrade normal tissue. Transin (the rat homologue to the human metalloproteinase, stromelysin) is prominently expressed at sites of tissue invasion [8]. Transin is a proteoglycanase which is also the major activator of collagenase. These enzymes are presumably critical in the breakdown of cartilage in the diseased joint [7, 34]. Of note, this enzyme was originally isolated on the basis of high expression in fibroblasts transformed by viruses. Transin has subsequently been shown to be highly expressed in invasive tumors, leading to the suggestion that high level expresion of this enzyme connotes an invasive phenotype for the cell [30]. Increased transin expression is one of the earliest detectable histological changes in the joints of SCW treated Lewis rats [8]. Intense expression of this metalloproteinase is also noted *before* the onset of clinically apparent arthritis in subchondral osteoclasts and in the chondrocytes adjacent to fibroblast-like cells staining for transin [8]. This observation suggests that some of cell-cell interaction by paracrine mechanisms is operative very early in the course of the disease. These observations may be relevant to humans because RA synovium also expresses abundant amounts of transin/stromelysin, while low amounts of this metalloproteinase are expressed in the noninvasive synovium from patients with osteoarthritis [7].

Autocrine/Paracrine/Neuroendocrine Regulatory Mechanisms

As noted above, the aggressive behavior of synovial fibroblast-like cells is dependent on the inflammatory milieu of the SCW arthritic joint. A search for the cytokines/growth factors that stimulate and inhibit the synovial pathology has implicated a wide variety of factors. These factors are derived from activated cells including infiltrating macrophages, lymphocytes, mast cells, platelets, endothelial cells, and the connective tissue cells themselves.

Extensive studies of the effects of various growth factors on the growth of synovial fibroblasts from patients with RA and Lewis with SCW arthritis under anchorage-dependent and -independent conditions have been reported [25, 36, 40]. Platelet-derived growth factor (PDGF) is consistently the most potent growth promoting factor studied and is probably the most important mitogenic growth factor in SCW and rheumatoid synovium. Epidermal growth factor (EGF) stimulates growth poorly alone, but strongly synergizes with PDGF. The heparin binding growth factors, acidic and basic fibroblast growth factors (aFGF, bFGF), also show stimulatory effects, but are potentially more important for their angiogenic effects [36]. Angiogenesis is a prominent feature of the destructive process in both SCW arthritis and human RA. Immunohisto-chemical localization has shown markedly increased levels of aFGF in SCW arthritis and RA. It is expressed at low or negligible levels in normal rats or patients with osteoarthritis [40].

Transforming growth factor-beta (TGF-β), predominantly type 1, inhibits anchorage-dependentand -independent growth of fibroblast-like synoviocytes [25, 36]. Several cell types including activated macrophages, lymphocytes, and fibroblast-like cells themselves secrete TGF-β in inflammatory synovium [25]. TGF-β stimulates production of collagen and inhibits production of collage-nase and stromelysin in fibroblast-like synoviocytes. This cytokine also has effects on the function of immune cells including macrophages and T cells. It inhibits IL-1 and IL-2 dependent T cell proliferation, inhibits cytotoxic T cell generation, and may deactivate macrophages, although stimulatory effects on macrophages have also been described [25]. Therefore, TGF-β may be an im-portant regulatory growth factor that modulates the effects of other stimulatory growth factors and immune and inflammatory cells in the arthritic joint.

IL-1, interferon-γ (IFN-γ), and tumor necrosis factor-α (TNF-α) are only weak, if at all, directly mitogenic for synovial fibroblasts. They do, however, have important local and systemic effects [36]. IL-1 and TNF-α increase production of the matrix degrading enzyme collagenase and stimulate the production of the proinflammatory prostaglandin E_2. The capacity of IL-1 to stimulate prostaglandin E_2 production in rheumatoid synovial fibroblasts is strikingly potentiated by PDGF [36]. Another important effect of IL-1 is the effect on the central nervous system. There are receptors for IL-1 in the brain through which IL-1 stimulates an apparently important counter-regulatory loop involving the HPA axis. The subsequent increase in glucocorticoid production appears to be an important mechanism for limiting inflammation induced self injury [47, 48]. As discussed above, this feedback loop is profoundly blunted in Lewis rats.

Streptococci and RFs

Streptococci and rheumatoid factors are frequently linked in the literature. For example, although SCW injection in Lewis rats induces only low titers of RF [60, 61], it is well known that SCW may induce high titers of RF in mice and rabbits [58]. In addition, persistent streptococcal infections in humans are commonly associated with RF, and patients with juvenile and adult forms of RA have elevated antibody titers to SCW [2].

Several interesting studies have been reported pursuing these observations. For example, repeated immunization of mice with isolated IgM or IgG RFs produces an anti-peptidoglycan polysaccharide response, indicating that RF could act as an anti-idiotype to anti-peptidoglycan polysaccharide [21]. Moreover, two groups have shown that RFs bear the conformational internal image of streptococcal Fc binding proteins. This again suggests that RFs could arise as antibodies to the idiotypic determinants on antibodies to microbial Fc binding proteins. Alternatively, microbial Fc binding proteins may present IgG to the immune system in such a way that the Fc fragment of IgG becomes specifically immunogenic [9, 33, 42]. These additional data support, although do not prove, the hypothesis that streptococcal or related cell wall antigens may play a role in the pathogenesis of selected cases of RA. Continued investigation is clearly indicated.

References

1. Allen JB, Blatter D, Calandra GB, Wilder RL (1983) Sex hormonal effects on the severity of streptococcal cell wall-induced polyarthritis in the rat. Arthritis Rheum 26:560–563
2. Allen JB, Malone DG, Wahl SM, Calandra GB, Wilder RL (1985) Role of the thymus in streptococcal cell wall-induced arthritis and hepatic granuloma formation. Comparative studies of pathology and cell wall distribution in athymic and euthymic rats. J Clin Invest 76:1042–1056
3. Anderle SK, Allen JB, Wilder RL, Eisenberg RA, Cromartie WJ, Schwab JH (1985) Measurement of streptococcal cell wall in tissue of rats resistant or susceptible to cell wall-induced chronic erosive arthritis. Infect Immun 49:836–837
4. Arnold MH, Tyndall A (1989) Poststreptococcal reactive arthritis. Ann Rheum Dis 48:686–688
5. Biesecker G, Koffler D (1988) Resistance to experimental autoimmune myasthenia gravis in genetically inbred rats. Association with decreased amounts of in situ acetylcholine receptor-antibody complexes. J Immunol 140:3406–3410
6. Bolton C, Flower RJ (1989) The effects of the anti-glucocorticoid RU 38486 on steroid-mediated suppression of experimental allergic encephalomyelitis (EAE) in the Lewis rat. Life Sci 45:97–104
7. Case JP, Lafyatis R, Remmers EF, Kumkumian GK, Wilder RL (1989) Transin/stromelysin in rheumatoid synovium. A transformation-associated metalloproteinase secreted by phenotypically invasive synoviocytes. Am J Pathol 135:1055–1064
8. Case JP, Sano H, Lafyatis R, Remmers EF, Kumkumian GK, Wilder RL (1989) Transin/stromelysin expression in the synovium of rats with experimental erosive arthritis. In situ localization and kinetics of expression of the transformation-associated metalloproteinase in euthymic and athymic Lewis rats. J Clin Invest 84:1731–1740
9. Christensen P, Schroder AK (1990) Possible role of microbial IgG Fc-binding proteins in rheumatoid arthritis. Agents Actions 29:88–94
10. Clark RL, Cuttino JT, Anderle SK, Cromartie WM, Schwab JH (1979) Radiologic analysis of arthritis in rats after systemic injection of streptococcal cell wall. Arthritis Rheum 22:25–35

11. Cromartie WJ, Craddock JC, Schwab JH, Anderle SK, Yang CH (1977) Arthritis in rats after systemic injection of streptococcal cells or cell walls. J Exp Med 146:1585–1602
12. Dalldorf FG, Anderle SK, Brown RR, Schwab JH (1988) Mast cell activation by group A streptococcal polysaccharide in the rat and its role in experimental arthritis. Am J Pathol 132:258–264
13. Damjanovic M, Jankovic BD (1989) Experimental autoimmune oophoritis. I. Inhibition of fertility in rats isoimmunized with homogenates of ovary. Am J Reprod Immunol 20 (1):1–8
14. De Cunto C, Giannini EH, Fink CW, Brewer EJ, Person DA (1988) Prognosis of children with poststreptococcal reactive arthritis. Pediatr Infect Dis J 7:683–688
15. DeJoy SQ, Ferguson-Chanowity KM, Sapp TM, Oronsky AL, Lapierre LA, Zabriskie JB, Kerwar SS (1990) M protein deficient streptococcal cell walls can induce acute and chronic arthritis rats. Cell Immunol 125:526–534
16. DeJoy SQ, Ferguson-Chanowity KM, Sapp TM, Zabriskie JB, Oronsky AL, Kerwar SS (1989) Streptococcal cell wall arthritis. Passive transfer of disease with a T cell line and crossreactivity of streptococcal cell wall antigens with *Mycobacterium tuberculosis.* J Exp Med 170:369–382
17. Dua HS, Liversidge J, Forrester JV (1989) Immunomodulation of experimental autoimmune uveitis using a rat anti retinal S-antigen specific monoclonal antibody: evidence for a species difference. Eye 3:69–78
18. Gibofsky A, Zabriskie JB (1988) Acute rheumatic fever: clinical and immunopathologic aspects. In: Espinosa L, Goldberg D, Arnett F, Alacron G (eds) Infections in the rheumatic diseases. Grune and Stratton, Inc, New York, pp 367–373
19. Geratz JD, Pryzwansky KB, Schwab JH, Anderle SK, Tidwell RR (1988) Supression of streptococcal cell wall-induced arthritis by a potent protease inhibitor, bis(5-amidino-2-benzimidazolyl)methane. Arthritis Rheum 31(9):1156–1164
20. Haraoui B, Wilder RL, Allen JB, Sporn MB, Helfgott RK, Brinckerhoff CE (1985) Dose-dependent suppression by the synthetic retinoid, 4-hydroxyphenyl retinamide, of streptococcal cell wall-induced arthritis in rats. Int J Immunopharmacol 7:903–916
21. Johnson PM, Smalley HB (1988) Idiotypic interactions between rheumatoid factors and other antibodies. Scand J Rheumatol [Suppl] 75:93–96
22. Kallen B, Nilsson O (1989) Age as a factor determining susceptibility for experimental autoimmune encephalomyelitis in the rat. Int Arch Allergy Appl Immunol 90:16–19
23. Kleinau S, Larsson P, Bjork J, Holmdahl R, Klareskog L (1989) Linomide, a new immunomodulatory drug, shows different effects on homologoous versus heterologous collagen-induced arthritis in rats. Clin Exp Immunol 78:138–142
24. Lafyatis R, Remmers EF, Roberts AB, Yocum DE, Sporn MB, Wilder RL (1989) Anchorage-independent growth of synoviocytes from arthritic and normal joints. Stimulation by exogenous platelet-derived growth factor and inhibition by transforming growth factor-beta and retinoids. J Clin Invest 83:1267–1276
25. Lafyatis R, Thompson NL, Remmers EF, Flanders KC, Roche NS, Kim S-J, Case JP, Sporn MB, Roberts AB, Wilder RL (1989) Transforming growth factor-beta production by synovial tissues from rheumatoid patients and streptococcal cell wall arthritic rats. Studies on secretion by synovial fibroblast-like cells and immunohistologic localization. J Immunol 143:1142–1148
26. Lehman TJA, Allen JB, Plotz PH, Wilder RL (1983) Polyarthritis in rats following the systemic injection of *Lactobacillus casei* cell walls in aqueous suspension. Arthritis Rheum 26:1259–1265
27. Lehman TJA, Allen JB, Plotz PH, Wilder RL (1984) *Lactobacillus casei* cell wall-induced arthritis in rats: cell wall fragment distribution and persistence in chronic arthritis-susceptible LEW/N and resistant F344/N rats. Arthritis Rheum 27:939–942
28. Liebert UG, Linington C, ter Meulen V (1988) Induction of autoimmune reactions to myelin basic protein in measles virus encephalitis in Lewis rats. J Neuroimmunol 17:103–118
29. Lohse AW, Manns M, Dienes HP, Meyer zum Buschenfelde KH, Cohen IR (1990) Experimental autoimmune hepatitis: disease induction, time course and T-cell reactivity. Hepatology 11:24–30

30. Matrisian LM, Bowden GT, Kreig P, Furstenburger G, Brian J-P, Leroy P, Breathnack R (1986) The mRNA coding for the secreted protease transin is expressed more abundantly in malignant than in benign tumors. Proc Natl Acad Sci USA 83:9413–9417
31. Moody KD, Barthold SW, Terwilliger GA, Beck DS, Hansen GM, Jacoby RO (1990) Experimental chronic Lyme borreliosis in Lewis rats. Am J Trop Med Hyg 42:165–174
32. Moore TL, El-Najdawi E, Dorner RW (1989) Antibody to streptococcal cell wall peptidoglycan-polysaccharide polymers in sera of patients with juvenile rheumatoid arthritis but absent in isolated immune complexes. J Rheumatol 16(8):1069–1073
33. Nardella FA, Oppliger IR, Stone GC, Sasso EH, Mannik M, Sjoquist J, Schroder AK, Christensen P, Johansson PJ, Bjork L (1988) Fc epitopes for human rheumatoid factors and the relationships of rheumatoid factors to the Fc binding proteins of microorganisms. Scand J Rheumatol [Suppl] 75:190–198
34. Okada Y, NagaseH, Harris ED (1986) A metalloproteinase from human rheumatoid synovial fibroblasts that digests connective tissue matrix components: purification and characterization. J Biol Chem 261:6742–6745
35. Regan DR, Cohen PL, Cromartie WJ, Schwab JH (1988) Immunosuppressive macrophages induced by arthropathic peptidoglycan-polysaccharide polymers from bacterial cell walls. Clin Exp Immunol 74:365–370
36. Remmers EF, Lafyatis R, Kumkumian GK, Case JP, Roberts AB, Sporn MB, Wilder RL (1990) Cytokines and growth regulation of synoviocytes from patients with rheumatoid arthritis and rats with streptococcal cell wall arthritis. Growth Factors 2:179–188
37. Renz J, Gentz U, Schmidt A, Dapper T, Nain M, Gemsa D (1989) Activation of macrophages in an experimental rat model of arthritis induced by *Erysipelothrix rhusiopathiae*. Infect Immun 57:3172–3180
38. Ridge SC, Zabriskie JB, Oronsky AL, Kerwar SS (1985) Streptococcal cell wall arthritis: studies with nude (athymic) inbred LEW rats. Cell Immunol 96:231–234
39. Ridge SC, Zabriskie JB, Osawa H, Diamantstein , Oronsky AL, Kerwar SS (1986) Administration of group A streptococcal cell walls to rats induces an interleukin-2 deficiency. J Exp Med 164:327–332
40. Sano H, Forough R, Maier JA, Case JP, Jackson A, Engleka K, Maciag T, Wilder RL (1990) Detection of high levels of heparin binding growth factor-1 (acidic fibroblast growth factor) in inflammatory arthritic joints. J Cell Biol 110:1417–1426
41. Sartor RB, Anderle SK, Rifai N, Goo DAT, Cromartie WJ, Schwab JH (1989) Protracted anemia associated with chronic, relapsing systemic inflammation induced by arthropathic peptidoglycan-polysaccharide polymers in rats. Infect Immun 57:1177–1185
42. Schroder AK, Gharavi AE, Christensen P (1988) Molecular interactions between human IgG, IgM rheumatoid factor and streptococcal IgG Fc receptors. Int Arch Allergy Appl Immunol 86:92–96
43. Schwab JH, Allen JB, Anderle SK, Daldorf F, Eisenberg R, Cromartie WJ (1982) Relationship of complement to experimental arthritis induced in rats with streptococcal cell walls. Immunology 46:83–88
44. Schwab JH, Ohanian SH (1967) Degradation of streptococcal cell wall antigens in vivo. J Bacteriol 94:1346–1352
45. Severijnen AJ, Hazenberg MP, van de Merwe JP (1988) Induction of chronic arthritis in rats by cell wall fragments of anaerobic coccoid rods isolated from the faecal flora of patients with Crohn's disease. Digestion 39:118–125
46. Spector TD (1989) Sex hormone measurements in rheumatoid arthritis. Brit J Rheum 28 (suppl I):62–68
47. Sternberg EM, Hill JM, Chrousos GP, Kamilaris T, Listwak SJ, Gold PW, Wilder RL (1989) Inflammatory mediator-induced hypothalamic-pituitary-adrenal axis activation is defective in streptococcal cell wall arthritis-susceptible Lewis rats. Proc Natl Acad Sci USA 86:2374–2378
48. Sternberg EM, Young WS, Bernardini R, Calogero AE, Chrousos GP, Gold PW, Wilder RL (1989) A central nervous system defect in biosynthesis of corticotropin-releasing hormone is associated with susceptibility to streptococcal cell wall-induced arthritis in Lewis rats. Proc Natl Acad Sci USA 86:4771–4775

49. Teuscher C, Zhou ZZ, Zheng Y, Hickey WF (1989) Actively induced experimental allergic orchitis in Lewis-resistant (Le-R) rats: reversibility of disease resistance by immunization with *Bordetella pertussis*. Cell Immunol 119:233–238

50. van Berlo MF, Warringa R, Wolswijk G, Lopes-Cardoza M (1989) Vulnerability of rat and mouse brain cells to murine hepatitis virus (JHM-strain): studies in vivo and in vitro. QLIA 2:85–93

51. van den Broek MF (1989) Streptococcal cell wall-induced polyarthritis in the rat. Mechanisms for chronicity and regulation of susceptibility. APMIS 97:861–878

52. van den Broek MF, Hogervorst EJ, van Bruggen MC, van Eden W, van der Zee R, van den Berg WB (1989) Protection against streptococcal cell wall-induced arthritis by pretreatment with the 65-kD mycobacterial heat shock protein. J Exp Med 170:449–466

53. van den Broek MF, van Bruggen MC, Stimpson SA, Severijnen AJ, van de Putte LB, van den Berg WB (1990) Flare-up reaction of streptococcal cell wall induced arthritis in Lewis and F344 rats: the role of T lymphocytes. Clin Exp Immunol 79:297–306

54 van den Broek MF, van Bruggen MC, van de Putte LB, van den Berg WB (1988) T cell responses to streptococcal antigens in rats: relation to susceptibility to streptococcal cell wall-induced arthritis. Cell Immunol 116:216–229

55. Vandenbark AA, Hashim GA, Celnik B, Galang A, Li XB, Heber KE, Offner H (1989) Determinants of human myelin basic protein that induce encephalitogenic T cells in Lewis rats. J Immunol 143:3512–3516

56. Wahl SM, Allen JB, Dougherty, Ebequoz V, Pluznik D, Wilder RL, Hand AR, Wahl LM (1986) T lymphocyte dependent evolution of bacterial cell wall induced hepatic granulomas. J Immunol 137:2199–2209

57. Wahl SM, Hunt DA, Allen JB, Wilder RL, Paglia L, Hand AR (1986) Bacterial cell wall-induced hepatic granulomas. An in vivo model of T cell dependent fibrosis. J Exp Med 163:884–902

58. Wilder RL (1987) Proinflammatory microbial products as etiologic agents of inflammatory arthritis. Rheum Dis Clin N Am 13:293–306

59. Wilder L (1988) Animal models of reactive arthritis. In: Espinosa L, Goldberg D, Arnett F, Alarcon G (eds) Infections in the rheumatic diseases. Grune and Stratton, Inc, New York, pp 311–316

60. Wilder RL (1988) Experimental animal models of chronic arthritis. In: Goodacre J, Dick WC (eds) Immunopathogenetic mechanisms of arthritis. MTP Press Ltd, London, pp 157–173

61. Wilder RL (1988) Streptococcal cell wall–induced polyarthritis in rats. In: Greenwald E, Diamond H (eds) Animal models for the rheumatic diseases. CRC Press, Boca Raton, pp 33–40 (CRC Handbook)

62. Wilder RL (1988) Streptococcal cell-wall-induced arthritis in rats: an overview. Int J Tissue React 10:1–5

63. Wilder RL, Allen JB (1985) Regulation of susceptibility to bacterial cell wall-induced arthritis in rats. Arthritis Rheum 28:1318–1319

64. Wilder RL, Allen JB, Hansen C (1987) Thymus-dependent and -independent regulation of Ia antigen expression in situ by cells in synovium of rats with streptococcal cell wall-induced arthritis. Differences in site and intensity of expression in euthymic, athymic, and cyclosporin A-treated LEW and F344 rats. J Clin Invest 79:1160–1171

65. Wilder RL, Allen JB, Wal LM, Calandra GB, Wahl SM (1983) The pathogenesis of group A streptococcal cell wall-induced polyarthritis in the rat. Arthritis Rheum 26:1442–1451

66. Wilder RL, Calandra GB, Garvin AJ, Wright KD, Hansen CT (1982) Strain and sex variation in the susceptibility to streptococcal cell wall-induced polyarthritis in the rat. Arthritis Rheum 25:1064–1072

67. Yocum DE, Allen JB, Wahl SM, Calandra GB, Wilder RL (1986) Inhibition by cyclosporin A of streptococcal cell wall-induced arthritis and hepatic granulomas in rats. Arthritis Rheum 29:262–273

68. Yocum DE, Lafyatis R, Remmers EF, Schumacher HR, Wilder RL (1988) Hyperplastic synoviocytes from rats with streptococcal cell wall-induced arthritis exhibit a transformed phenotype that is thymic-dependent and retinoid inhibitable. Am J Pathol 132:38–48

69. Yocum DE, Wilder RL, Dougherty S, Klippel JH, Pillemer S, Wahl SM (1990) Immunologic parameters of response in patients with rheumatoid arthritis treated with cyclosporin A. Arthritis Rheum 33:1310–1316
70. Zhang Y, Barkas T, Juillerat M, Schwendimann B, Wekerle H (1988) T cell epitopes in experimental autoimmune myasthenia gravis of the rat: strain-specific epitopes and cross-reaction between two distinct segments of the alpha chain of the nicotinic acetylcholine receptor *(Torpedo californica).* Eur J Immunol 18:551–557
71. Ziegler M, Ziegler B, Kohnert KD, Kloting I (1988) Genetic control of susceptibility to severe hyperglycaemia evoked by CFA/SZ-induced immune response against beta cells in various rat strains. Biomed Biochem Acta 47:337–342
72. Zimmer MJ, Dales S (1989) In vivo and in vitro models of demyelinating diseases. XXIV. The infectious process in cyclosporin A treated Wistar Lewis rats inoculated with JHM virus. Microb Pathog 6:7–16

Caprine Arthritis-Encephalitis*

E. Peterhans[1], B. Pohl[1], R. Zanoni[1], and S. Lazary[2]

[1]Institute of Veterinary Virology and [2]Institute of Animal Husbandry, University of Berne, Länggass-Strasse 122, CH-3012 Berne, Switzerland

Introduction

Caprine arthritis-encephalitis (CAE) is a disease in goats which occurs worldwide [3]. Interest in this disease has increased in recent years mainly for two reasons. CAE virus, also referred to as caprine lentivirus, is a member of the same subfamily as the viruses causing AIDS, the human immunodeficiency viruses (HIV) [14, 76]. CAE, along with other lentiviral infections of domestic animals, shares some of the features of AIDS, such as a long and variable incubation time and lifelong persistence, but differs by not causing immunodeficiency. Moreover, the economic losses caused by CAE have become more obvious and CAE eradication programs have been established in several countries. In this article, we shall consider an additional aspect of CAE, namely the possibility of using this disease as a model for arthritis in humans. This possibility is suggested by the fact that arthritis is the hallmark of CAE. We shall review basic properties of the virus, the disease symptoms and pathological alterations, the epidemiology, and the main aspects of the pathogenesis of CAE. In the concluding section, we shall discuss the possible use of CAE as a model in the study of the mechanisms involved in the pathogenesis of human arthritis.

CAE Virus

CAE virus belongs to the *Lentivirinae* subfamily of retroviruses [57, 38, 81]. Its genome consists of a dimer of positive-stranded RNA (i. e., the RNA is of the same polarity as mRNA) of approximately 9200 nucleotides [14, 76]. The

---

* This work was supported by the Swiss National Science Fund, Grant 31-28810.90 (EP) and 3.879-0.88 (SL).

Smolen, Kalden, Maini (Eds.)
Rheumatoid Arthritis
© Springer-Verlag Berlin Heidelberg 1992

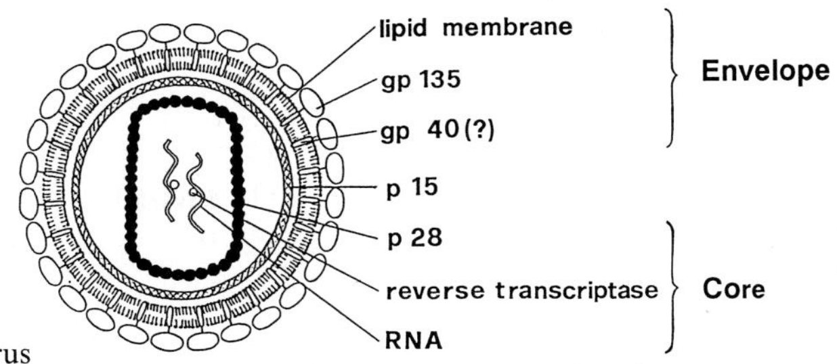

Fig. 1. Structure of CAE virus

Table 1. Subfamily Lentivirinae

Virus	Host	Isolated by
Maedi-visna virus	Sheep	Sigurdsson et al. (1957)
Equine infectious anemia virus	Horses	Kobayashi (1961)
Bovine immunodeficiency virus	Cattle	Van Der Maaten et al. (1972)
Caprine arthritis-encephalitis virus	Goats	Crawford et al. (1980)
Human immunodeficiency virus type 1	Humans	Barré-Sinoussi et al. (1983)
Simian immunodeficiency virus	Monkeys	Daniel et al. (1985); Kanki et al. (1985)
Human immunodeficiency virus type 2	Humans	Clavel et al. (1986)
Feline immunodeficiency virus	Cats	Pedersen et al. (1987)

structure of CAE virus and the main structural proteins are indicated in Fig. 1. Lentiviruses have also been isolated from horses, cattle, monkies, cats, and humans (Table 1). The closest relatives of CAE virus are undoubtedly the sheep lentiviruses, Maedi-visna and ovine progressive pneumonia viruses [26, 39]. The main symptoms of maedi-visna are pneumonia and encephalitis [25]. Goats can be experimentally infected with maedi-visna virus and sheep are susceptible to CAE virus [64, 7, 65, 30]. Moreover, the American sheep lentivirus, ovine progressive pneumonia virus, differs substantially from maedi-visna virus in causing arthritis in a high proportion of infected sheep [24, 47]. The prevalence of lentiviral infection may differ markedly between goats and sheep kept on the same farm [52]. Moreover, in Australia, the sheep population has been reported to be free from maedi-visna despite the presence of a CAE virus-infected goat population [74, 33, 77]. Although these observations do not exclude that interspecies transmission can occur, they nevertheless argue against an important role under field conditions. The close relationship between CAE and maedi visna viruses is also reflected at the level of the genome [38, 14, 76] and has practical consequences in the serological diagnosis of infection. Antiviral antibodies in goats can be detected using antigen prepared from maedi-visna virus [17]. Importantly, neither CAE nor maedi-visna viruses have ever been reported to cause infection in humans.

Clinical Manifestations and Pathological Lesions of CAE

The disease "big knees" has been known for a long time, but its etiology remained obscure until 1980 [21]. It had been proposed that goat arthritis was a hereditary affliction [12]. The fact that CAE is spread mainly via colostrum and milk from mother to kid easily explains this interpretation [2, 32]. However, very recent evidence suggests that there may indeed exist a genetically determined predisposition to disease, albeit not to infection [71]. The main clinical manifestations of CAE are arthritis, encephalitis, and mastitis [21, 80, 84, 46, 13]. The latter has long been overlooked but seems to be a significant economical factor because of a reduction in milk production which has been estimated to be 5%–10% [75, 52]. Interestingly, only 25%–30% of naturally infected animals develop clinically detectable arthritis and/or mastitis [23, 52]. Most often, arthritis is detected visually from the enlargement of the carpal joint (Fig. 2). For obvious reasons, it is difficult to say whether arthritis is painful for the animal, but judged by the observation that animals may live for years with arthritis without showing severe lameness, one would suspect that arthritic goats do not experience acute pain. Typically, lesions develop slowly over months to years which is reflected in a higher prevalence of disease in older animals (Table 2). Possibly, the absence of acute lameness relates to the slow development of lesions. As an incidental consequence of the slow course of disease, goat owners get used to having in their herds animals with big knees and generally do not consider this to be a major health problem [52]. In contrast to arthritis, encephalitis takes a faster course. It begins with weakness mainly of the hind legs and may progress to quadriplegia within 2–3 weeks. Animals remain perceptive and do not develop fever unless infected with other microorganisms. Those with uncomplicated encephalitis may recover if nursed carefully. In contrast to arthritis, encephalitis is observed mainly in young

Table 2. Prevalence of carpitis[a] in goats of different age groups

Age (months)	Animals (number) 1614	Carpitis	
		Positive ($n = 375$)	Negative ($n = 1239$)
1– 6	214	8 (4%)	206 (96%)
7–12	240	31 (13%)	209 (87%)
>12	1160	336 (29%)	824 (71%)

[a] Diagnosed by palpation.

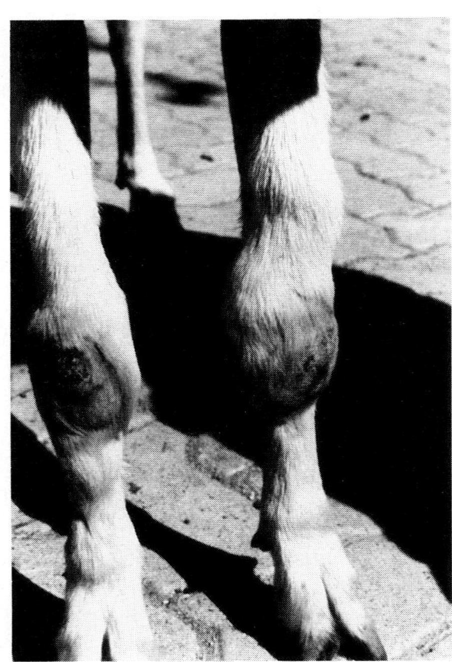

Fig. 2. Carpitis and pericarpitis in a goat infected with CAE virus. Note marked swelling of carpal joint and surrounding tissue

animals of less than 6 months of age, and its prevalence shows remarkable variation. For example, in some herds several cases have been reported simultaneously [18], while elsewhere encephalitis is rare [52]. It seems possible that strain differences may contribute to differences in the clinical symptoms of infection with CAE virus [13]. Interestingly, the arthritic goats from which CAE virus was originally isolated belonged to a group of animals in which encephalitis had been studied previously [18, 21], and this led to the acronym "CAE".

The carpal joint is the preferential site of arthritis in goats infected with CAE virus. The reason for this is not known, but recently the interesting suggestion was made that repeated mild trauma resulting from frequent kneeling during feeding may account for the high frequency of carpitis in CAE [9]. It is important to note that arthritis may also be observed in other sites, such as the tarsal and femorotibial joints [80]. Advanced arthritis, in particular carpitis, is easily detected by inspection of the animals (Fig. 2). The joint is markedly enlarged with swelling extending into the subcutis of the surrounding tissue, tendon sheaths, and bursae. Gross pathological changes include excessive synovial fluid with occasional fibrin tags and modestly increased numbers of lymphocytes, plasma cells, and macrophages [80, 13]. Synovial necrosis and mineralization may be seen in advanced disease. Histopathologically, synovitis, proliferation of synovial lining cells with formation of villi, and subsynovial mononuclear cell infiltrates with only few polymorphonuclear leukocytes are prominent. Destruction of underlying bone tissue is seen in advanced disease.

Examination by X-ray reveals extensive mineralization in the joint and bursal capsules extending into the tendons and tendon shafts. The changes in brain and mammary gland are characterized essentially by extensive mononuclear inflammation [20, 1, 22, 84, 13].

Genetic Aspects

The manifestation of clinical arthritis in families of Toggenburg breed goats was studied by Büchi et al. [12]. At that time, without any knowledge of the virological etiology of the disease, the authors found clearly increased susceptibility in certain lines.

In recent years, a class I caprine leukocyte alloantigen system (CLA), encoded by the major histocompatibility complex (MHC), has been serologically characterized in goats [70]. In humans, certain MHC gene products occur at increased frequency in patients afflicted by various forms of arthritis. It was therefore of general interest to study the distribution of CLA alleles in arthritis affected goats [71]. In this study, the distribution of CLA alleles in goats from four different breeds ($n = 546$) affected by CAE virus induced arthritis was investigated and compared breed for breed with those of infected but clinically healthy controls ($n = 402$). There was no correlation between alleles of the MHC and presence of antiviral antibodies, but clinically affected animals showed differences in frequencies of some of the CLA specificities. After correction of the ordinary p values for number of observed alleles, only the CLA Be7 specificity in the Saanen breed showed a significant deviation at the 0.05 probability level. Animals of the Saanen breed carrying this specificity are less prone to develop arthritis after CAE infection than goats lacking this specificity. Eleven groups (multiple case families or half-sibling groups with at least two informative diseased offspring/group) were analyzed for manifestation of the disease and segregation of parental haplotypes. The results of the maximum likelihood test of association ($p < 0.005$) and the calculated high log score value of 5.70 give evidence for linkage between the locus encoding the determined class I CLA alleles and a hypothetical locus (i) coding for genes responsible for arthritis resistance/susceptibility. The particular class I CLA allele associated with the disease susceptibility varied from family to family. These data provide evidence that CAE virus induced arthritis in the goat is genetically influenced by the MHC system; they also suggest that susceptibility/resistance genes are not directly associated with the determined class I gene products but rather are in close genetic linkage.

Epidemiology

Since disease symptoms are seen only in a minority of animals, testing for antiviral antibody is the method of choice for the detection of CAE. Infection with CAE virus is very widespread in most countries [3]. In Switzerland, a recent survey showed that over 60% of the goat population have antibody to CAE virus [52]. Interestingly, CAE has not been detected in countries which never imported goats from Europe, suggesting that the virus may have evolved in Europe [3]. As a rule, more intensive goat farming practices are correlated with a higher prevalence of infection. In particular, goat milk farms have been reported to show the highest prevalence of infection, possibly due to the habit of feeding colostrum and milk from single infected does to groups of kids [31]. Horizontal transmission also leads to the spread of infection. Most available evidence suggests that intrauterine transmission of virus to the fetus may not occur [2]. As with other lentiviral infections, the virus persists lifelong. The eradication programs established in several countries take into account the epidemiological features of CAE (which are similar to those of maedi-visna in sheep). In essence, kids are removed from their infected mothers immediately after birth and are reared in separate herds. The virus-containing colostrum and milk are replaced either by that from CAE-free does or the kids are fed cow's colostrum and milk. Testing for antiviral antibody is used to assure that all animals in the new herd are free from infection with CAE virus [2, 32, 6, 34]. The obvious advantage of this scheme is that valuable genetic material can be preserved and in fact several CAE-free kids can be obtained from infected does. In our experience, this method of eradication is successful if the measures are strictly adhered to.

Pathogenesis

The pathogenesis of CAE has many fascinating aspects, such as the lifelong persistence, the unique tropism for joints, and the mechanisms resulting in the formation of lesions in the infected animal.

The precise mechanism of viral entry into susceptible animals has not been determined. Virus present in colostrum is thought to enter from the intestinal tract via uptake of intact infected macrophages into the bloodstream or via initial infection of intestinal lining cells [42]. Sialic acids of the viral surface glycoprotein seem to be important in protecting the virus against proteases present in the intestinal fluid and have been shown to protect the virus against neutralization by antiviral antibodies [42]. As in other lentiviral infections, there may be a lag time of several weeks (in some cases even months) before detectable antiviral antibodies are formed [2], but in most animals these antibodies do not neutralize the virus [48, 61]. In addition, neutralizing antibodies are of extremely narrow specificity [61]. As an additional mechanism which may contribute to the escape of the virus from immune control, neutralization sensitive epitopes of CAE virus have been shown to undergo antigenic variation in infected goats [35, 55] and also in cultured cells [16]. In vivo, CAE virus infects primarily cells of the mononuclear lineage [58, 5]. The way in which the virus interacts with these cells also contributes to persistence. Thus, circulating monocytes in blood may harbor the viral genome but little or no viral protein is produced due to a restriction of viral replication at the level of RNA transcription. After migration into tissue and maturation to macrophages, viral protein and infectious virus are produced, but a unique mechanism curtails viral replication also at this stage. Lymphocytes release a lentivirus specific interferon which inhibits viral multiplication and also decreases the rate at which monocytes mature to macrophages, thereby making these cells less permissive for viral replication. Moreover, expression of MHC class II antigen is enhanced by the lentivirus specific interferon, facilitating interaction with lymphocytes. Other cytokines released from lymphocytes and mononuclear phagocytes promote inflammation [83, 63]. Overall, this process ensures the presence of a large number of host cells and at the same time limits virus production. The restriction of virus replication in monocytes also protects these cells from immune attack because no viral antigens are expressed at the surface of the latently infected cells. This situation has aptly been referred to as the "trojan horse mechanism" indicating that the virus is not "seen" by the immune system [67].

The unique tropism for joints, the mammary gland and the central nervous system is not understood in detail. However, recent studies with the closely related maedi-visna virus demonstrated that the long terminal repeat (LTR) of the viral genome may play a role in cell and tissue tropism. Using transgenic mice carrying LTR-CAT (chloramphenicol acetyltransferase) constructs, it was shown that enzyme activity was expressed in cells of the monocyte-macrophage lineage and correlated with maturation to macrophages. Moreover, CAT activity was also observed in lymphocytes, suggesting that these cells may potentially allow the replication of visna virus. Expression was also observed in brain tissue but the CAT-positive cells were not identified. The experiments also showed that expression of CAT activity can be induced by phorbol myristate acetate [73], which, like maturation to macrophages, is known to result in activation of c-*fos* [69, 56]. The product of this oncogene combines with the cellular DNA-binding proteins JUN and AP-1 which then interact with AP-1 binding sites on DNA [36]. Interestingly, AP-1 binding sites have recently been demonstrated on proviral DNA of visna virus [41, 37]. These observations suggest a mechanism for the activation of viral replication that is observed when monocytes differentiate to macrophages [5, 59, 60].

How does the virus cause the arthritic lesions? In certain types of cultured cells, CAE virus causes cytopathic effects characterized by syncytia formation [57]. However, there is little or no evidence that the virus destroys its host cells in vivo [1, 22]. In fact, it was reported that maedi-visna virus (which is more cytopathic than CAE virus in vitro) fails to kill cultured macrophages [59]. As an alternaive possibility, the host's immune system, rather than the virus itself, may cause the lesions. Different from certain arthritides caused by other microorganisms (e. g., mycobacteria), autoimmune reactions triggered by molecular mimicry or other mechanisms have not been demonstrated in CAE [79]. However, there are several lines of evidence suggesting that the immune system plays a detrimental role in the development of arthritis. Thus, immunosuppressive treatment was shown to ameliorate the course of disease [19], while vaccination with inactivated virus prior to infection and challenge of persistently infected goats with infectious virus aggravated arthritis [53]. The observation that immunosuppression decreased the formation of lesions but did not alter the amount of detectable virus suggests that virus multiplication per se does not significantly contribute to the development of lesions. The presence of a high concentration of antiviral antibody, predominantly of the IgG1 subtype [43], and directed mainly against viral surface glycoprotein is indicative of an active local immune response at the site where the arthritic lesions develop [44]. Macrophages isolated from synovial fluid of infected goats showed higher rates of cell division than those isolated from uninfected animals [45], and the presence of CAE virus augmented the mitogenic response of T lymphocytes of uninfected goats to concanavalin A in vitro [29]. Moreover, arthritis induced with methylated human serum was exacerbated by concurrent infection with CAE virus [8]. Based on these observations, two alternative explanations were proposed for the formation of the arthritic lesions in CAE. McGuire suggested that the antiviral immune response was mainly responsible [54], while Banks and colleagues put more emphasis on the nonspecific augmentation of the immune response [9]. These two explanations are not mutually exclusive. Thus, as outlined above, cell activation may also lead to the activation of viral multiplication via AP-1 binding sites [73]. Viral infection may also perpetuate the inflammatory response by mechanisms such as enhanced Ia antigen expression in macrophages, and stimulation of proliferation of macrophages and T lymphocytes [45, 9]. It seems likely that cytokines play an important role in this process. To date, the presence of high concentrations of interferon in synovial fluids of arthritic goats has been reported, but this type of interferon seems to differfrom the lentivirus specific interferon described by Narayan and co-workers [82, 62]. It has been shown in other systems that certain cytokines (e. g., interleukin-1 and tumor necrosis factor) can promote proliferation of synovial fibroblasts and cartilage destruction. Determination of the spectrum of cytokines present in arthritic joints could therefore promote our understanding of the mechanisms of lesion formation. While cytokines are likely to be important in the regulation of chronic inflammation, it is unclear how the virus promotes chronic inflammation. Stimulation by viral antigen and alterations in the expression of cytokine genes in virus infected macrophages are two obvious mechanisms which could explain the persistent inflammation. We have studied the first of these mechanisms by monitoring luminol-dependent chemiluminescence in various types of phagocytes in the presence of viral antigen. Luminol-dependent chemiluminescence reflects the generation of reactive oxygen species (ROS) produced by phagocytic cells [4]. ROS play

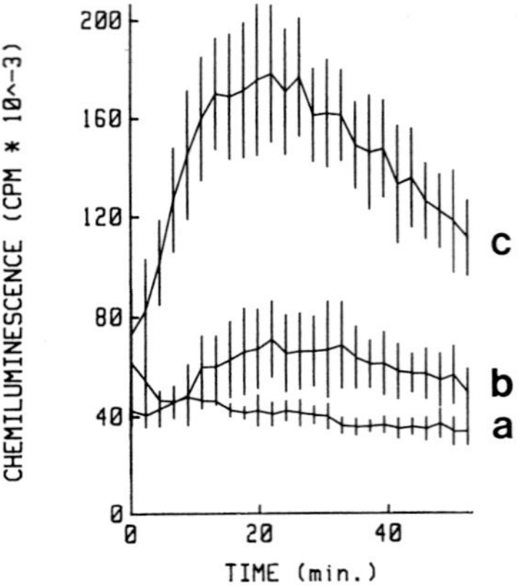

Fig. 3. The induction of chemiluminescence in sheep monocytes by antibody-coated maedi-visna virus. Lamb carpal cells infected with maedi-visna virus were detached from plastic culture flasks by incubation with 0.15% EDTA and incubated for 10 min at 37°C with heat-inactivated (56°C/30 min) serum obtained from a sheep infected with maedi-visna virus as indicated by a positive ELISA test for antiviral antibody. The cells were subsequently washed twice and added to mononuclear cells (1.5×10^6/0.75 ml/vial, containing approximately 1.5×10^5 monocytes) suspended in Hanks' saline supplemented with 2.5 mM glucose. To enhance chemiluminescence (CL), luminol was added to a final concentration of 5 μM. CL was measured in a modified liquid scintillation spectrometer and recorded on line with a computer as previously described [68]. Each point represents the mean $\pm$ SD of three replicate samples. *a,* cells not incubated with serum; *b,* cells incubated with serum from a noninfected sheep and *c* cells infected from an infected sheep. Noninfected cells coated with either immune or nonimmune serum failed to induce CL (results not shown)

multiple roles in inflammatory diseases. Some oxygen species such as ·OH are highly toxic by directly attacking proteins, lipids, and nucleic acids, but more indirect effects (e. g., via inactivation of protease inhibitors resulting in increased protease activity) also contribute to tissue destruction [40]. We have previously shown that certain paramyxoviruses which cause cell fusion at physiological pH are capable of activating ROS generation in phagocytes in the absence as well as presence of antiviral antibodies. Activation of cellular ROS generation in the absence of antiviral antibody is mediated by an interaction of the viral surface glycoproteins with the phagocyte's plasma membrane while antibody-dependent activation is mediated via Fc receptors [68]. To investigate the effect of lentiviral antigen on ROS generation, we infected lamb carpal cells with virus and added infected cells (known to have viral antigens on their surface) to various populations of phagocytes (Fig. 3). These experiments, which for technical reasons were done with sheep lentivirus, clearly showed that antiviral antibodies are required for triggering ROS generation. Thus, viral antigen bound to antiviral antibody could represent a factor promoting local inflammation in joints. It seems possible that immune complexes could contribute to the formation of arthritic lesions by other mechanisms, such as activation of cytokine secretion, e. g., tumor necrosis factor [28].

CAE: A Model for Rheumatoid Arthritis?

CAE shares some features with rheumatoid arthritis, but there are also some clear differences (see Table 3 and this volume). The main one is that CAE is caused by a well-known virus but the mechanism by which the arthritic lesions are caused are largely unknown. In contrast, many pathogenetic features of rheumatoid arthritis are known, but its cause is still a matter of debate. As outlined above, the symptoms of CAE are, in general, more benign than those of rheumatoid arthritis, and this may relate to the different composition of the inflammatory cells observed in the two arthritides. Polymorphonuclear leukocytes predominate at least in the acute phase of rheumatoid arthritis, while CAE is characterized by mononuclear inflammation. It seems possible, but not proven, that the virtual absence of polymorphonuclear leukocytes may explain why cartilage destruction is less prominent in CAE than in rheumatoid arthritis. It would be of interest to compare the cytokine and arachidonate metabolite profiles since differences in the chemotactically active components could explain the composition of the inflammatory cell population in arthritic joints.

Table 3. Comparison of CAE with rheumatoid arthritis

Parameter	CAE	Rheumatoid arthritis
Infectious agent	CAE virus	Several viruses and other microorganisms suspected
Genetic predisposition	Demonstrated	Demonstrated
Type of inflammation	Mononuclear	Mononuclear, but also neutrophils present
Cells in synovial fluid	Mononuclear	Predominantly neutrophils
Cytokines in synovial fluid	Interferon (gamma?; others unknown)	IL-1, TNF-α, IL-6, GM-CSF
Arachidonate metabolites in synovial fluid	Unknown	Several metabolites demonstrated
Clinical Parameters		
Early lesions	Large joints, symmetric	Small joints, symmetric (finger, toes)
Development	Slow-chronic-intermittent	Intermittent
Pain	Little evidence	Severe in acute phase
Fever	Absent	In acute phase
nonarthritic manifestation	Mamma (brain, lung)	Severe eye, lung fibrosis disease
Serology		
Rheumatoid factor	Not demonstrated	Majority of patients

IL-1, interleukin-1; TNF-α, tumor necrosis factor-α; GM-CSF, granulocyte/macrophage colony-stimulating factor

In contrast to rheumatoid arthritis, rheumatoid factors or other autoantibodies have not been detected in serum or synovial fluid of arthritic goats [85]. Although it is clear that CAE virus is the cause of arthritis in goats, it is not quite clear how the virus maintains the chronic inflammation. As outlined in the section on the pathogenesis of CAE, viral antigen is only infrequently detected in arthritic joints and virus isolation was not successful at all times after initial establishment of the inflammation [49]. These features of lentiviral infection suggest that the search for viruses or other infectious causes should be intensified in human rheumatoid arthritis, perhaps including more sensitive techniques such as the polymerase chain reaction (PCR), capable of detecting incomplete genome sequences and minor mRNA populations [11].

The above considerations illustrate that CAE, although not identical to rheumatoid arthritis in humans, could well serve as a useful model to better understand some of its features. The fact that the inflammation observed in CAE lacks some of the features of rheumatoid arthritis should not preclude its use as a model but should rather encourage it. The possibilities to modulate arthritis in goats have not been explored. In particular "up-regulation" by supplementation of the joint with cytokines or arachidonate metabolites chemotactic for polymorphonuclear leukocytes would provide insight into the role of these cells in the formation of lesions. Moreover, the recent demonstration that CAE exacerbates concomitant arthritis induced by methylated human serum shows the role a preexisting inflammation can have in a process characterized mainly by inflammation with polymorphonuclear leukocytes. Another essentially untapped possibility is the use of CAE to explore novel antiinflammatory drugs in a "natural" arthritis. In addition to giving valuable insight into the mechanisms involved in arthritis and possible therapeutic approaches, such studies are likely to provide important information on the effects that such modulation may have on viral gene expression. Thus, CAE could be a model from which rheumatologists as well as virologists could learn.

Acknowledgements. We thank Drs. T. W. Jungi and B. Rey for stimulating discussions.

References

1. Adams DS, Crawford TB, Klevjer-Anderson P (1980) A pathogenetic study of the early connective tissue damage of viral arthritis-encephalitis. Am J Pathol 99:257–278
2. Adams DS, Klevjer-Anderson P, Carlson JL, McGuire TC (1983) Transmission and control of caprine arthritis-ecephalitis virus. Am J Vet Res 44:1670–1675
3. Adams DS, Oliver RE, Ameghino E, DeMartini JC, Verwoerd DW, Houwers DJ, Waghela S, Gorham JR, Hyllseth B, Dawson M, Trigo FJ (1984) Global survey of serological evidence of caprine arthritis-encephalitis virus infection. Vet Rec 115:493–495
4. Allen RC (1986) Phagocytic leukocyte oxygenation activities and chemiluminscence: a kinetic approach to analysis. Methods Enzymol 133:449–493

5. Anderson LW, Klevjer-Anderson P, Liggitt HD (1983) Susceptibility of blood-derived monocytes and macrophages to caprine arthritis-encephalitis virus. Infect Immun 41:837–840
6. Balcer T, Stucki M, Krieg A, Zwahlen R (1985) Caprine-retrovirus infection: experience with a pilot sanitation program in Swiss goat herds. In: Sharp JM, Hoff-Jorgensen R (eds) Slow viruses in sheep, goats and cattle. ECSC-EEC-EAEC, Brussels, Luxembourg, pp 253–264
7. Banks KL, Adams DS, McGuire TC, Carlson J (1983) Experimental infection of sheep by caprine arthritis-encephalitis virus and goats by progressive pneumonia virus. Am J Vet Res 44:2307–2311
8. Banks KL, Jacobs CA, Michaels FH, Cheevers WP (1987) Lentivirus infection augments concurrent antigen-induced arthritis. Arthritis Rheum 30:1046–1053
9. Banks KL, Jutila MA, Jacobs CA, Michaels FH (1989) Augmentation of lymphocyte and macrophage proliferation by caprine arthritis-encephalitis virus contributes to the development of progressive arthritis. Rheum International 9:123–128
10. Barre-Sinoussi F, Chermann JC, Rey F, Nugeyre MT, Chamaret S, Gruest J, Dauguet C, Axler-Blin C, Vezinet-Brun F, Rouzioux C, Rozenbaum W, Montagnier L (1983) Isolation of a T-lymphotrophic retrovirus from a patient at risk for acquired immune deficiency syndrome (AIDS). Science 220:868–871
11. Bell J (1989) The polymerase chain reaction. Immunol Today 10:351–355
12. Büchi HF, Le Roy HL, Böni A (1962) Über das Auftreten von Polyarthritis bei der Species *Capra hircus,* ein medizinisch-genetisches Problem. Z Rheumaforsch 21:88–98
13. Cheevers WP, Knowles DP, Mc Guire TC, Cunningham DR, Adams DS, Gorham JR (1988) Chronic disease in goats orally infected with two isolates of the caprine arthritis-encephalitis lentivirus. Lab Invest 58:510–517
14. Chiu IM, Yaniv A, Dahlberg JE, Gazit A, Skuntz SF, Tronick SR, Aaronson SA (1985) Nucleotide sequence evidence for relationship of AIDS retrovirus to lentiviruses. Nature 317:366–368
15. Clavel F, Guetard D, Brun-Vezinet F, Chamaret S, Rey MA, Santos-Ferreira MO, Laurent AG, Dauguet C, Katlama C, Rouzioux C, Klatzmann D, Champalimaud JL, Montagnier L (1986) Isolation of a new human retrovirus from West African patients with AIDS. Science 233:343–346
16. Clements JE, Gdovin SL, Montelaro RC, Narayan O (1988) Antigenic variation in lentiviral diseases. Ann Rev Immunol 6:139–159
17. Coackley W, Smith VW, Houwers DJ (1984) Preparation and evaluation of antigens used in serological tests for caprine syncytial retrovirus antibody in sheep and goat sera. Vet Microbiol 9:581–586
18. Cork LC, Hadlow WJ, Crawford TB, Gorham JR, Piper RC (1974) Infectious leukoencephalomyelitis of young goats. J Infect Dis 129:134–141
19. Cork LC, Narayan O (1980) Pathogenesis of goat viral leukoencephalomyelitis-arthritis. Proceedings 31st Annual Meeting, American College of Veterinary Pathologists, p 115
20. Cork LC, Narayan O (1980) The pathogenesis of viral leukoencephalomyelitis -arthritis of goats. I. Persistent viral infection with progressive pathologic changes. Lab Invest 42:596–602
21. Crawford TB, Adams DS, Cheevers WP, Cork LV (1980) Chronic arthritis in goats caused by a retrovirus. Science 207:997–999
22. Crawford TB, Adams DS, Sande RD, Gorham JR, Henson JB (1980) The connective tissue component of the caprine arthritis-encephalitis syndrome. Am J Pathol 100:443–454
23. Crawford TB, Adams DS (1981) Caprine arthritis-encephalitis: clinical features and presence of antibody in selected goat populations. J Am Vet Med Ass 178:713–719
24. Cutlip RC, Lehmkuhl HD, Wood RL, Brogden KA (1985) Arthritis associated with ovine progressive pneumonia. Am J Vet Res 46:65–68
25. Cutlip RC, Lehmkuhl HD, Schmerr MJF, Brogden KA (1988) Ovine progressive pneumonia (maedi-visna) in sheep. Vet Microbiol 17:237–250

26. Dahlberg JE, Gaskin JM, Perk K (1981) Morphological and immunological comparison of caprine arthritis encephalitis and ovine progressive pneumonia viruses. J Virol 39:914–919
27. Daniel MD, Letvin NL, King NW, Kannagi M, Sehgal PK, Hunt RD, Kanki PJ, Essex M, Desrosiers RC (1985) Isolation of T-cell tropic HTLV-III-like retrovirus from macaques. Science 228:1201–1204
28. Debets JMH, Van der Linden CJ, Dieteren IM, Leeuwenberg JFM, Buurman WA (1988) Fc-receptor cross-linking induces rapid secretion of tumor necrosis factor (cachectin) by human peripheral blood monocytes. J Immunol 141:1197–1201
29. DeMartini JC, Banks KL, Greenlee A, Adams DS (1983) Augmented T lymphocyte response and abnormal B lymphocyte numbers in goats chronically infected with the retrovirus causing caprine arthritis-encephalitis. Am J Vet Res 44:2064–2069
30. Dickson J, Ellis T (1989) Experimental caprine retrovirus infection in sheep. Vet Rec 125:649
31. East NE, Rowe JD, Madewell BR, Floyd K (1987) Serologic prevalence of caprine arthritis-encephalitis virus in California goat dairies. J Am Vet Med Assoc 190:182–186
32. Ellis T, Robinson W, Wilcox G (1983) Effect of colostrum deprivation of goat kids on the natural transmission of caprine retrovirus infection. Aust Vet J 60:326–329
33. Ellis T, Robinson W, Wilcox G (1983) Characterization, experimental infection and serological response to caprine retrovirus. Aust Vet J 60:321–325
34. Ellis TM, Robinson WF (1984) Studies on a control programme for caprine arthritis encephalitis virus infection. Les maladies de la chevre, Niort (France), 9–11 Oct. 1984, Les Colloques de l' INRA 28:651–654
35. Ellis TM, Wilcox GE, Robinson WF (1987) Antigenic variation of caprine arthritis-encephalitis virus during persistent infection of goats. J Gen Virol 68:3145–3152
36. Franza BR, Rauscher FJ, Josephs SF, and Curran T (1988) The fos complex and fos-related antigens recognize sequence elements that contain AP-1 binding sites. Science 239:1150–1153
37. Gabuzda DH, Hess JL, Small JA, Clements JE (1989) Regulation of the visna virus long terminal repeat in macrophages involves cellular factors that bind sequences containing AP-1 sites. Mol Cell Biol 9:2728–2733
38. Gazit A, Yaniv A, Dvir M, Perk K, Irving SG, Dahlberg JE (1983) The caprine arthritis-encephalitis virus is a distinct virus with in the lentivirus group. Virology 124:192–195
39. Gogolewski RP, Adams DS, McGuire TC, Banks KL, Cheevers WP (1985) Antigenic cross-reactivity between caprine arthritis-encephalitis, visna and progressive pneumonia viruses involves all virion-associated proteins and glycoproteins. J Gen Virol 66:1233–1240
40. Halliwell B, Gutteridge JMC (1989) Free radicals in biology and medicine, 2nd edn. Clarendon Press, Oxford, England
41. Hess JL, Small JA, Clements JE (1989) Sequences in the visna virus long terminal repeat that control transcriptional activity and respond to viral trans-activation – involvement of AP-1 sites in basal activity and trans-activation. J Virol 63:3001–3015
42. Huso DL, Narayan O, Hart GW (1988) Sialic acids on the surface of caprine arthritis-encephalitis virus define the biological properties of the virus. J Virol 62:1974–1980
43. Johnson GC, Barbet AF, Klevjer-Anderson P, McGuire TC (1983) Preferential immune response to virion surface glycoproteins by caprine arthritis-encephalitis virus-infected goats. Infect Immun 41:657–665
44. Johnson GC, Adams DS, McGuire TC (1983) Pronounced production of polyclonal immunoglobulin G 1 in the synovial fluid of goats with caprine arthritis-encephalitis virus infection. Infect Immun 41:805–815
45. Jutila MA, Banks KL (1988) Increased macrophage division in the synovial fluid of goats infected with caprine arthritis-encephalitis virus. J Infect Dis 157:1193–1202
46. Kennedy-Stoskopf S, Narayan O, Strandberg JD (1985) The mammary gland as a target organ for infection with caprine arthritis-encephalitis virus. J Comp Pathol 95:609–617
47. Kennedy-Stoskopf S (1989) Pathogenesis of lentivirus-induced arthritis – a review. Rheum International 9:129–136

48. Klevjer-Anderson P, McGuire TC (1982) Neutralizing antibody response of rabbits and goats to caprine arthritis-encephalitis virus. Infect Immun 38:455–461
49. Klevjer-Anderson P, Adams DS, Anderson W, Banks KJ, McGuire TC (1984) Sequential study of virus expression in retrovirus-induced arthritis of goats. J Gen Virol 65:1519–1525
50. Kobayashi K (1961) Studies on the cultivation of equine infectious anemia virus in vitro. II. Propagation of the virus in horse bone marrow culture. Arch Ges Virusforsch (Arch Virol) 11:189–201
51. Kanki PJ, McLane MF, King Jr NW, Letvin NL, Hunt RD, Sehgal P, Daniel MD, Desrosiers RC, Essex M (1985) Serologic identification and characterization of a macaque T-lymphotrophic retrovirus closely related to HTLV-III. Science 228:1199–1201
52. Krieg A, Peterhans E (1990) Die caprine Arthritis-Encephalitis in der Schweiz: epidemiologische und klinische Untersuchungen. Schweiz Arch Tierheilk 132:345–352
53. McGuire TC, Adams TS, Johnson GC, Klevjer-Anderson P, Barbee DD, Gorham JR (1986) Acute arthritis in caprine arthritis-encephalitis virus challenge exposure of vaccinated or persistently infected goats. Am J Vet Res 47:537–540
54. McGuire TC (1987) The immune response to viral antigens as a determinant of arthritis in caprine arthritis-encephalitis virus infection. Vet Immunol Immunopathol 17:465–470
55. McGuire TC, Norton LK, O'Rourke KI, Cheevers WP (1988) Antigenic variation of neutralization-sensitive epitopes of caprine arthritis-encephalitis lentivirus during persistent arthritis. J Virol 62:3488–3492
56. Mitchell RL, Zokas L, Schreiber RD, and Verma IM (1985) Rapid induction of the expression of proto-oncogene *fos* during human monocytic differentiation. Cell 40:209–217
57. Narayan O, Clements JE, Strandberg JD, Cork LC, Griffin DE (1980) Biological characterization of the virus causing leukoencephalitis and arthritis in goats. J Gen Virol 50:69–79
58. Narayan O, Wolinsky JS, Clements JE, Standberg JD, Griffin DE, Cork LC (1982) Slow virus replication: the role of macrophages in the persistence and expression of visna viruses of sheep and goats. J Gen Virol 59:345–356
59. Narayan O (1983) Role of macrophages in the immunopathogenesis of visna-maedi of sheep. Immunology of nervous system infections. Prog Brain Res 59:233–235
60. Narayan O, Kennedy-Stoskopf S, Sheffer D, Griffin DE, Clements JE (1983) Activation of caprine arthritis-encephalitis virus expression during maturation of monocytes to macrophages. Infect Immun 41:67–73
61. Narayan O, Sheffer D, Griffin DE, Clements J, Hess J (1984) Lack of neutralizing antibodies to caprine arthritis-encephalitis lentivirus in persistently infected goats can be overcome by immunization with inactivated *Mycobacterium tuberculosis.* J Virol 49:349–355
62. Narayan O, Sheffer D, Clements JE, Tennekoon G (1985) Restricted replication of lentiviruses. Visna viruses induce a unique interferon during interaction between lymphocytes and infected macrophages. J Exp Med 162:1954–1969
63. Narayan O, Zink Ch (1988) Role of macrophages in Lentivirus infections. Adv Vet Sci Comp Med 32:129–148
64. Oliver RE, McNiven RA, Julian AF (1982) Experimental infection of sheep and goats with caprine arthritis-encephalitis virus. New Zealand Vet J 30:158–159
65. Oliver R, Cathcart A, McNiven R, Poole W, Robati G (1985) Infection of lambs with caprine arthritis encephalitis virus by feeding milk from infected goats. Vet Rec 116:83
66. Pedersen NC, Ho EW, Brown ML, Yamamoto JK (1987) Isolation of a T-lymphotropic virus from domestic cats with an immuodeficiency-like syndrome. Science 235:790–793
67. Peluso R, Haase A, Stowring L, Edwards M, Ventura P (1985) A Trojan horse mechanism for the spread of visna virus in monocytes. Virology 147:231–236
68. Peterhans E, Jungi Th, Bürge Th, Grob M, Jörg A (1988) Phagocyte chemiluminescence. In: Rice-Evans C, Halliwel B (eds) Free radicals, methology and concepts. Richelieu Press, London, pp 309–334

69. Rauscher FJ III, Cohen DR, Curran T, Bos TJ, Vogt PK, Bohmann D, Tijian R, Franza BR Jr (1988) Fos-associated protein p 39 is the product of the *jun* protooncogene. Science 240:1010–1016
70. Ruff G (1987) Investigations on the caprine leukocyte antigen (CLA) system. Dissertation No 8468, Swiss Federal Institute of Technology Zürich, Switzerland
71. Ruff G, Lazary S (1988) Evidence for linkage between the caprine leucocyte antigen (CLA) system and susceptibility to CAE virus-induced arthritis in goats. Immunogenetics 28:303–309
72. Sigurdsson B, Thormar H, Palsson PA (1961) Cultivation of visna virus in tissue culture. Arch ges Virusforsch (Arch Virol) 10:368–381
73. Small JA, Bieberich C, Ghotbi Z, Hess J, Scangos GA, Clements JE (1989) The visna virus long terminal repeat directs expression of a reporter gene in activated macrophages, lymphocytes, and the central nervous systems of transgenic mice. J Virol 63:1891–1896
74. Smith VW, Dickson J, Coackley W, Carman H (1985) Response of merino sheep to inoculation with a caprine retrovirus. Vet Rec 117:61–63
75. Smith MC, Cutlip R (1988) Effects of infection with caprine arthritis-encephalitis virus on milk production in goats. J Am Vet Med Ass 193:63–67
76. Sonigo P, Alizon M, Staskus K, Klatzmann D, Cole S, Danos O, Retzel E, Thiollais P, Haase A, Wain-Hobson S (1985) Nucleotide sequence of the visna lentivirus: relationship to the AIDS virus. Cell 42:369–382
77. Surman PG, Daniels E, Dixon BR (1987) Caprine arthritis-encephalitis virus infection of goats in South Australia. Aust Vet J 64:266–271
78. Van Der Maaten MJ, Boothe AD, Seger CL (1972) Isolation of a virus from cattle with persistent lymphocytosis. J Natl Cancer Inst 52:1649–1657
79. Winfield JB (1989) Stress proteins, arthritis and autoimmunity. Arthritis Rheum 32:1497–1504
80. Woodard JC, Gaskin JM, Poulos PW, MacKay RJ, Burridge MJ (1982) Caprine arthritis-encephalitis: clinicopathologic study. Am J Vet Res 43:2085–2096
81. Yaniv A, Dahlberg J, Gazit A, Sherman L, Chiu I-M, Tronick SR, Aaronson SA (1986) Molecular cloning and physical characterization of integrated equine infectious anemia virus: molecular and immunologic evidence of its close relationship to caprine lentiviruses. Virology 154:1–8
82. Yilma T, Owens S, Adams DS (1988) High levels of interferon in Synovial fluid of retrovirus-infected goats. J Interferon Res 8:45–50
83. Zink MC, Narayan O, Kennedy PGE, Clements JE (1987) Pathogenesis of visna/maedi and caprine arthritis-encephalitis: new leads on the mechanism of restricted virus replication and persistent inflammation. Vet Immunol Immunopathol 15:167–180
84. Zwahlen R, Aeschbacher M, Balcer Th, Stucki M, Wyder-Walther M, Weiss M, Steck F (1983) Lentivirusinfektionen bei Ziegen mit Carpitis und interstitieller Mastitis. Schweiz Arch Tierheilk 125:281–299
85. Zwahlen R, Spaeth PJ, Stucki M (1985) Histological and immunopathological investigations in goats with carpitis/pericarpitis. In: Sharp JM, Hoff-Jorgensen (eds) Slow viruses in sheep, goats and cattle. ECSC-EEC-EAEC, Brussels, Luxembourg, pp 239–248

Oncogenes and Retroviruses in Rheumatoid Arthritis

G. Stransky, R. E. Gay, A. Trabandt, W. K. Aicher, S. R. Barnum,
and S. Gay

Division of Clinical Immunology and Rheumatology, Department of Medicine,
University of Alabama at Birmingham, Birmingham, AL 35294, USA

Rheumatoid arthritis is a chronic systemic disorder of currently still unknown etiology. Its most serious and debilitating consequences are derived from the destruction of affected joints. An exceedingly large number of reports have described the histopathologic lesions in the rheumatoid joint. However, the interpretation of these observations must be carefully guarded because of the static nature of the studies and the usually advanced stage of joint destruction.

The nature of the previously mentioned studies make it difficult to define and characterize the early events in the pathogenesis of rheumatoid arthritis. This problem might be overcome to some extent by the use of appropriate animal models which are suitable for the detailed study of selected pathogenetic mechanisms found or seen in the early stages of joint disease [1]. The MRL/l mouse strain, which has previously served as a useful model for the study of spontaneous systemic lupus erythematosus (SLE) [2–4], spontaneously develops a destructive arthropathy of the hind limbs [5]. In addition, high levels of circulating rheumatoid factors are found in the sera of these animals making this murine disease a useful model for human rheumatoid arthritis and allowing a detailed and systemic study of early occurring tissue injury in the rheumatoid joint [6].

The pathological changes observed in the diseased joints of MRL/l mice can be divided into three distinct stages [7]. The first stage consists of synovial cell proliferation in the joint recesses. The second stage is characterized by continued proliferation of transformed-appearing synoviocytes which closely resemble immature mesenchymal cells. The ultrastructural morphology of these cells reveals the typical characteristics of fibroblastic type B synoviocytes [8]. The earliest destructive changes occur in this stage and consist of cartilage lesions and/or marginal erosions of subchondral bone. These erosions are restricted to areas contiguous with the proliferating transformed synovial lining cells which became attached to the underlying articular matrix and subsequently invaded it. The final stage is characterized by a diminution of synovial hyperplasia, extensive cartilage destruction, formation of scar tissue, and a moderate infiltration of the synovial stroma with inflammatory cells. Through-

Smolen, Kalden, Maini (Eds.)
Rheumatoid Arthritis
© Springer-Verlag Berlin Heidelberg 1992

out the progression of disease, there is a striking dissociation between the presence of inflammatory cells and the degree of joint destruction.

Interestingly, the early stages of the MRL/l mouse arthropathies resemble the early stages of rheumatoid arthritis as described by Fassbender [9]. These early stages of rheumatoid arthritis, characterized by the presence of trans-formed-appearing proliferating synovial lining cells seen in close contact with erosive joint defects, appear distinct from more advanced stages of disease which are generally characterized by infiltration with T lymphocytes [10].

The observations that early erosions of articular structures in the MRL/l arthropathies and human rheumatoid arthritis occur in areas contiguous with proliferating transformed-appearing synovial lining cells suggest a decisive role for these cells in the development of joint destruction. Therefore, it may be assumed that initial synovial cell proliferation and tissue breakdown do not necessarily depend on the presence of inflammatory cells and their mediators.

The capacity to proliferate and become attached to other tissue components and the ability to show local invasiveness and exert destructive properties was attributed to "tumor-like" characteristics of synoviocytes in human rheumatoid arthritis [11–14]. The molecular and cellular basis for the change in the biological behavior of these cells, which is reflected by an altered phenotypical appearance, is not understood. Therefore, present studies on the basic mechanisms regulating cellular proliferation, transformation, and signaling mechanisms for the production of enzymes at the molecular level should yield detailed insight into the cellular basis of joint destruction [15–17].

In recent years evidence has accumulated that basic cellular processes such as proliferation, differentiation, and the capability to respond to activating signals underlie the control exerted by a group of genes called cellular oncogenes [18]. Cellular oncogenes (c-*onc*) are defined as sequences in the mammalian genome showing a various degree of homology to viral oncogenes (v-*onc*) [19]. Viral oncogenes are the transforming sequences in the genome of certain retroviruses that are responsible for the malignant transformation of cells and which cause tumors in animals [20]. At the present time studies concerning the basic role of oncogenes in the regulation of cellular processes are increasing extensively.

Data concerning the role of oncogenes in rheumatoid arthritis are very limited and generally restricted to observations derived from studies on oncogene expression in peripheral blood mononuclear cells in non-rheumatoid autoimmune diseases. In these studies, samples from patients with rheumatoid arthritis served as controls [21, 22]. Increased levels of c-*myc* and c-*myb* could be demonstrated in these samples, whereas the amnount of c-*fos* was decreased.

Since cellular oncogenes code for proteins that may act as growth factors, cell surface receptors for growth factors, molecules for the delivery of intracellular messages, or nuclear proteins with regulatory functions, our laboratory has searched for a possible involvement of oncogenes and their products in the pathogenesis of rheumatoid arthritis. Within the large number of oncogenes that have been identified so far, our studies have focused on those associated with cellular activation and proliferation (*myc, myb, fos*) and the synthesis of connective tissue matrix degrading enzymes (*fos, ras*) [23–25].

The c-*myc* oncogene is the cellular homologue of the transforming gene of the avian myelocytomatosis virus 29 [26, 27]. It is located on chromosome 8 in humans [28] and encodes a protein with a molecular mass of 65–68 kDa [29]. This protein is found in the nucleus where it is associated with small ribonucleoprotein particles [30]. c-*myc* is present in varying amounts in all cell types, with the highest levels in hematopoietic organs such as thymus and spleen [31]. The role of c-*myc* has been studied thoroughly in normal human peripheral blood mononuclear cells and cultured murine 3T3 fibroblasts [20, 31, 32]. In resting peripheral blood mononuclear cells, c-*myc* is almost undetectable [21, 22]. In general, antigenic or mitogenic stimulation induces a marked increase in c-*myc* mRNA within 1–3 h [21, 33–37], which succeeds the transient increase of c-*fos* detected 10 min after stimulation. After reaching its peak 5 h after stimulation, the level of c-*myc* persists for approximately 18 h and then decreases to its baseline level. The same pattern of increased c-*myc* expression is seen in cultured 3T3 fibroblasts after mitogenic stimulation with platelet-derived growth factor (PDGF) [33, 38]. The ordered expression of c-*fos* and c-*myc* occurs early after stimulation and is a general feature of cellular activation and proliferation [39]. The transcription of these cellular oncogenes precedes the cell cycle dependent changes of DNA and RNA [21]. The properly regulated expression of c-*fos* and c-*myc* seems to exert important control on the cell in its passage through the cell cycle, most likely by positive regulation of other genes [31, 32]. In light of these findings, the expression of c-*myc* in synovial cells of rats with experimental erosive arthritis [40] and in rheumatoid joints [23–25] indicates an activated state of these cells at the site of cartilage and bone destruction.

The c-*myb* oncogene has been identified as the cellular homologue of the transforming gene of the avian myeloblastosis virus [41]. It has been mapped to chromosome 6 in humans and codes for a protein with a molecular mass of 45 kDa which, like the c-*myc* protein, is localized in the nucleus where it is associated with the nuclear matrix [42]. c-*myb* is expressed predominantly by hematopoietic cells and by thymocytes [43, 44]. In immature cortical thymo-cytes a high amount of c-*myb* can be found which is transcribed in a cell cycle independent manner, whereas in more mature lymphoid cells its decrease is associated with a change in its regulation, from constitutive cell cycle independent expression to a cell cycle regulated expression [45]. This down-regulation of c-*myb* is thought to be a necessary event during lymphocyte differentiation [43, 44]. Normal resting peripheral blood mononuclear cells have very low amounts of c-*myb* mRNA [22], whereas mitogenic stimulation leads to an increase of c-*myb* in lymphocytes [21]. The rise of c-*myb* mRNA level precedes the increase in cellular RNA and DNA content in the cell cycle [21]. Moreover, it has been suggested that its inappropriately high expression may be capable of blocking cellular differentiation [46, 47]. Therefore, c-*myb* ex-pression seems to be closely correlated with the regulation of cellular differentiation and proliferation [45]. The deregulation in the expression of cellular oncogenes may account for the phenotypical alterations of synovio-cytes exhibiting morphological characteristics of transformed cells [17]. This hypothesis is supportd by the immunohistochemical demonstration of elevated levels of c-*myb* in proliferating transformed-appearing synoviocytes of patients with rheumatoid arthritis [24].

The c-*fos* oncogene is the cellular homologue of the transforming gene of the Finkel-Biskins osteosarcoma virus. It codes for a DNA binding phosphopro-tein with a molecular mass of 55 kDa which is also localized in the nucleus [48]. The expression of c-*fos* is transient and has been studied in normal human peripheral blood mononuclear cells and cultured 3T3 fibroblasts [20, 31, 32]. Mitogenic and antigenic stimulation of peripheral blood mononuclear cells results in an increase in the level of c-*fos* mRNA within minutes [21], which reaches its peak 1 h after stimulation and finally decreases to baseline levels after 3 h. A similar pattern of c-*fos* expression is observed in cultured 3T3 fibroblasts, where the mitogenic stimulation with PDGF is followed within 30 min by a transient increase of c-*fos* expression [49, 50].

However, the role of c-*fos* does not seem to be limited to an association with cellular proliferation. Recent studied have elucidated the function of c-*fos* as a "master regulatory gene" controlling the activation of other genes [51]. c-*fos* exerts this regulatory function in close collaboration with another oncogene, c-*jun*. The latter is the cellular homologue of the transforming gene of the avian sarcoma virus 17 [52]. It codes for a protein with nuclear localization, presumably the transcription factor AP-1 [53], which forms a complex with the c-*fos* protein [54]. c-*fos*/c-*jun* has been shown to be essential for the activation of the transcription of other genes by binding to gene promoter regions [55]. Moreover, it has been reported that the promoter region of the gene coding for collagenase is under the control of c-*fos* [56]. In this region, the DNA sequence has been identified to which c-*fos* binds, thus exerting its control activity [56]. A similar DNA sequence has been shown to exist for stromelysin, another enzyme involved in the degradation of extracellular matrix molecules [57]. In histologi-cal studies of the rheumatoid joint, type B synoviocytes have been identified as the source for the production of stromelysin [58]. The presence of c-*fos* in synoviocytes at the site of rheumatoid joint destruction [24] suggests an activated state for these cells associated with the production of proteolytic enzymes such as collagenase and stromelysin.

Other studies have shown additional evidence for the existence of a close connection between the elevated production of proteolytic enzymes and the increased expression of cellular oncogenes. The *ras* oncogene encodes p21, a protein with a molecular mass of 21 kDa, which is anchored to the inner surface of the cell membrane and serves as a messenger molecule for the transduction of exogenous signals from cell surface receptors into the cell [59, 60]. Cell culture experiments have revealed a close correlation between the expression of *ras* and the production of proteinases with the capability of degrading extracellular matrix molecules. The transfection of *ras* oncogene into 3T3 fibroblasts led to a detectable increase in the level of the mRNA for procathepsin L [61]. Procathepsin L is the precursor form of cathepsin L, the most active lysosomal cysteine proteinase [62]. Cathepsin L degrades the N-terminal nonhelical portion of type I collagen [63], intact basement membranes [64], and fibronectin [65]; moreover, its specificity for collagen types II, IX and XI has been determined [106]. The importance of cysteine proteinases in the breakdown of extracellular matrix molecules is supported by the recent finding that metalloproteinases, the group of enzymes collagenases belong to, are not involved in the phagocytosis and intracellular digestion of collagen fibrils by fibroblasts [66]. In addition, osteoclasts have been shown to degrade type I collagen of bone by an entirely collagenase independent pathway [67]. In this regard, there is now increasing evidence that noncollagenase proteinases may play a key role in the breakdown of extracellular matrix molecules also in arthritic disease. In the experimental ovalbumin induced arthritis in rabbits, cathepsin L was detected in synovial lining cells, fibroblasts, and macrophages [68]. In addition, fibroblasts derived from the diseased joints of MRL/l mice were shown to contain elevated levels of cathepsin L mRNA [69]. The recent finding of significant amounts of cathepsin, L mRNA in synoviocytes from patients with rheumatoid arthritis suggests that this proteinase may play a major role in the tissue breakdown in human destructive joint disease [25, 70]. Support for this hypothesis comes from the immunohistochemical demonstration of *ras* protein in the cytoplasm of proliferating synoviocytes [23–25]. The same studies have also shown that *ras* oncogene expression is not limited to the sites of joint destruction, but also occurs in the vascular cells of proliferating synovial blood vessels [25]. This finding is especially of interest in light of the fact that elevated levels of another basement membrane-degrading enzyme, type IV collagenase, have been detected in *ras* transfected human bronchial epithelial cells and in *ras* transformed mouse fibroblasts [71, 72]. The effect of this increased type IV collagenolytic activity is substantiated by the finding that the intravenous injection of 3T3 fibroblasts, which had been transfected either with tumor DNA or with *ras* oncogene, led to the spontaneous development of metastasis in nude mice [73]. With respect to the expression of *ras* in rheumatoid vascular structures, it is likely that a *ras* induced type IV collagenase may be responsible for the alteration of basement membranes resulting in an increased vascular permeability and accumulation of T lymphocytes and macrophages characteristic for the inflamed rheumatoid synovium [74].

The increased *ras* expression in proliferating synoviocytes is important not only in conjunction with the secretion of proteolytic enzymes. Cell culture experiments have revealed the cooperation of oncogenes such as *ras* and *myc* in the transformation of primary fibroblasts [75, 76]. The combined activity of these two oncogenes could account for the transformed phenotype of synoviocytes in rheumatoid arthritis [15, 24, 25].

The importance of oncogenes and their products in the regulation of cellular growth and proliferation is further substantiated by the close association between PDGF and the c-*sis* oncogene. PDGF is a glycoprotein with a molecular mass of 30 kDa consisting of two chains [77]. Its A-chain is the protein product of a gene located on chromosome 7 [78], whereas the precursor form of the B-chain is encoded by a separate gene on chromosome 22 [79]. This

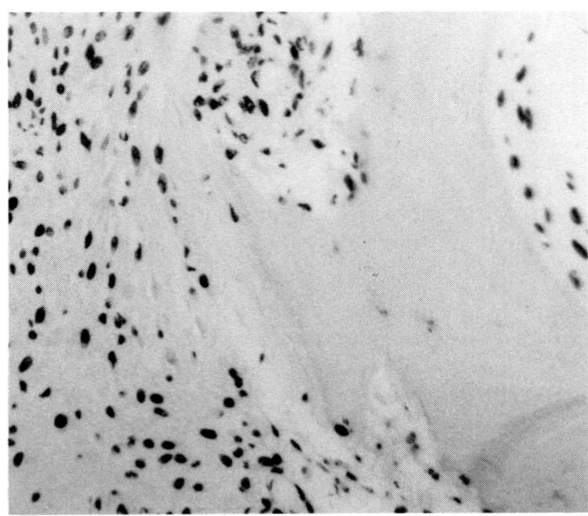

Fig. 1. Proliferating synovial lining cells at the site of invasion and bone destruction in a patient with rheumatoid arthritis. Section stained with monoclonal antibody against PDGF, visualized by black silver enhanced gold label ($\times$ 150)

particular gene has been identified as the c-*sis* oncogene, which is the cellular homologue of the transforming gene of the simian sarcoma virus [80]. PDGF acts as a potent mitogen for connective tissue cells in vitro [81, 82] and leads to a marked increase of c-*myc* mRNA levels in cultured 3T3 fibroblasts [33]. Platelets, monocytes/macrophages, megakaryocytes, and endothelial cells have been shown to be able to produce PDGF [82–85]. As normal plasma is devoid of circulating PDGF, tissue-bound cells have to be considered as the main source for the secretion of this molecule [82]. From this finding it may be concluded that mainly cells situated in close vicinity to PDGF-producing cells are under the influence of this molecule [82]. Due to the fact that activated macrophages have been shown to produce PDGF [84] they may be considered as a candidate for the secretion of this molecule in rheumatoid joints [82, 86]. In this regard it is of interest that PDGF can also be detected in proliferating synovial lining cells, especially at the site of joint destruction (Fig. 1). PDGF exerts its stimulatory activity by binding to a receptor molecule located on the surface of the cell membrane [87]. Normal synoviocytes do not have detectable PDGF receptors, whereas synovial cells from rheumatoid arthritis joints express considerable amounts of this receptor on their surface [86]. In rheumatoid joints, the presence of PDGF receptors on synoviocytes was found to be especially prominent at sites of extensive cellular proliferation and local degradation of articular cartilage [86].

Additional support for the importance of these observations comes from studies evaluating the growth characteristics of transformed cells cultures. Among certain other features, the most consistent and reliable sign of transformed cellular growth was found to be the ability to grow in soft agar or agarose, under "anchorage-independent" conditions [88–91]. Synoviocytes derived from patients with rheumatoid arthritis could grow under such conditions in the beginning, but lost this ability after a few passages when grown

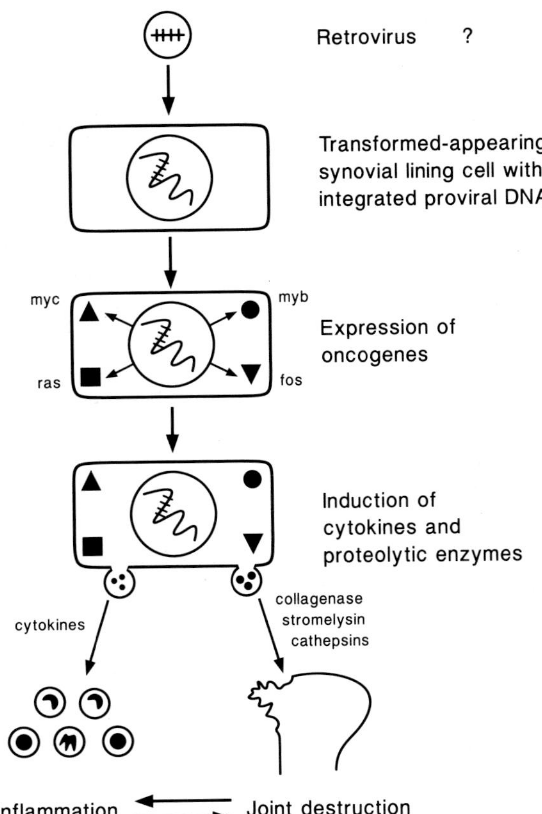

Fig. 2. Hypothesis on the molecular mechanisms of joint destruction in rheumatoid arthritis

in media with PDGF. In contrast, synoviocytes cultured in media lacking PDGF failed to exhibit anchorage-independent growth through multiple passages [13]. From these observations it may be concluded that the expression of the c-*sis* oncogene with its concomitant production of PDGF participates in the maintenance of a transformed phenotype of synoviocytes in the rheumatoid joint.

Based on the transformed-appearing phenotype of rheumatoid synovial lining cells also in tissue culture and the elevated expression of oncogenes at the site of joint destruction, our laboratory searched for the presence of retroviral sequences [15].

Evidence for the possible involvement of a retroviral agent in the development of an arthritic disease has come from studies concerning the pathogenesis of chronic arthritis in animals. The caprine arthritis-encephalitis virus, an animal retrovirus, has been found to be the etiological agent for the development of chronic arthritis in goats [92]. Indeed, the presence of a retrovirus in the pathogenesis of rheumatoid arthritis could explain the expression of oncoproteins with the induction of cytokines and proteases involved in rheumatoid joint destruction, as illustrated in Fig. 2.

Up to now the search for the presence of a retrovirus in human rheumatoid arthritis has been inconclusive. Despite the use of a variety of virological methods, no retrovirus has been detected in peripheral blood mononuclear cells, mononuclear cells of synovial effusions, or synoviocytes [93–97]. Furthermore, circulating antibodies against the human T-lymphotropic virus type I, II, and III could not be detected in sera from patients with rheumatoid arthritis [98].

A number of morphological observations have, however, pointed to the possible involvement of a viral agent in the development of human rheumatoid arthritis. Virus-like particles, inclusion bodies, and structures resembling nucleocapsids have been found in endothelial cells, pericytes, or macrophages of synovial tissues from patients with rheumatoid arthritis [99–102]. These observations are supported by the immunohistochemical demonstration of human T-lymphotropic virus type I related antigenicity in proliferating synoviocytes from patients with early stages of rheumatoid arthritis [103]. Due to the absence of circulating antibodies against human T-lymphotropic virus type I in the sera of these patients, this observation is likely to be interpreted as a form of cross-reactivity with a currently undefined antigen of possible retroviral origin, present in the rheumatoid joint. This concept of cross-reactivity gains additional support from the finding that human rheumatoid factor-positive sera contain antibodies which bind to a synthetic human T-lymphotropic virus type I derived peptide [104]. The recent observation of virus-like particles in synovial fluid from patients with rheumatoid arthritis [105, 107] makes the search for a possible retroviral origin of human arthritis an exciting challenge in the ongoing attempt to elucidate the molecular mechanisms of erosive joint destruction.

References

1. Klareskog L (1989) What can we learn about rheumatoid arthritis from animal models? Springer Semin Immunopathol 11:315–333
2. Murphy ED, Roths JB (1978) Autoimmunity and lymphoproliferation: induction by mutant gene *lpr* and acceleration by a male-associated factor in strain BXSB mice. In: Rose NR, Bigazzi RE, Warner NL (eds) Genetic Control of Autoimmune Disease. Elsevier/North-Holland, New York, pp 207–219
3. Theofilopoulos AN, Dixon FJ (1981) Etiopathogenesis of immune SLE. Immunol Rev 55:179–216
4. Andrews BS, Eisenberg RA, Theofilopoulos AN, Izui S, Wilson CB, McConahey PJ, Murphy ED, Roths JB, Dixon FJ (1978) Spontaneous murine lupus-like syndromes. J Exp Med 148:1198–1215
5. Hang L, Theofilopoulos AN, Dixon FJ (1982) A spontaneous rheumatoid arthritis-like disease in MRL/1 mice. J Exp Med 155:1690–1701
6. Koopman WJ, Gay S (1988) The MRL-lpr/lpr mouse. A model for the study of rheumatoid arthritis. Scand J Rheumatol 75(S):284–289

7. O'Sullivan FX, Fassbender H-G, Gay S, Koopman WJ (1985) Etiopathogenesis of the rheumatoid arthritis-like disease in MRL/l mice. I. The histomorphologic basis of joint destruction. Arthritis Rheum 28:529–536
8. Tanaka A, O'Sullivan FX, Koopman WJ, Gay S (1988) Etiopathogenesis of rheumatoid arthritis-like disease in MRL/l mice: II. Ultrastructural basis of joint destruction. J Rheumatol 15:10–16
9. Fassbender H-G (1983) Histomorphological basis of articular cartilage destruction in rheumatoid arthritis. Coll Relat Res 3:141–155
10. Gay S, Koopman WJ (1989) Immunopathology of rheumatoid arthritis. Curr Opin Rheumatol 1:8–14
11. Fassbender H-G, Simmling-Annefeld M, Stofft E (1980) Transformation der Synovialzellen bei rheumatoider Arthritis. Verh Dtsch Ges Pathol 64:193–212
12. Harris ED (1989) Pathogenesis of rheumatoid arthritis. In: Kelley WS, Harris ED, Rudy S, Sledge CB (eds) Textbook of Rheumatology. WB Saunders, Philadelphia, pp 905–942
13. Lafyatis R, Remmers EF, Roberts AB, Yocum DE, Sporn MB, Wilder RL (1989) Anchorage-independent growth of synoviocytes from arthritic and normal joints. J Clin Invest 83:1267–1276
14. Sano H, Forough R, Maier JA, Case JP, Jackson A, Engelka K, Maciag T, Wilder RL (1990) Detection of high levels of heparin binding growth factor-1 (acidic fibroblast growth factor) in inflammatory arthritic joints. J Cell Biol 110:1417–1426
15. Gay S, Gay RE (1989) Cellular basis and oncogene expression of rheumatoid joint destruction. Rheumatol Int 9:105–113
16. Krane SM, Conca W, Stephenson ML, Amento EP, Goldring MB (1990) Mechanisms of matrix degradation in rheumatoid arthritis. Ann N Y Acad Sci 580:340–354
17. Ritchlin CT, Winchester RJ (1989) Potential mechanisms for coordinate gene activation in the rheumatoid synoviocyte: implications and hypotheses. Springer Semin Immunopathol 11:219–234
18. Sibbitt WL (1988) Oncogenes, normal cell growth, and connective tissue disease. Annu Rev Med 39:123–133
19. Bishop JM (1983) Cellular oncogenes and retroviruses. Annu Rev Biochem 52:301–354
20. Burck KB, Liu ET, Larrick JW (1988) Oncogenes. An introduction to the concept of cancer genes. Springer, New York
21. Klinman DM, Mushinski JF, Honda M, Ishigatsubo Y, Mountz JD, Raveche ES, Steinberg AD (1986) Oncogene expression in autoimmune and normal peripheral blood mononuclear cells. J Exp Med 163:1292–1307
22. Boumpas DT, Tsokos GC, Mann DL, Eleftheriades EG, Harris CC, Mark GE (1986) Increased proto-oncogene expression in peripheral blood lymphocytes from patients with systemic lupus erythematosus and other autoimmune diseases. Arthritis Rheum 29:755–760
23. Gay S, Tanaka A, Tarkowski A, Gay RE, Fassbender H-G (1988) Expression of oncogenes *ras* and *myc* in proliferating synovial lining cells in rheumatoid arthritis. Arthritis Rheum 31(S):R40
24. Gay S, Huang G, Ziegler B, Fassbender H-G, Gay RE (1989) Expression of *myb, myc, ras* and *fos* oncogenes in synovial cells of patients with rheumatoid arthritis (RA) or osteoarthritis (OA). Arthritis Rheum 32(S):R39
25. Trabandt A, Aicher W, Gay RE, Sukhatme V, Nilson-Hamilton M, Hamilton RT, McGhee JR, Fassbender H-G, Gay S (1990) Expression of the collagenolytic and ras-induced cysteine proteinase cathepsin L and proliferation-associated oncogenes in synovial cells of MRL/l mice and patients with rheumatoid arthritis. Matrix 10:349–361
26. Watson DK, Psallidopoulos MC, Samuel KP, Dalla-Favera R, Papas TS (1983) Nucleotide sequence analysis of human c-*myc* locus, chicken homologue, and myelocytomatosis virus MC 29 transforming gene reveals a highly conserved gene product. Proc Natl Acad Sci USA 80:3642–3645
27. Colby WW, Chen EY, Smith DH, Levinson AD (1983) Identification and nucleotide sequence of a human locus homologous to the v-*myc* oncogene of avian myelocytomatosis virus MC 29. Nature 301:722–725

28. Dalla-Favera R, Bregni M, Erikson J, Patterson D, Gallo RC, Croce CM (1982) Human c-*myc* oncogene is located on the region of chromosome 8 that is translocated in Burkitt's lymphoma cells. Proc Natl Acad Sci USA 79:7824–7827
29. Watt RA, Shatzman AR, Rosenberg M (1985) Expressin and characterization of the human c-*myc* DNA-binding protein. Mol Cell Biol 5:448–456
30. Spector DL, Watt RA, Sullivan NF (1987) The v- and c-*myc* oncogene protein colocalize in situ with small ribonucleoprotein particles. Oncogene 1:5–12
31. Boumpas DT, Mark GE, Tsokos GC (1986) Oncogenes and autoimmunity. Anticancer Res 6:491–498
32. Boumpas DT, Eleftheriades EG, Barez S, Tsokos GC (1988) Oncogene expression and regulation in normal lymphocytes and lymphocytes from patients with autoimmune diseases. Anticancer Res 8:977–984
33. Kelly K, Cochran BH, Stiles CD, Leder P (1983) Cell specific regulation of the c-*myc* gene by lymphocyte mitogens and platelet derived growth factor. Cell 35:603–610
34. Smeland EB, Beiske K, Ek B, Watt R, Pfeifer-Ohlsson S, Blomhoff HK, Godal T, Ohlsson R (1987) Regulation of c-*myc* transcription and protein expression during activation of normal human B cells. Exp Cell Res 172:101–109
35. Reed JC, Alpers JD, Nowell PC, Hoover RG (1986) Sequential expression of proto-oncogenes during lectin-stimulated mitogenesis of normal human lymphocytes. Proc Natl Acad Sci USA 83:3982–3986
36. Kelly K, Siebenlist U (1988) Mitogenic activation of normal T cells leads to increased initiation of transcription in the c-*myc* locus. J Biol Chem 263:4828–4831
37. Reed JC, Nowell PC, Hoover RG (1985) Regulation of c-*myc* mRNA levels in normal human lymphocytes by modulators of cell proliferation. Proc Natl Acad Sci USA 82:4221–4224
38. Armelin HA, Armelin MCS, Kelly K, Stewart T, Leder P, Cochran BH, Stiles CD (1984) Functional role for c-*myc* in mitogenic response to platelet-derived growth factor. Nature 310:655–660
39. Müller R, Bravo R, Burckhardt J (1984) Induction of c-*fos* gene and protein by growth factors precedes activation of c-*myc*. Nature 312:716–720
40. Case JP, Sano H, Lafyatis R, Remmers EF, Kumkumian GK, Wilder RL (1989) Transin/stromelysin expression in the synovium of rats with experimental erosive arthritis. J Clin Invest 84:1731–1740
41. Gonda TF, Bishop JM (1983) Structure and transcription of the cellular homolog (c-*myb*) of the avian myeloblastosis virus transforming gene (v-*myb*). J Virol 46:212–220
42. Klempnauer KH, Symonds G, Evan G, Bishop JM (1984) Subcellular localization of proteins encoded by oncogenes of avian myeloblastosis virus and avian leukemia virus E 26 and by the chicken c-*myb* gene. Cell 37:537–547
43. Gonda TJ, Sheiness DK, Bishop JM (1982) Transcripts from the cellular homologs of retroviral oncogens: distribution among the chicken tissues. Mol Cell Biol 2:617–624
44. Sheiness D, Gardinier M (1984) Expression of proto-oncogene (proto-*myb*) in hemapoietic tissues of mice. Mol Cell Biol 4:1206–1212
45. Thompson CB, Challoner PB, Neiman PE, Groudine M (1986) Expression of the c-*myb* proto-oncogene during cellular proliferation. Nature 319:374–380
46. Clarke MF, Kukowska-Latallo JF, Westin E, Smith M, Prochownik EV (1988) Constitutive expression of a c-*myb* cDNA blocks Friend murine erythroleukemia cell differentiation. Mol Cell Biol 8:884–892
47. Gonda TJ, Ramsay RG, Johnson GR (1989) Murine myeloid cell lines derived by in vitro infection with recombinant c-*myb* retroviruses express myb from rearranged vector proviruses. EMBO J 8:1767–1775
48. Curran T, Miller AD, Zokas L, Verma IM (1984) Viral and cellular fos proteins: a comparative analysis. Cell 36:259–268
49. Greenberg ME, Ziff EB (1984) Stimulation of 3T3 cells induces transcription of the c-*fos* proto-oncogene. Nature 311:433–438
50. Kruijer W, Cooper JA, Hunter T, Verma IM (1984) Platelet-derived growth factor induces rapid but transient expression of the c-*fos* gene and protein. Nature 312:711–716

51. Marx J (1987) The *fos* gene as master "switch". Science 237:854–856
52. Vogt PK, Bos TJ, Doolittle RT (1987) Homology between the DNA-binding domain of the GCN4 regulatory protein of yeast and the carboxy-terminal region of a protein coded for by the oncogene *jun.* Proc Natl Acad Sci USA 84:3316–3319
53. Bohmann D, Bos TJ, Admon A, Nishimura T, Vogt PK, Tjian R (1987) Human proto-oncogene c-*jun* encodes a DNA binding protein with structural and functional properties of transcription factor AP-1. Science 238:1386–1392
54. Gentz R, Rauscher FJ, Abate C, Curran T (1989) Parallel association of fos and jun leucine zippers juxtaposes DNA binding domains. Science 243:1695–1699
55. Chiu R, Boyle WJ, Meek J, Smeal T, Hunter T, Karin M (1988) The c-*fos* protein interacts with c-*jun*/AP-1 to stimulate transcription of AP-1 responsive genes. Cell 54:541–552
56. Schönthal A, Herrlich P, Rahmsdorf HF, Ponta H (1988) Requirement for *fos* gene expression in the transcriptional activation of collagenase by other oncogenes and phorbol esters. Cell 54:325–334
57. Angel P, Imagawa M, Chiu R, Stein B, Imbra RJ, Rahmsdorf HJ, Jonat C, Herrlich P, Karin M (1987) Phorbol ester-inducible genes contain a common cis element recognized by a common TPA-modulated transacting factor. Cell 49:729–739
58. Okada Y, Takeuchi N, Tomita K, Nakanishi I, Nagase H (1989) Immunolocalization of matrix metalloproteinase 3 (stromelysin) in rheumatoid synovioblasts (B cells): correlation with rheumatoid arthritis. Ann Rheum Dis 48:645–653
59. Barbacid M (1987) Ras genes. Annu Rev Biochem 56:779–827
60. Santos E, Nebreda AR (1989) Structural and functional properties of ras proteins. FASEB J 3:2151–2163
61. Denhardt DT, Greenberg AH, Egan SE, Hamilton RT, Wright JA (1987) Cysteine proteinase cathepsin L expression correlates closely with the metastatic potential of H-*ras*-transformed murine fibroblasts. Oncogene 2:55–59
62. Barrett AJ, Kirschke H (1981) Cathepsin B, cathepsin H, and cathepsin L. Methods Enzymol 80:535–561
63. Kirschke H, Kembhavi AA, Bohley P, Barrett AJ (1982) Action of rat liver cathepsin L on collagen and other substrates. Biochem J 201:367–372
64. Maciewicz RA, Wardale RJ, Etherington DJ, Paraskeva C (1989) Immunodetection of cathepsins B and L present in and secreted from human pre-malignant and malignant colorectal tumor cell lines. Int J Cancer 43:478–486
65. Rozhin J, Wade RL, Honn KV, Sloane BF (1989) Membrane-associated cathepsin L: a role in metastasis of melanomas. Biochem Biophys Res Commun 164:556–561
66. Everts V, Hembry RM, Reynolds JJ, Beertsen W (1989) Metalloproteinases are not involved in the phagocytosis of collagen fibrils by fibroblasts. Matrix 9:266–276
67. Delaisse JM, Eeckhout Y, Vaes G (1984) In vivo and in vitro evidence for the involvement of cysteine proteinases in bone resorption. Biochem Biophys Res Commun 125:441–447
68. Etherington DJ, Taylor MAJ, Henderson B (1988) Elevation of cathepsin L levels in the synovial lining of rabbits with antigen-induced arthritis. Br J Exp Pathol 69:281–289
69. Trabandt A, Aicher W, Stewart T, Gay RE, Sukhatme V, Gay S (1989) Expression of cathepsin L mRNA, a major *ras* oncogene transcript, in rheumatoid synovial cells of MRL/1 mice. Arthritis Rheum 32(S):S 143
70. Trabandt A, Aicher W, Gay RE, Sukhatme V, Gay S (1990) Expession of cathepsin L mRNA, a major *ras* oncogene transcript, in synovial cells of patients with rheumatoid arthritis. Arthritis Rheum 33(S):R12
71. Collier IE, Wilhelm SM, Eisen AZ, Marmer BL, Grant GA, Seltzer JL, Kronberger A, He C, Bauer EA, Goldberg GI (1988) H-*ras* oncogene transformed bronchial epithelial cells (TBE-1) secrete a single metalloprotease capable of degrading basement membrane collagen. J Biol Chem 263:6579–6587
72. Spinucci C, Zucker S, Wieman JM, Lysik RM, Imhof B, Ramamurthy N, Liotta LA, Nagase H (1988) Purification of a gelatin degrading type IV collagenase secreted by *ras* oncogene transformed fibroblasts. J Natl Cancer Inst 80:1416–1420

73. Thorgeirsson UP, Turpeenniemi-Hujanen T, Williams JE, Westin EH, Heilman CA, Talmadge JE, Liotta LA (1985) NIH/3T3 cells transfected with human tumor DNA containing activated *ras* oncogenes express the metastatic phenotype in nude mice. Mol Cell Biol 5:259–262
74. Ziff M (1989) Pathways of mononuclear cell infiltration in rheumatoid synovitis. Rheumatol Int 9:97–103
75. Land H, Parada LF, Weinberg RA (1983) Tumorigenic conversion of primary embryo fibroblasts requires at least two cooperating oncogenes. Nature 304:596–602
76. Richards CA, Short SA, Thorgeirsson SS, Huber BE (1990) Characterization of a transforming N-*ras* gene in the human hepatoma cell line Hep G2: additional evidence for the importance of c-*myc* and *ras* cooperation in hepatocarcinogenesis. Cancer Res 50:1521–1527
77. Johnsson A, Heldin CH, Westermark B, Wasteson A (1982) Platelet-derived growth factor: identification of constituent polypeptide chains. Biochem Biophys Res Commun 104:66–74
78. Betsholtz C, Johnsson A, Heldin CH, Westermark B, Lind P, Urdea MS, Eddy R, Shows TB, Philpott K, Mellor AL, Knott TJ, Scott J (1986) cDNA sequence and chromosomal localization of human platelet-derived growth factor A-chain and its expression in tumour cell lines. Nature 320:695–699
79. Dalla-Favera R, Gallo RC, Giallongo A, Croce CM (1982) Chromosomal localization of the human homolog (c-*sis*) of the simian sarcoma virus *onc* gene. Science 218:686–688
80. Waterfield MD, Scrace GT, Whittle N, Stroobant P, Johnsson A, Wasteson A, Westermark B, Heldin CH, Huang JS, Deuel TF (1983) Platelet-derived growth factor is structurally related to the putative transforming protein p28 of simian sarcoma virus. Nature 304:35–39
81. Heldin CH, Wasteson A, Westermark B (1985) Platelet-derived growth factor. Mol Cell Endocrinol 39:169–187
82. Ross R, Raines EW, Bowen-Pope DF (1986) The biology of platelet-derived growth factor. Cell 46:155–169
83. Dicorleto PE, Bowen-Pope DF (1983) Cultured endothelial cells produce a platelet-growth factor-like protein. Proc Natl Acad Sci USA 80:1919–1923
84. Martinet Y, Bitterman PB, Mornex JF, Grotendorst GR, Martin GR, Crystal RG (1986) Activated human monocytes express the c-*sis* proto-oncogene and release a mediator showing PDGF-like activity. Nature 319:158–160
85. Shimokado K, Raines EW, Madtes DK, Barrett TB, Benditt EP, Ross R (1985) A significant part of macrophage-derived growth factor consists of at least two forms of PDGF. Cell 43:277–286
86. Rubin K, Terracio L, Rönnstrand L, Heldin CH, Klareskog L (1988) Expression of platelet-derived growth factor receptors is induced on connective tissue cells during chronic synovial inflammation. Scand J Immunol 27:285–294
87. Yarden Y, Escobedo JA, Kuang WJ, Yang-Feng TL, Daniel TO, Tremble PM, Chen EY, Ando ME, Harkins RN, Francke U, Fried VA, Ullrich A, Williams LT (1986) Structure of the receptor for platelet-derived growth factor helps define a family of closely related growth factor receptors. Nature 323:226–232
88. Freedman VH, Shin S (1974) Cellular tumorigenicity in nude mice: Correlation with cell growth in semi-solid medium. Cell 3:355–359
89. Neugut AI, Weinstein IB (1979) The use of agarose in the determination of anchorage independent growth. In Vitro 15:351–355
90. Colburn NH, Vorder Bruegge WF, Bates JR, Gray RH, Rossen JD, Kelsey WH, Shimada T (1978) Correlation of anchorage-independent growth with tumorigenicity of chemically transformed mouse epidermal cells. Cancer Res 38:624–634
91. Cifone MA, Fidler IJ (1980) Correlation of patterns of anchorage-independent growth with in vivo behavior of cells from a murine fibrosarcoma. Proc Natl Acad Sci USA 77:1039–1043
92. Crawford TB, Adams DS, Cheevers WP, Cork LC (1980) Chronic arthritis in goats caused by a retrovirus. Science 207:997–999

93. Spruance SL, Richards OC, Smith CB, Ward JR (1975) DNA polymerase activity of cultured rheumatoid synovial cells. Arthritis Rheum 18:229–235
94. Norval M, Hart H, Marmion BP (1979) Viruses and lymphocytes in rheumatoid arthritis. I. Studies on cultured rheumatoid lymphocytes. Ann Rheum Dis 38:507–513
95. Hart H, Norval (1980) Search for viruses in rheumatoid macrophage-rich synovial cell populations. Ann Rheum Dis 39:159–163
96. Galeazzi M, Tuzi T, Amici C, Benedetto A (1986) Rheumatoid arthritis and human T cell lymphotrophic retroviruses. Arthritis Rheum 29:1533–1534
97. Pelton BK, North M, Palmer RG, Hylton W, Smith-Burchnell C, Sinclair AL, Malkovsky M, Dalgleish AG, Denman AM (1988) A search for retrovirus infection in systemic lupus erythematosus and rheumatoid arthritis. Ann Rheum Dis 47:206–209
98. Panayi GS, Dalgleish AG (1986) Retroviruses in rheumatoid arthritis. Ann Rheum Dis 45:439
99. Neumark T, Farkas K (1970) Nuclear bodies in rheumatoid synovium. Ann Rheum Dis 29:653–659
100. Györkey F, Sinkovics JG, Min KW, Györkey P (1972) A morphologic study on the occurrence and distribution of structures resembling viral nucleocapsids and collagen diseases. Am J Med 53:148–158
101. Neumark T, Hollos I, Farkas K (1973) Virus-like particles in rheumatoid synovium. Scand J Rheumatol 2:21–28
102. Schumacher HR (1975) Synovial membrane and fluid morphologic alterations in early rheumatoid arthritis: microvascular injury and virus-like particles. Ann N Y Acad Sci 256:39–64
103. Ziegler B, Gay RE, Huang G, Fassbender H-G, Gay S (1989) Immunohistochemical localization of HTLV-I p19- and P24-related antigens in synovial joints of patients with rheumatoid arthritis. Am J Pathol 135:1–5
104. Blomberg J, Fölsch G, Nilsson I, Fäldt R (1985) Immunoglobulin G antibodies binding to a synthetic peptide deduced from the nucleotide sequence of the env gene of HTLV I in patients with leukemia and rheumatoid arthritis, HLA sensitized persons and blood donors. Leuk Res 9:1111–1116
105. Stransky G, Moreland LW, Gay RE, Gay S (1990) Virus-like particles (VLP) in synovial fluids from patients with rheumatoid arthritis (RA). Arthritis Rheum 33(S):S143
106. Maciewicz RA, Wotton SF, Etherington DJ, Duance VC (1990) Susceptibility of the cartilage collagens type II, IX and XI to degradation by the cysteine proteinases, cathepsin B and L. FEBS Lett 269:189–193
107. Stransky G, Aicher WK, Gay RE, Gay S (1991) Characterization of virus-like particles (VLP) derived from patients with rheumatoid arthritis (RA). Arthritis Rheum 34(S):S177

Are Retroviruses Involved in the Pathogenesis of Autoimmune Diseases?

E. F. Krapf

Institute of Clinical Immunology and Rheumatology, Department of Internal Medicine III, Friedrich Alexander University Erlangen-Nürnberg, Krankenhausstrasse 12, W-8530 Erlangen, FRG

Introduction

Large portions of mammalian genomes consist of DNA sequences originally derived from retroviruses during ontogenesis. The majority of these retroviral sequences are non-infectious. However, during the past few years, evidence has been gained for the hypothesis that retroviral sequences or their products might play a role in the pathogenesis of autoimmune diseases (Table 1). The question

Table 1. Indications for retroviruses in autoimmune diseases

Reference	Indication
Melors and Mellors [25a]	Anti-type C-RV antibodies in SLE patients
Okamoto et al. [27]	Antibodies against endogenous RV-polymerase in human SLE
Rucheton et al. [38]	Antibodies against p30 gag in patients with SLE and MCTD
Shirai et al. [42]	Anti-gp70 antibody is correlated with autoantibody production and SLE-like disease in mice
Denman, 1986:	Unusual interferons are found in SLE and AIDS patients
Olsen et al. [28]	HTLV 1 antigenic determinants expressed in PBL of SLE patients
Keene, 1987:	U1 RNP-associated p70 contains the immunodominant epitope of p30 gag : p30 gag provokes autoantibodies
Volk et al. [49b]	The number of activated CD5$^+$ B cells is elevated in SLE and AIDS patients
Via et al. [49a]	Autoreactive B cell clones may be triggered by viruses and maintained by defective CTL
Reddy et al. [36a]	Amplification and molecular cloning of HTLV 1 sequences from DNA of multiple sclerosis patients
Talal et al. [46, 47]	Thirty percent of patients with primary Sjögren's syndrome and 36% of SLE patients show antibody reactivity against p24 core protein of HIV I[a]

[a] Was not confirmed by Krapf et al. [20] Venables (personal communication) and Krieg (personal communication)

Smolen, Kalden, Maini (Eds.)
Rheumatoid Arthritis
© Springer-Verlag Berlin Heidelberg 1992

Table 2. Immunologic features in HIV 1-infected persons (modified from [54])

Follicular hyperplasia
Loss of dendritic cells
Progressive lymphoid atrophy
Hypergammaglobulinemia
Circulating immune complexes
Acid-labile serum interferon
Increased lymphokine production
Depletion of CD 4 lymphocytes
Impaired alpha IF production
Antibodies against myelin basic protein in sera and cerebrospinal fluid

Table 3. Rheumatic manifestations of human immunodeficiency virus infection (according to [10a])

Arthralgias
Reactive arthritis
    HLA B 27-related Reiter's syndrome
    Non-HLA B 27-related Reiter's syndrome
HIV-associated arthropathy
Psoriatic arthritis
Polymyositis, dermatomyositis
Sjögren's syndrome
Necrotizing vasculitis
Septic arthritis
Other connective tissue disorders

now arises whether newly discovered infectious retroviruses might induce autoimmune diseases. Many autoimmune features of HIV 1 infection point to this possibility (Table 2, 3).

Several authors have discovered that endogenous or exogenous retroviruses might indeed be involved in the pathogenesis of autoimmune diseases: A silent but persistent viral infection or the activation of endogenous retroviruses may affect many parameters of immune function, and especially retroviral expression is associated with several features of autoimmunity in animal models. The association of antiviral activity with autoimmune diseases and particularly the role of retroviruses in the pathogenesis of human autoimmune diseases remains unclear. Nevertheless, there is considerable circumstantial evidence for the involvement of retroviruses in the etiopathogenic mechanisms of autoimmune diseases and this will be summarized in the first section of the paper. Reports on our experiments addressing this problem follow.

Retroviruses
in Experimental and Clinical Autoimmune Diseases

Experimental Models

Among animal models, an endogenous avian leukosis virus (ev 22) has recently been found to be integrated into the genomes of obese chickens with spontaneous autoimmune thyroiditis [53]. Retrovirus-like particles have been detected in pancreatic islet beta cells of non-obese diabetic mice [11, 23], and retroviral C-type particles have been identified in islet cells of mice genetically susceptible to low-dose streptozocin-induced diabetes [1].

In both the mouse and man, tissue-specific and age-dependent expression of retroviral transcripts have been reported [17, 29]. These RNAs might encode proteins which may have the potential to activate or suppress immune cell functions. A synthetic peptide with 17 amino acids homologous to a highly conserved region of the transmembrane protein TM [22] (formerly called p 15E), to envelope proteins of HTLV, and to a protein encoded by an endogenous C-type human retroviral DNA has been shown to inhibit monocyte-mediated killing by inactivation of IL-1 [18]. This example of a profound immunosuppression gained further support from experiments outlined by Krieg et al., who not only showed the expression of the transmembrane protein but were also able to block the expression and transcription by antisense oligonucleotides to the endogenous MCF envelope gene. The antisense oligonucleotides induced activation of spleen-derived lymphocytes or inhibited the blocking effects of MCF-derived polypeptides: oligonucleotides complementary to the MCF initiation site significantly increased RNA synthesis in cultured DBA/2 spleen cells. In contrast, oligonucleotides complementary to other retroviral sequences including the initiation sequences of ecotropic and xenotropic viruses did not bind to complementary mRNA. Therefore, they did not inhibit translation of the genes and did not show any effect in these experiments. Krieg et al. suggested that the stimulation of lymphocytes by antisense oligonucleotides to viral sequences might reflect the former suppression of lymphocyte activation due to endogenous retroviruses [21].

In man, RNA is transcribed from endogenous retroviral sequences in healthy donors, especially in placental tissues and cell lines [16, 35, 36]. These endogenous sequences have open reading frames that could potentially encode several retroviral proteins. In addition, apparent retroviral particles have been observed budding from human placenta [10, 14, 15]. No studies of endogenous retroviral expression in patients with SLE or other autoimmune diseases have yet been reported. Despite the volume of data demonstrated in mouse models, and in spite of the fact that it was recently possible to show reverse transcriptase activity in supernatants of lymphocyte cultures from SLE patients [12], the role of retroviruses, whether endogenous or exogenous, or their possible immunoregulatory proteins remains unclear at present.

Antigens and Antibodies to Retroviruses

In spite of many attempts, with the exception of HIV1 infection, the demonstration of infectious particles in autoimmune diseases has not been possible [30]. Since HIV infections are not regarded as autoimmune diseases, we are still waiting for convincing evidence to prove the existence of infectious particles in autoimmunity. However, p24 core antigen was demonstrated in vitro in the supernatant of lymphocyte cultures from SLE patients coincubated with allogeneic donor lymphocytes in five of 12 cases, including two cases where this phenomenon could be reproduced in different blood samples of the same patient. Additionally, in one of the culture supernatants borderline reverse transcriptase activity was determined (Baur and Krapf, manuscript in preparation). Furthermore, Gay (1990, personal communication) found retroviral sequences and particles in the synovial fluid of patients with rheumatoid arthritis.

SLE patients often show IgG and IgM antibody activity to different retroviruses [21, 43, 44, 59]. IgM, but no IgG, anti-HTLV1 was demonstrated [19] in patients with rheumatoid arthritis and SLE [19, 26]. Recently, antibodies against p24 gag of HIV1 were shown in 30% of patients with Sjögren's syndrome [46] and in 34% of patients with SLE by using recombinant p24 core protein, not only in enzyme-linked immunosorbent assays but also by the more specific Western blot technique [47]. Phillips and Olsen reported the existence of anti-HTLV1 antibodies in SLE patients' sera in ELISA and Western blots as well [28, 31]. In contrast to these findings, McDougal et al. obtained no evidence, applying Western blot techniques in SLE patients' sera, for the presence of antibodies specific for HTLV1, HTLV2, and HIV1, with the exception of one SLE patient who showed a reaction against p18 of HIV1 [25].

Autoantibodies reactive with antigens of small ribonucleoproteins, which can be demonstrated in many patients with SLE or mixed connective tissue disease, were shown to be cross-reactive with retroviral gag proteins [38]. Applying Western blot analysis and an antibody against p30 gag, Query and Keene [34] reported cross reactivity with a recombinant 70kD protein using synthetic polypeptides. The region of homology between the 70kD protein and p30 gag was shown to contain sites of amino acid homology, obviously including the site of crossreactivity. In addition, they demonstrated that rabbits immunized with retroviral p30 gag produced antibodies reactive also against human U1 snRNP. Epitope mapping experiments with synthetic polypeptides derived from the amino acid sequence of the recombinant 70kD fusion protein containing overlapping segments of this protein resulted in the demonstration of a polyclonal antibody response against multipe epitopes of 70kD [34]. The patients individually showed a somewhat different set of antibody specificities, similar to the data recorded by other authors concerning reactivity of autoimmune patients'sera against proteins or polynucleotides (W. Nürnberg 1989, personal communication). Therefore, it remains unclear whether the p30 gag homologous region of 70kD protein is a major or minor antigenic determinant. Furthermore, none of the rare known human endogeous or infectious retroviral gag sequences contains this region. Additional circumstantial evidence is the increased level of an unusual acid-labile alpha-interferon in the serum of SLE patients [40], similar to that demonstrated in patients with viral or retroviral infections. This may contribute to the immune abnormalities of SLE patients and could be triggered by a viral or retroviral infection [40].

Retroviral DNA and RNA in Human Autoimmune Diseases

In 1981 the first human endogenous retroviral sequences were cloned [24], and many of them have now been identified, classified, and partially characterized [5, 41]. Nevertheless, there are relatively few data based on molecular analysis of RNA and DNA concerning the involvement of retroviruses in the pathogenesis of human autoimmune diseases. Southern blot experiments using a 720-bp and a 942-bp probe for gag, derived from HIV 1 sequences, gave positive hybridization signals with DNA extracted from the thyroid glands of five patients with Grave's disease. Furthermore, DNA derived from peripheral blood mononuclear cells hybridized with a 720-bp gag HIV 1 probe in three of five patients with Grave's disease [7].

Indications of Retroviral Involvement in SLE

Biochemical Characterization of Plasma Nucleic Acids

A characteristic finding in SLE patients is circulating antigen-antibody complexes, especially those consisting of DNA and anti-DNA antibodies [20]. For the purification and characterization of nucleic acids from immune complexes in SLE patients, we used anti-doublestranded (ds) DNA antibodies from the patients and dsDNA anti-dsDNA immune complexes as tools for the preparation of the unknown antigens. The aim of our studies was to characterize the obviously immunogenic nucleic acids. Addressing the same problem, Pisetsky et al. [32] reported that bacterial DNA is recognized as foreign because of the presence of a different primary sequence rate, different secondary and tertiary structures, and higher-order conformations, but that is not usually present in human DNA and is unlikely to be involved in the pathogenesis of SLE. Other authors have shown that bacterial DNA differs from mammalian DNA in its content of pyrimidine clusters, patterns of base methylation, and, undoubtedly, in many of its coding sequences [8, 45, 50, 51]. Rozenberg-Arska et al. [37] reported that intracellular enzymes from mononucler cells can degrade bacterial chromosomal DNA but not plasmid DNA. This finding suggests the requirement for other effective mechanisms to remove these molecules and exclude or at least reduce transmission of genetic information that could promote pathogenicity. In this context it is worth mentioning that the involvement of plasmid-containing *Klebsiella* as a trigger mechanism for spondylitis ankylopoietica is also still under discussion [6].

In contrast to these investigators, we did not use DNA or RNA of bacterial or viral origin as antigens for affinity studies of anti-DNA antibodies. Instead, we investigaed immune complexes containing nucleic acid from the plasma of 20 patients with clinically active SLE. As controls we used three patients with Waldenström's disease, three with myasthenia gravis, three with rheumatoid arthritis, three with necrotizing vasculitis, one patient with pancreatitis, and one with mixed cryoglobulinemia II. From each patient up to 2.5 l of plasma were obtained by plasmapheresis; the protein concentration was roughly 50% of the usual concentration in patients' plasma. EDTA and NaN_3 (0.01%) were added immediately to the material to avoid bacterial contamination. The initial 250 ml of the plasmapheresis fluid were discarded to prevent contamination by nucleic acids from cell detritus.

All samples and the plasma specimens from 100 healthy controls were investigated for double-stranded nucleic acids by means of an ethidium bromide fluorescence staining test. All samples from the 20 SLE patients contained 30–400 ng/ml dsDNA equiv. of double-helical nucleic acids. In contrast, nucleic acids were not demonstrated in any of the 100 plasma samples from healthy controls in the plasmapheresis fluids, with the exception of the one patient with mixed cryoglobulinemia II. However, this nucleic acid seemed to be structurally different from that of patients with SLE [13]. HIV infection was ruled out in all patients.

As a first crude purification step, antigen-antibody complexes were precipitated with 5% polyethylene glycol 6000. The precipitates were redissolved in buffer and divided into two aliquots. The first one was used for the preparation of immunoglobulins [20], the second for the purification of nucleic acids. Fractions containing nucleic acids were extracted with phenol/chloroform, washed in diethylether, and precipitated with ethanol.

To remove contaminating polypeptides the pellets were dissolved in buffer and treated with proteinase K and again extracted with phenol, washed, and redissolved in buffer. Five of the 20 plasmapheresis specimens from SLE patients were digested with RNase.

When the plasma nucleic acids were examined by electron microscopy they showed tertiary structures similar to DNA supercoils, hairpins, and strand crosses. The length of the nucleic acids, as determined with an optometrical scanner, was up to 7 µm (Fig. 1).

The question of whether the nucleic acids purified from the plasma of SLE patients were derived from cell debris was answered by hybridization experiments with ^{32}P-labeled BLUR 12 DNA (*Bam*HI Linked Unique Repeats) recognizing highly repetitive *Alu* sequences of the human genome [9]. There was no hybridization with these highly dispersed sequences; therefore, the possiblity that the nucleic acids originated from mere random human DNA, released by cell rupture, was ruled out.

The size of the nucleic acids was determined by electrophoresis in 1% agarose gels. This revealed a high molecular weight, comigrating with 20 kbp

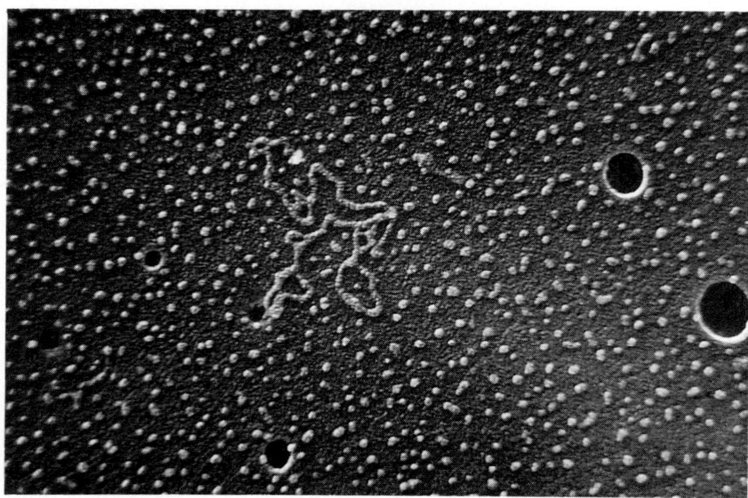

Fig. 1. Electron microscopy of tertiary-structured nucleic acids purified from the plasma of patients with SLE

linear dsDNA in all 20 patients. In some of the patients nucleic acids of lower molecular weight were also present [20]. These data roughly support the estimation of size by electron microscopy. Bacterial and Z-DNA induce cross-reactive anti-B-DNA antibodies in animals. Therefore, the possibility that the nucleic acids from SLE patients contained relevant amounts of highly methylated Z-DNA or bacterial DNA had to be examined [32, 48]. The degree of methylated desoxycytidines was about 1%, compared with about 4.5% for random human cellular DNA. Since Z-DNA is even more methylated than common B-DNA, it was ruled out. The same was true for bacterial DNA, which was demonstrated by cesium buoyant density gradient centrifugation [20]. HPLC analysis showed a considerably increased dG/dC content, as compared with human hepatocyte DNA. According to this analysis, CpG dinucleotides are fivefold enriched compared with random human DNA.

Taken together, these data suggest that the isolated plasma-derived DNA represents a eukaryotic nucleic acid species not originating from unselected human cellular DNA. Similarities to DNA structures of approximately 1 kbp which are involved in regulatory functions, termed *Hpa* II tiny fragments (HTF islands, CpG-rich islands) [4], are discussed elsewhere [20].

Biological Properties of Plasma Nucleic Acids

Rabbits were immunized with plasma nucleic acids from SLE patients, dsDNA, or synthetic polyriboguanylic acid, which is known to induce anti-dsDNA antibody activity in animals. All potential immunizing agents were used with and without methylated BSA as carrier. After 2 months, antibody reactivity against polyriboguanylic acid, dsDNA, and the plasma-derived nucleic acids was shown only in the animals immunized with polyribuguanylic acid or plasma-derived nucleic acids. No activity was obtained in rabbits immunized with dsDNA with or without methylated BSA [20]. In mice it was possible to induce monoclonal antibodies mainly of the IgM, but also of the IgG class. Surprisingly, two of the 15 monoclonal antibodies showed precipitating activity in the Farr assay [54].

To investigate possible cytotoxic or cytopathic effects, five cell lines were incubated for 72 h with nucleic acids purified from SLE patients' plasma. One of the cell lines, an EBV immortalized B cell line established from a normal human donor, had a significantly increased uridine uptake as compared with thymidine. Additionally, clear cytopathic effects were seen in this cell line only. Neither the control cell line which was sham incubated for 72 h nor any of the other cell lines reacted in this way. In addition, the B cell line showing cytopathic effects also reacted with an antiserum directed preferentialy against cells infected with feline leukemia virus. In Western blot experiments, SLE patients' sera reacted with new epitopes on the surface of the B cell line after coincubation with the plasma nucleic acids.

Molecular Characteristics of Plasma Nucleic Acids

In spite of the fact that the cesium buoyant density gradient showed heterogenous DNA and RNA, we cloned the DNA contents into M13 vectors and sequenced the plasma DNA insert by the dideoxy chain termination method [39]. The sequences were analyzed for base distribution and screened for sequence homologies using the MicroGenie DNA analysis program and the faster BESTFIT analysis program respectively [33]. Thirteen recombinant clones were selected and sequenced. Besides scanning for the dG/dC content, the presence of 5′-CpG-3′ dinucleotides, which occur in common human DNA at reduced rates, dinucleotide frequencies typical of eukaryotic DNA, and, most interestingly, homologies to known sequences were investigated. While the first results confirmed the biochemical features of nucleic acids, as mentioned above, the comparison with the known sequences revealed 81.6% sequence homology in 174 bp overlap to the gag pol region of HIV 1 in one clone, called E6 (Fig. 2). It should be stressed that none of the 20 SLE patients showed any clinical sign of HIV 2 infection or any ELISA and Western blot reactivity.

To exclude the possibility that this clone was unique for the patient from whom it was derived, dot blot experiments under high-stringency conditions were performed. The clone E6 was used as a probe for the nucleic acids from SLE patients and for the nucleic acids from the only other patient (mixed cryoglobulinemia II) with preparable amounts (> 20/ng/ml) of nucleic acids in his plasma. The radiolabeled E6 showed positive reactions only in SLE patients' nucleic acid preparations [13]. This indicates that this sequence is not unique, and similar sequences can be found in other patients with SLE.

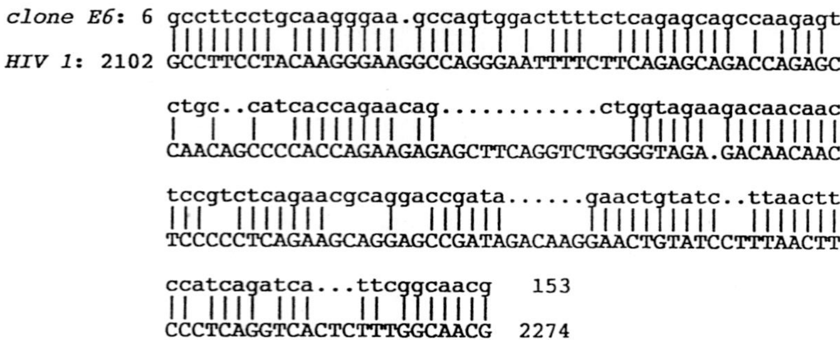

Fig. 2. Sequence of clone E6, derived from nucleic acids demonstrated in the plasma of SLE patients. Comparison with other DNA sequences (program: BESTFIT, databank: Genbank (NIH, Bilofsky et al., NAR 14 (1), 1–4, 1986, version 2/90) showed significant homology to several retroviruses. Best match: HIV 1 isolate HXB2 (percent identity: 81.633%, length: 174 bp overlap)

Indication of Retroviral Involvement

Southern blot experiments at moderate stringency probing genomic DNA with a radio-labeled oligonucleotide derived from E6 did reveal positive signals; however, they did not show any differences between SLE patients, patients with other chronic inflammatory diseases, and healthy controls. This finding was supported by DNA amplification techniques: polymerase chain reaction (PCR) was performed with E6-derived flanking primers, and no significant differences between several disease entities and healthy donors were shown. Yet the limited length of E6 attenuates these results. In contrast, in Hirt's supernatants containing an enriched fraction of episomal DNA, high amounts of E6-hybridizing material were demonstrated for SLE patients but not for healthy controls.

With regard to the Southern blots, experiments at higher stringency are under way. To overcome the technical problems of genomic DNA amplification with E6-derived flanking primers, PCR using conserved lentiviral sequences such as PPT (polypurine tract) and PBS (primer binding site) in combination with unique E6-derived primers without sequence homology to any known retrovirus will be performed.

Since on the level of genomic DNA no significant differences have been demonstrated so far, we questioned whether the expression of ubiquitous sequences might be the harmful event. Northern blot experiments using E6- and HIV 1-derived probes showed messenger RNA not only in the B cell line, initially coincubated with the plasma-derived nucleic acid from SLE patients, but also in two of seven EBV-immortalized B cell lines established from SLE patients. In contrast, no mRNA reacting with E6 was present in the EBV lines derived from ten healthy donors. These results correspond to the findings recently reported by Krieg et al. [21]. The expression of transmembrane proteins of some infectious type-C retroviruses suppresses lymphocyte activation [27, 42]. This suppression can be inhibited by antisense oligonucleotides [21].

Conclusion

In summary, convincing but circumstantial evidence has accumulated during the recent years for an involvement of endogenous and/or exogenous retroviruses in the pathogenesis of autoimmune diseases, e. g., as trigger mechanisms or co-factors. Autoimmune manifestations seen in HIV 1-infected patients and in animal models such as the caprine arthritis encephalitis virus infectio, which is similar to human rheumatoid arthritis [3], support this concept. The search for an etiologic agent is complicated by the possibility that a putative retrovirus may cause disease in only a subpopulation of those exposed. In some persons the virus could become dormant soon after infection but might still cause persistent altered immune reactivity, which may lead to autoimmune features later on. In other individuals, co-factors may be required to cause autoimmunity. Furthermore, it remains unclear whether SLE is one disease entity in this respect; therefore, in various patient subsets different agents might trigger the onset of the disease. The techniques used in our experiments are still inadequate. For example, DNA amplification gives no answer about repeated sequences, such as tandem repeats, which might be present in patients with chronic inflammatory diseases, or about the localization of the amplified product.

There is evidence suggesting that retroviruses play an important role, directly or indirectly, in autoimmune diseases, e. g., as trigger mechanisms, but more research is necessary to demonstrate this definitely. This research will benefit from impressive improvements that have been made in characterizing reagents and in techniques, especially in molecular biology, and may at least help to clarify the open questios and some of the contradictory results.

References

1. Appel MC, Rossini AA, Williams RM, Like AA (1978) Viral studies in streptozotocin-induced pancreatic beta cells. J Exp Med 163:87–100
2. Baltimore D (1985) Retroviruses and retrotransposons: The role of reverse transcription in shaping the eukaryotic genome. Cell 40:481A–482
3. Banks KL, Jacobs FH, Michaels FH, Cheevers WP (1987) Lentivirus infection augments concurrent antigen-induced arthritis. Arthritis Rheum 30:1046–1053
4. Bird AP (1986) CpG-rich islands and the function of DNA methylation. Nature 321:209–213
5. Bonner TI, O'Connell C, Cohen M (1982) Cloned endogenous retro-viral sequences from human DNA. Proc Natl Acad Sci USA 79:4709–4713

6. Cameron FH, Russel PS, Sullivan J, Geczy AF (1983) Is a Klebsiella plasmid involved in the etiology of ankylosing spondylitis in HLA 27 B-positive individuals? Hum Immunol 20:563–567

7. Ciampollilo A, Marini V, Mirakian R, Buscema M, Schulz T, Pujol-Borrell R, Bottazzo GF (1989) Retrovirus-like sequences in Graves disease: Implications for human autoimmunity. Lancet 1 (8647):1096–1100

8. Cheng SC, Herman G, Modrich P (1985) Extent of equilibrium perturbation of the DNA helix upon enzymatic methylation of adenine residues. J Biol Chem 260:191–194

9. Deininger PL, Jolly DJ, Rubin CM, Friedmann T, Schmidt CW (1981) Base sequence studies of 300 nucleotide renatured repeated human DNA clones. J Mol Biol 151:17–33

10. Dirksen ER, Levy JA (1977) Virus-like particles in placentas from normal individuals and patients with systemic lupus erythematosus. J Natl Cancer Inst 59:1187–1192

10a. Espinoza LR, Aguilar JL, Berman A, Gutierrez F, Vasey FB, Germain BF (1989) Rheumatic manifestations associated with human immunodeficiency virus infection. Arthritis Rheum 32(12):1615–1622

11. Fujita H, Fujino H, Nonaka K, Tarui S, Tochino Y (1984) Retro-virus-like particles in pancreatic B cells of NOD (non-obese diabetic) mice. Biomed Res 5:67–75

12. Harisdangkul V, Blakeslee JR, Olsen RG (1989) Isolation of an agent from SLE cell lines with properties of a retro-virus. Handbook and abstracts, Second Intl Conf on SLE:54

13. Herrmann M, Leitmann W, Krapf FE, Kalden JR (1989) Molecular characteristics and in vitro effects of nucleic acids from plasma of patients with systemic lupus erythematosus. J Cell Biochem, Suppl 12E:147–157

14. Imamura M, Philips PE, Mellors RC (1976) The occurrence and frequency of type C virus-like particles in placentas from patients with systemic lupus erythematosus and from normal subjects. Am J Pathol 83:383–394

15. Kalter SS, Helmke RJ, Heberling RL, Panigel M, Fowler AK, Strickland JE, Hellman A (1973) C-type particles in normal human placentas. J Natl Cancer Inst 50:1081–1084

16. Kato N, Pfeifer-Ohlsson S, Kato M, Larsson E, Rydnert J, Ohlsson R, Cohen M (1987) Tissue-specific expression of human provirus ERV3 mRNA in huam placenta: two of the three ERV3 mRNAs contain human cellular sequences. J Virol 61:2182–2191

17. Khan AS, Laigret F, Rodi CP (1987) Expression of mink cell focus-forming murine leukemia virus-related transcripts in AKR mice. J Virol 61:876–882

18. Kleinerman ES, Lachman LB, Knowles RD, Snyderman R, Cianciolo GJ (1987) A sysnthetic peptide homologous to the envelope proteins of retroviruses inhibits monocyte-ediated killing by inactivating interleukin 1. J Immunol 139:2329–2337

19. Kozak CAS (1985) Retroviruses as chromosomal genes in the mouse. Adv Cancer Res 44:295–336

20. Krapf F, Herrmann M, Leitmann W, Kalden JR (1989) Antibody binding of macromolecular DNA and RNA in the plasma of SLE patients. Clin Exp Immunol 75:336–342

21. Krieg AM, Gause WC, Courley MF, Steinberg AD (1989) A role for endogenous retroviral sequences in the regulation of lymphocyte activation. J Immunol 143:2448–2451

22. Leis J, Baltimore D, Bishop JM, Coffin J, Fleissner E, Goff SP, Oroszlan S, Robinson H, Skalka AM, Temin MM, Vogt V (1988) Standardized and simplified nomenclature for proteins common to all retroviruses. J Virol 62:1808–1809

23. Leiter EH, Fewell JW, Kuff EL (1986) Glucose induces intraintestinal type A retroviral gene transcription and translation in pancreatic beta cells. J Exp Med 163:87–100

24. Martin MA, Bryan T, Rasheed S, Khan AS (1981) Identification and cloning of endogenous retroviral sequences present in human DNA. Proc Natl Acad Sci USA 78:4892–4896

25. McDougal JS, Kennedy MS, Kalyanaraman VS, McDuffie FC (1985) Failure to demonstrate (cross-reacting) antibodies to human T-lymphotrophic viruses in patients with rheumatic disease. Arthritis Rheum 28:1170–1174

25a. Mellors RC, Mellors JW (1978) Type C RNA virus-specific antibody in human systemic lupus erythematosus demonstrated by enzymeimmunoassay. Proc Natil Acad Sci 75(5):2463–2467
26. Morse HC III, Chused TM, Boehm-Truitt M, Mathieson BJ, Sharrow SO, Hartley JW (1979) XenCSA: cell surface antigens related to the major glycoproteins (gp70) of xentotropic murine leukemia viruses. J Immunol 122:443–454
27. Okamoto T, Tamura T, Takano T (1983) Evidencein patients with systemic lupus erythematosus of the presence of antibodies against RNA-dependent DNA polymerase of baboon endogenous virus. Clin Exp Immunol 54:747–755
28. Olsen RG, Tarr MJ, Mathes LE, Whisler R, Plessis DD, Schulz EJ, Blakeslee JR (1987) Serological and virological evidence of human T-lymphotrophic virus in systemic lupus erythematosus. Med Microbiol 176:53–64
29. Ono T, Cutler RG (1978) Age-dependent relaxation of gene repression: Increase of endogenous murine leukemia virus-related and globin-related RNA in brain and liver of mice. Proc Natil Acad Sci USA 75:4431–4435
30. Phillips PE, Christian CL (1985) Infections agents in chronic rheumatic diseases. In Arthritis and Allied Conditions, 10th edn. D. J. McCarty, ed. Philadelphia, Lea & Febiger pp 431–449
31. Phillips PE, Johnston SL, Runge LA, Moore JL, Poiesz BJ (1986) High IgM antibody to human T-lymphotropic virus type 1 in systemic lupus erythematosus. J Clin Immunol 3:234–241
32. Pisetsky DS, Grudier JP, Gilkeson GS (1990) A role for immunogenic DNA in the pathogenesis of systemic lupus erythematosus. Arthritis Rheum 33:153–159
33. Queen C, Korn LJ (1984) A comprehensive sequence analysis program for the IBM personal computer. Nucleic Acid Res 12:581–599
34. Query CC, Keene JD (1987) A human autoimmune protein associated with U1 RNA contains a region of homology that is cross-reactive p30 gag antigen. Cell 51:211–220
35. Rabson B, Steele PE, Garon CF, Martin MA (1983) mRNA transcripts related to full-length endogenous retriviral DNA in human cells. Nature (London) 306:604–607
36. Rabson AB, Hamagishi Y, Steele PE, Tykocynski M, Martin MA (1985) Characterization of human endogenous retroviral envelope RNA transcripts. J Virol 56:176–178
36a. Reddy EP, Sandberg-Wollheim M, Mettus RV, Ray PE, DeFreitas E, Koprowski H (1989) Amplification and molecular cloning of HTLV-I sequences from DNA of multiple sclerosis patients. Science 243(4890):529–533
37. Rozenberg-Arska M, van Strijp JAG, Hoekstra WPM, Verhoef J (1984) Effect of human polymorphonuclear and mononuclear leukocytes on chromosomal and plasmid DNA of Escherichia coli. J Clin Invest 73:1254–1262
38. Rucheton M, Graafland H, Fanton H, Ursule L, Ferrier P, Larsen CJ (1985) Presence of circulating antibodies against gag-gene MuLV proteins in patients with autoimmune connective tissue disorders. Virology 144:468–480
39. Sanger F, Nicklen S, Coulson R (1977) DNA sequencing with chain terminating inhibitors. Proc Natl Sci 74:5463–5467
40. Schattner A (1988) Review: Interferons and autoimmunity. Am J Med Sci 295:532–544
41. Shih A, Misra R, Rush MH (1989) Detection of multiple, novel reverse transcriptase coding sequences in human nucleic acids: relation to primate retroviruses. J Virol 63:64–75
42. Shirai T, Ohta K, Kohno A, Furukawa F, Yoshida H, Maruyama K, Hirose S (1986) Naturally occurring antibody response to DNA is associated with the response to retroviral gp70 in autoimmune New Zealand mice. Arthritis Rheum 29:242–250
43. Steele PE, Martin MA, Rabson AB, Bryan T, O'Brien SJ (1986) Amplifcation and chromosomal dispersion of human endogenous retroviral sequences. J Virol 59:545–550
44. Stoye J, Coffin J (1985) Endogenous viruses. In RNA Tumor Viruses Vol. 2 suppleent. R. Weiss, N. Teich, H. Varmus and J. Coffin, eds. New York: Cold Spring Harbor Laboratory. pp 357–404

45. Szybalski W, Kubinski H, Sheldrick P (1966) Pyrimidine clusters on the transcribing strand of DNA and their possible role in initiation of RNA synthesis. Cold Spring Harbor Symp Quant Biol 31:123–127
46. Talal N, Dauphinée MJ, Dang H, Alexander SS, Hart DJ, Garry RF (1990a) Detection of serum antibodies to retroviral proteins in patients with primary Sjögren's syndrome (Autoimmunity exocrinopathy) Arthritis Rheum 33:774–781
47. Talal N, Garry RF, Schur PH, Alexander S, Dauphinee MJ, Livas IH, Ballester A, Takei M, Dang H (1990b) A conserved idiotype and antibodies to retroviral proteins in systemic lupus erythematosus. J Clin Invest 85(6):1866–1871
48. Trifonov EN, Konopka AK, Jovin TM (1985) Unusual frequencies of certain alternating purine-pyrimidine runs in natural DNA sequences: relatin to Z-DNA. FEBS Lett 185(1):197–202
49. Varmus H, Swanstrom L (1985) Replication of retroviruses. In RNA Tumor Viruses, Vol. 2, supplement. R. Weiss, N. Teich, H. Varmusand J. Coffin, eds. New York: Cold Spring Harbor Laboratory pp 75–134
49a. Via CS, Stanley JD, Weatherly BR, Lang P, Shearer GM (1988) Altered threshold for the induction of graft-versus-host immunodeficiency following murine cytomegalovirus infection. Host and donor contributions. Transplantation 46(29):298–302
49b. Volk HD, Koyka I, Schmidt R, Baumgarten R, Breustedt W, Sönnichsen N, von Baehr R (1988) Changes in the subsets of lymphocytes and monocytes in the peripheral blood of individuals infected with HIV-1. AIFO 6:350–354
50. Wells RD (1988) Unusual DNA structures. J Biol Chem 263:1095–1098
51. Wells RD, Blakesly RW, Hardies SC, Horn GJ, Tarson JE, Selsing E, Burd JF, Chan HW, Dodgson JB, Jensen KF, Nes IF, Wartell RM (1977) The role of DNA structure in genetic regulation. CRC Crit Rev Biochem 4:305–340
52. Wold RT, Young FE, Tan EM, Farr RS (1968) Deoxyribonucleic acid antibody: a method to detect its primary interaction with deoxyribonucleic acid. Science 161:806–807
53. Ziemiecki A, Kromer G, Mueller RG, Hala K, Wick G (1988) ev 22, a new endogenous avian leukosis virus locus found in chickens with spontaneous autoimmune thyroiditis. Arch Virol 100:267–71
54. Ziegler JL, Stites DP (1986) Hypothesis: AIDS is an autoimmune disease directed at the immune system and triggered by a lymphotrophic retrovirus. Clin Immunol Immunopathol 41(3):305–313

Epstein-Barr Virus and Rheumatoid Arthritis

M. Lotz[1] and J. Roudier[2]

[1] Department of Medicine, University of California, San Diego, La Jolla, CA 92093, USA
[2] Université d'Aix Marseille II, Faculté de Médecine, Boulevard Jean Moulin, Marseille 13005, France

Introduction

Research on the role of Epstein-Barr virus (BV) in the pathogenesis of rheumatoid arthritis (RA) has been an exciting topic for the past 15 years. The use of EBV as a probe for cellular and humoral immune responses has contributed to our current understanding of RA. However, it is still difficult to assign a definitive role to EBV in the pathogenesis of RA.

This chapter will summarize EBV biology, the interaction between EBV and infected cells, normal immune responses to EBV, the role of EBV in human disease, and the potential link between EBV and RA.

EBV Biology

Structure of the Virus

EBV is a double-stranded DNA virus. Its natural host is the human [1]. The EBV genome, which is 180 kilobases (Kb) long, was the first herpesvirus which was completely sequenced. Open reading frames (ORF) on the genome are identified by the name (letter) of the *Bam*H1 fragment to which they map, followed by the direction (rightward or leftward) of transcription and the rank of the ORF in the direction on the fragment. Thus, BALF4 designates the fourth leftward reading frame starting within *Bam*H1 fragment A. The EBV genome encodes approximately 80 proteins and 30 of these have been identified, either by expression or by sequence comparison with known proteins from other herpesviruses [2].

Smolen, Kalden, Maini (Eds.)
Rheumatoid Arthritis
© Springer-Verlag Berlin Heidelberg 1992

Infected Cells

Primary EBV infection begins in epithelial cells of the oropharnyx where the virus can fully replicate. The virus can also spread to B cells where it does not replicate very well [3].

Cycles

The *replicative* or *lytic cycle* occurs in epithelial cells and to a lesser extent in B cells. It includes rounds of infection, virus replication, cell death, virus release, and infection of new cells. The *latent cycle* is the nonproductive infection of B cells. Latently infected B cells can proliferate indefinitely and secrete immuno-globulins (Ig) in vitro [3]. They express a limited set of EBV encoded proteins, which are antigenic [4]. The virus also activates cellular genes that include growth factors [5–7] and cell surface receptors [8–10].

EBV Encoded Antigens

EBV encoded antigens were initially detected in EBV-infected cells by immunofluorescence techniques and this resulted in the identification of groups of antigenic complexes that are expressed in latent or lytic infection. The replicative cycle antigens, defined by immunofluorescence (IF), are the early antigen (EA), the viral capsid antigen (VCA), and the membrane antigen (MA) [11, 12].

The antigens expressed during latent cycle are the EBV nuclear antigen (EBNA) [13], the latent membrane antigens (LMP) [14], and the terminal proteins (TP) [15, 16]. The individual proteins that constitute these complexes and the corresponding ORFs have been identified. Table 1 summarizes current knowledge of well characterized antigenic proteins expressed in latent and lytic cycles and their relation to the IF patterns.

Functional and Phenotypic Changes in EBV Infected Cells

The principal targets for EBV infection are human B cells and epithelial cells. Infection of cultured human epithelial cells has been difficult [17, 18] and thus information on functional changes in these cells is limited. LMP and EBNA-1 are the only EBV encoded proteins known to be expressed in infected epithelial cells. As an alternative approach to infection with the virus, a human epithelial cell line has recently been transfected with LMP [19]. This resulted in enhanced expression of adhesion receptors and of the CD40 antigen, surface molecules which are also induced by EBV in B cells. In addition, transfected cells were not

Table 1. EBV proteins expressed in the latent or replicative cycle

IF defined antigen	Identified protein	EBV ORF[a]
Latent cycle		
EBNA	EBNA-1 72 kDa	BKRF1
	EBNA-2	BYRF1
	EBNA-3	BERF1
	EBNA-4	BERF2
	EBNA-5	IR1
	EBNA-6	BERF4
LMP		Terminal repeat
TP		Terminal repeat
Replicative cycle		
EA-D	50 kDa	BMLF1
	54 kDa	BMRF1
EA-R	85 kDa glycoprotein	BORF2
VCA	gp110	BALF4
	p150	BCLF1
MA	gp85	BXLF2
	gp350–220	BLLF1

IF, immunofuorescence; ORF, open reading frame; EBNA, Epstein-Barr nuclear antigen; LMP, latent membrane antigens; TP, terminal proteins; EA-D, early antigen-diffuse; EA-R, early antigen-restricted; VCA, viral capsid antigen; MA, membrane antigen
[a] See text for definition of ORFs

able to differentiate. This blockage at an immature stage is also observed in nasopharyngeal carcinoma cells and may represent a virus induced change that is important in tumorigenesis.

EBV binding and possibly infection has also been demonstrated for T cells [20]. Specific binding of EBV was demonstrated to immature human thymocytes. The virus can infect these cells based on the presence of episomal EBV DNA and EBNA-1 expression in these cells. EBV induces thymocyte proliferation in synergy with IL-2 [20a]. However, only limited information is available on the mechanisms and consequences of their infection by EBV. The interaction between EBV and host cells is best characterized for B lymphocytes.

The Virus Receptor

The first step in the interaction of EBV target cells is the binding of the virus to its receptor, which has been identified on B cells as complement receptor type 2 (CR2, CD21) [21–23]. The binding site on EBV has been mapped to an epitope near the N-terminus of the viral capsid protein gp350/220, which is similar to the binding motif on complement component C3d, the natural ligand for CR2. This binding of EBV to CR2 has been confirmed in several different assays. It was shown that antibodies to CR2 [24], soluble CR2 [25], and peptides representing the binding motif on gp350/220 [26] inhibit EBV binding or infection of the cells. Since the virus contains multiple binding sites for CR2, it is possible that the resulting cross-linking of CR2 is one component required for the B cell proliferative response that is seen after infection. This is consistent with the enhancing effects of C3d, solid-phase C3d peptides, and antibody cross-linking of CR2 on B cell proliferation [27]. EBV binding to CR2, however, is not sufficient to induce proliferation, since UV-inactivated EBV promotes resting cells into the early stages of the cell cycle only [28]. EBV binding induces phosphorylation of CR2, which is presumably mediated by a protein kinase that is activated by EBV [29].

EBV binding to epithelial cells has been demonstrated [30]. However, the EBV receptor on epithelial cells has not yet been identified. Epithelial cells carry membrane proteins which are antigenically related to CR2. Still, only some anti-CR2 antibodies recognize proteins on both B cells and epithelial cells while several anti-CR2 antibodies that bind to B cells do not stain epithelial cells. Immunoprecipitation of surface molecules with antibodies to CR2 revealed proteins of different sizes in epithelial cells as compared to B cells [31].

The nature of a potential EBV receptor on T cells has not been established either. Binding of the virus to mature T cells and some T cell lines has been demonstrated, but the virus did not enter the cells [20]. Furthermore, binding to T cells was not inhibited by antibodies to CR2. However, when EBV was introduced into T cells by implantation of CR2 into T cell membranes [32] and by transfection of EBV DNA [33], it was able to express its genes and transform the cells. EBV appears to be able to infect T cells in vivo, since EBV-positive T cells have been detected in chronic active EBV infection of children [34] and adults [35]. It is possible that this is related to the infection of immature thymocytes with EBV which appear to differ from mature T cells with respect to the EBV binding characteristics and the fact that the virus can infect them [20a].

Activated monocytes also express CR2 or CR2-like molecules [36, 37]. At present it is not known whether EBV can bind to these cells and induce expression of its own or of cellular genes.

It is possible that this apparent heterogeneity of EBV receptors is related to the presence of variants of CR2 which have been described [38, 39].

Expression of Viral Genes in Latently Infected Cells

Upon CR2 binding, the virus is internalized and undergoes a critical change in the structure of its DNA, which characteristic of latent infection [40]. Within the virion, the viral DNA is present in a linear form. As early as 20 h after infection of primary B cells, EBV DNA can be detected as covalently closed circular episomes. At the same time, infected cells express the activation antigen CD23. The expression of CD23 together with the presence of episomal EBV DNA identifies B cells that will be immortalized. Circularization of the viral genome is essential for the maintenance of latency and growth transformation.

The expression of viral genes during primary and latent infection of B cells is rather limited. It includes the latent membrane proteins LMP, the nuclear antigens EBNA-1, EBNA-2, EBNA-3, EBNA-4, EBNA-6 and EBNA-5, and TP [13–16].

Of these EBV proteins, EBNA-2 and LMP have been implicated in the regulation of cell growth [3]. Some of their effects are closely related since EBNA-2 up-regulates the expression of LMP [41]. Studies of EBV strains which express different levels and forms of EBNA-2 [42, 43] and transfection experiments [44] suggest that EBNA-2 is essential EBV component in inducing phenotypic and functional changes in B cells.

Phenotypic Changes in Infected B Cells

EBNA-2 and LMP have been shown to increase B cell expression of CD 23 (Fcε Receptor II). Transfection of LMP in EBV-negative Burkitt's lymphoma cells also increased the expression of CD 40. This surface molecule is probably involved in B cell growth regulation since it is homologous to the nerve growth factor receptor. Additional membrane molecules that are induced include CD 71, the transferrin receptor, and the adhesion receptors LFA-1, ICAM-1 and LFA-3. LMP also increases the expression of vimentin, the cytoskeletal protein that connects LMP to the cytoskeleton [9, 10].

EBV Induced B Cell Proliferation and Transformation

The Early Proliferative Response
Within 2–3 days after primary EBV infection, B cells start to proliferate [45]. This response is independent of accessory cells and T cells. It involves the majority of B cells as indicated by the expression of EBNA in approximately 90% of the cells 2 days after infection [40]. Moderate increases in this early response can be induced by the addition of T cell conditioned media [46]. From the cells that show early proliferation, only a small proportion (1–5%) is transformed into continuously growing lymphoblasts [47]. This frequency is not increased by T cell conditioned media nor by the presence of irradiated T lymphocytes as feeder cells [46].

The early increase in DNA synthesis is associated with activation of CR 2 and requires virus entry and the expression of EBNA-2 [40].

In contrast to the limited information about proliferation during this early phase, growth regulation of transformed cells has been studied in more detail.

Autocrine Growth Factors

Analysis of secretory products of EBV infected and transformed B cells has shown that EBV stimulates the production of growth factors [5–7]. These findings have been further examined to define the role of autocrine growth factors in EBV transformed lymphoblasts.

In low density cultures addition of the cytokines interleukin-1 (IL-1) and IL-6 can increase proliferation [48, 49]. These findings are in contrast to the inability of these cytokines to directly stimulate normal resting B cells and are related to additional EBV induced activation events in the lymphoblasts. Factors such as IL-1 or IL-6 that stimulate growth of EBV infected cells may be important in pathological conditions, in which they are present in high concentrations. Thus, EBV transformed cells that are induced to express increased levels of IL-6 form colonies in soft agar and tumors in nude mice [50], malignant features that are usually not seen with EBV lymphoblasts. IL-6 may play a similar role in humans. This cytokine is overexpressed in conditions that are associated with an increased frequency of EBV related lymphoprolifera-tions such as immunodeficiencies [51] or immunosuppression after organ transplantation [52].

The soluble form of the membrane antigen CD23 has been found in some studies to stimulate the growth of EBV infected B cels [53]. However, other reports failed to detect such effects [54].

Additional growth promoting factors are produced by EBV transformed B cell lines and most of these activities may reside in a population of small (<5 kDa) molecules [6].

Hematopoietic growth factors also regulate growth of EBV infected B cells. Granulocyte-macrophage colony stimulating factor (GM-CSF) increases the frequency of B cells that spontaneously grow out from peripheral blood mononuclear cells (PBMC) obtained from EBV-positive donors [55]. GM-CSF also stimulates proliferation of already established EBV lymphoblastoid cell lines. This observation is remarkable considering the lack of GM-CSF receptors and action on normal B cells and EBV-negative B cell lymphomas.

In contrast, IL-3 inhibits outgrowth of lymphoblastoid cells. This probably occurs via indirect mechanisms [55], since the IL-3 effect is inhibited by antibodies to tumor necrosis factor-α (TNFα) and interferon-γ (IFNγ). These cytokines also inhibit the activation of primary B cells by EBV [56, 57]. It is not known whether CSFs can serve as autocrine regulators of EBV transformed B cells since production of IL-3 and GM-CSF has not been reported. For CSF1/G-CSF, which is produced by these cells [7], it is not known whether it affects their function.

Collectively these studies demonstrate that during EBV induced immortali-zation, the virus stimulates the production of growth factors and modulates the responsiveness to them. The viral components responsible for this action are EBNA and LMP, and their effect may in part be mediated through deregulated expression of oncogenes.

Oncogenes

EBNA-2 increases mRNA levels for c-*fgr* which encodes a growth factor receptor-associated tyrosine kinase of the *src* gene family [58]. This has been demonstrated by transfection experiments with EBNA-2. All EBV transformed B cells and in vitro EBV infected Burkitt's lymphoma cells express c-*fgr* [59]. The P3HR1 strain of EBV, which is deficient in the ORF for EBNA-2, does not induce c-*fgr*. This may in part explain the inability of this EBV strain to transform B cells.

The *BCl-2* gene, whose product participates in signal transduction from growth factor receptor(s), is expressed at relatively low levels in EBV transformed B cells. High levels of this protein induced by transfection conferred a moderate growth advantage to the cells, but did not render the cells tumorigenic in nude mice [60].

The oncogenes *myc* and *ras* appear to have more striking effects on cell growth. The myc protein is involved in the regulation of cell cycle progression. In EBV-negative Burkitt's cells *myc* mRNA levels decrease during stationary growth phase and this down-regulation is blocked after EBV infection [61]. This EBV effect on *myc* expression was related to an increase im mRNA stability and could also be induced by the P3HR1 strain of EBV, indicating that it is not a function of EBNA-2. EBV transformed B cells also show increased c-*myc* mRNA stability. Thus, this may be one important mechanism in the induction and maintenance of growth transformation by EBV. Overexpression of c-*myc* induced by transfection of lymphoblastoid cell lines (LCL) fully transformed the cells and led to tumor formation [62]. Similar to the effects of *myc,* the expression of the *ras* oncogene resulted in sustained growth of LCL. In addition, *ras* also induced differentiation of LCL, resulting in a completely transformed and terminally differentiated phenotype of the tumor cells [63].

Resistance to Antiproliferative Control Mechanisms

A distinct property of EBNA-2 is important for the outgrowth of lymphoblasts. While normal B cells are sensitive to the antiproliferative effects of IFN, LCL are resistant to growth inhibition by class I IFN [57]. Aman and Gabein have recently shown that EBNA-2 and EBNA-5 are responsible for this phenomenon [64]. Thus, EBNA-2 confers a growth advantage to the infected cells and provides a mechanism to escape control mechanisms. Transforming growth factor-β (TGFβ) is a potent inhibitor of normal B cell proliferation [65], but, during EBV induced transformation, B cells become resistant to this factor [66]. The mechanism of resistance to TGFβ is unknown, but it is of interest that a similar change occurs during transformation of T cells by human T cell leukemia virus-1 HTLV-1 (Lotz et al., to be published).

EBV Induced B Cell Differentiation

Associated with EBV induced B cell proliferation is the induction of B cell differentiation and polyclonal production of antibodies. The specificity of the antibodies induced by EBV reflects the B cell donor's preexisting repertoire and includes autoantibodies. Studies with normal volunteers that had been immunized with tetanus toxoid (TT) showed that their B cells produced antibodies to TT after in vitro stimulation with EBV [67]. The isotype of the antibodies was related to the phenotype of the infected B cells. Cells expressing the CD5 antigen IgM antibodies; CD5-negative cells secreted predominantly IgG. In addition, the CD5-positive cells produced low affinity autoantibodies against single-stranded DNA and rheumatoid factor (RF). In earlier studies Fong et al. [68] had demonstrated that EBV induces high levels of RF in B cells from RA patients and the secretion of IgM was enhanced in cells that probably corresponded to the CD5-positive subset. In contrast to these effects of EBV on CD5-positive B cells from normal donors or RA patients, EBV does not appear to infect or transform CD5-positive chronic lymphocytic leukemia B cells [69]. Chronic lymphocytic leukemia B cells express CR2 and should thus be able to bind EBV. The mechanism that is responsible for the resistance of these cells to EBV infection is unknown, and its identification will provide further insight into the activation of B cells and in particular of CD5-positive B-cells.

Attempts have been made to analyze whether EBV preferentially infects or stimulates certain subsets of B cells. It appers that cells that are preactivated and express early activation markers are EBV responsive [70]. Other criteria such as size and density may also allow identification of cells susceptible to EBV infection [71]. In addition to mature B cells EBV also infects pre-B cells that have not yet rearranged their Ig genes and do not express CD20 [72].

EBV induces proliferation and the secretion of IgA, IgM, and IgG in pure populations of B cells without requiring the presence of monocytes or T cells as accessory cells [73]. This implies that the virus provides signals that are usually a function of cytokines and cell-cell interactions and has led to speculations about a role for EBV in the polyclonal antibody production that is seen in RA and other diseases. One exception to this accessory cell independent induction of B cell differentiation by EBV is the production of IgE. In cultures of pure B cells infected by the virus, levels of IgE are not detectable but can be induced by the addition of IL-4 [74]. However, this cytokine has only modest stimulatory effects on the other Ig isotypes and on EBV induced B cell proliferation. This may suggest that all signals needed for the production of other isotypes and for the induction of proliferation are expressed by the infected cells but that IL-4, or an IL-4-related signal which is required for IgE secretion, is not induced by EBV.

Immune Response to EBV in Normal Adults

Continuous immune surveillance is required to control EBV infection which persists in a latent form in the majority of adults. This is clearly documented by the reactivation of EBV infection in patients with immunodeficiencies.

In interpretations of antibody or T cell responses to EBV encoded proteins, one must consider that a response detected against a particular antigen is not necessarily effective in preventing initial infection or in controlling the number of virus infected cells in vivo [75]. Although significant progress has been made in using certain EBV antigens as models in vitro, the information on relevant targets of an effective immune response in vivo is still limited.

Target Antigens in Antibody Responses

Antibody Response Against Lytic Cycle Antigens (EA, VCA, MA). During infectious mononucleosis, antibodies are generated against the replicative antigens of EBV. The target antigens include the 50 kDa and the 85 kDa proteins of EA, the 350 kDa and the 85 kDa proteins of MA, and the 110 kDa glycoprotein of VCA [76]. In vitro studies with mouse monoclonal antibodies suggest that antibodies directed at the gp 350 and the gp 85 component of the MA carry virus neutralizing activity [77, 78].

Antibody Response Against Latent Infection Antigens. Antibodies against EBNA-1 and EBNA-2 appear early after infectious mononucleosis. Anti EBNA-1 antibodies recognize predominantly a glycine-alanine repeat sequence and cross-react with many different human cellular proteins [79–81].

Target Antigens in T Cell Responses

Studies to define target antigens for T cell recognition of EBV infected B cells have been performed in cytotoxicity or T cell proliferation assays. These responses are functions of T cells that bear the $\alpha\beta$ T cell receptor and are HLA class I or class II restricted [75]. T cells that express the $\gamma\delta$ antigen receptor can also exert cytotoxic activity against EBV infected lymphoblasts, but this response is not restricted by the known HLA class I and class II antigens [82].

T Cell Response Against Latent Cycle Antigens. HLA-restricted cytotoxic T cells directed at EBNA-2, EBNA-3 and [83], and EBNA-6 [84] have recently been identified. For EBNA-2 the antigenic epitope has been localized to the N-terminus 100 amino acid fragment [83]. In the case of EBNA-3 the epitope has precisely been mapped to a site contained in a 15 amino acid peptide [85]. This peptide served as a recognition element for EBV specific cytotoxic T lympho-cytes (CTL) when presented on autologous, i. e. HLA identical, target cells. With a peptide from LMP is was possible to induce CTL. This peptide, however did not act as a target for CTL recognition [86].

T cells capable of proliferating in response to peptides from EBNA-1 have been isolated from the blood of patients with past EBV infection [87].

T Cell Response Against Lytic Antigens. T cells proliferating in response to the 350 kDa component of MA and the 110 kDa component of VCA were detected in the blood of patients with latent EBV infection [88–90]. T cells specific for MA gp350 can inhibit the outgrowth of EBV B cells in vitro [91]. Vaccination of cottontop tamarins with gp350 has been shown to prevent EBV induced lymphomas [92]. Thus, gp350 is likely to be the target of an efficient immune response.

Interferons

IFNs represent a first-line defense against EBV during primary and latent infection. The release of IFNα is the earliest detectable response to in vitro EBV infection of PBMC from donors with [93] or without prior exposure to EBV (unpublished). This release of IFNα originates predominantly from the infected B cells. It appears that natural killer (NK) cells, as defined by the expression of the Leu7/CD57 antigen, also participate in the production of IFNα, but the mechanism of IFNα induction in NK cells during in vitro EBV infection is unknown.

The production of IFNγ occurs later, first detectable after 48 h and maximal by day 5. It requires prior production of IL-1 and IL-2. IFNγ is exclusively produced by T cells and this occurs in the absence of monocytes, suggesting that the infected B cells can serve as antigen presenting cells and provide sufficient levels of IL-1 to T cells.

The role of IFNs in controlling EBV infection has been well-established [94–96]. Prior exposure of B cells to any of the three types of interferon protects the cells from virus infection as indicated by inhibition of early EBV induced proliferation, B cell differentiation, and prevention of outgrowth of lymphoblastoid cell lines [57]. Some qualitative differences have been observed between the IFN subtypes. IFNγ appears to inhibit B cell proliferation even when added after viral infection, while IFNα and IFNβ are most effective when they are used for preincubation of the cells. One possible explanation for this difference may be that IFNγ is a regulator of B cell differentiation, a function that IFNα and IFNβ do not express. An alternative hypothesis is based on the recent identification of the EBV receptor, CR2, as one of the B cell receptors for class I IFN (IFNα and IFNβ) [97]. In these studies it was demonstrated that the motif that is responsible for C3d binding to CR2 is not only present on EBV gp350/220 but also on IFNα. Remarkably, this structure is conserved among most of the 23 known IFNα subtypes. These results raise the possibility that IFNα can interfere with EBV infection by blocking virus binding to its receptor or internalization in addition to the classical IFN induced antiviral state.

Viral Interference with Immune Responses

EBV utilizes several mechanisms to interfere with antiviral host defense responses. Similar observations have been obtained for other viruses including adenoviruses, cytomegalovirus and the human T lymphotropic retroviruses HIV and HTLV-1.

Binding to Interferon Receptor

While the receptor protein that binds IFNγ has been purified in different species and the corresponding genes been cloned, the receptor that presumably binds both IFNα and IFNβ has long been an enigma. Although the gene for a presumptive class I IFN receptor has been cloned, the corresponding protein bound only the subtype IFNαD and was not able by itself to mediate IFN effects [98]. In binding studies with different natural and synthetic ligands, Delcayre et al. [97] have recently shown that the EBV receptor also serves as a receptor for IFNα or B cells. Thus, occupancy of CD21 by EBV provides virus entry into the B cell and, at the same time, prevents binding of IFNα, thereby blocking the first line of the antiviral immune response.

Interleukin-10

A novel cytokine, cytokine synthesis inhibitory factor (CSIF)/IL-10, has recently been identified in culture supernatants from B cells. The unique biological activity of this factor is inhibition of IFNγ production in T cells. Other biological effects of this cytokine on T cells and mast cells have now been reported. In murine systems it seems that B cells, in particular the CD5-positive subset, are the major source of IL-10. A very surprising observation was made after the nucleotide sequence of this cytokine had been identified. The EBV BCRFI ORF and IL-10 have 90% sequence homology [99]. Comparison of the biological activities of the product of the EBV ORF and IL-10 revealed that both share the inhibition of IFNγ production (99a). The 10% divergence of the EBV product conserved the activity to inhibit IFNγ synthesis, the effect EBV utilizes to block an important component of the antiviral host defense response.

Molecular Mimicry

HLA D Molecules. The EBNA-6 protein, encoded by the BERF4 ORF, contains a sixfold repeat of the GPPAA amino acid sequence found in the third hypervariable region of the HLA DQB3.2 allele of DQβ (now designated DQB1 0302). The gp110 protein encoded by the BALF4 ORF contains the EQKRAA sequence and the LEQKR sequence, both found in the third hypervariable region of the DRβ1 chain of HLA-Dw4 (now designated as DRB1 0401) which carries susceptibility to RA [89]. Thus, important T cell epitopes present on HLA-D histocompatibility molecules are expressed by EBV proteins. In the HLA-DR4 haplotype, where both DQB1 and DRB1 0401 can be expressed, this might constitute a mechanism to escape the host cellular immune response.

Other Host Proteins. Antibodies to EBNA-1 cross-react with many different human cellular proteins [81]. The molecular basis of such cross-reactivity is currently being analyzed by isolating cross-reactive human cell proteins from expression librairies (Rhodes et al., to be published).

Type II collagen contains several sites of amino acid homology with EBNA-5. To assess the significance of these homologies it will be necessary to analyze whether immune responses are generated against these epitopes and whether they are indeed involved in molecular mimicry.

EBV and Human Diseases

Infectious Mononucleosis

Demonstration that primary infection by EBV causes infectious mononucleosis (IM) was first provided by Henle's laboratory, where a technician seroconverted during the course of this IM [100].

Primary infection by EBV in the first decade of life, as occurs in populations with poor hygiene conditions, causes no pathology. For reasons which are still unclear, primary infection in the second decade of life, as seen in economically developed countries, causes IM [101].

Burkitt's Lymphoma and Nasopharyngeal Carcinoma

Burkitt's lymphoma (BL) is the malignant proliferation of EBV infected B cells which usually carry a c-*myc*/Ig locus translocation. The reasons why the malignant B cells escape immune control are unknown [102]. Possible explanations include the lack of expression of the latent antigens EBNA-2 to -6 and LMP by BL cells and the low expression of HLA antigens on their surface [103].

Nasopharyngeal carcinoma (NPC) is the proliferation of a poorly differentiated epithelial cell that is infected by EBV. Pathogenetic mechanisms that potentially contribute to NPC are the ability of the LMP protein (with EBNA-1, one of the two EBV proteins detectabe in NPC cells) to inhibit epithelial cell differentiation [19]. Recently, a particular genetic background, involving genes linked to HLA-B17 and HLA-Bw46, has been noted to have a high frequency of HLA haplotype sharing between NPC affected twins [104].

EBV Associated Lymphoproliferative Diseases
in the Immunocompromised Host

The three major conditions in which reactivation of latent EBV infection and EBV associated malignancies occur are the use of immunosuppressive drugs in transplant recipients, inherited immunodeficiencies, and HIV infection.

Transplant Recipients
EBV induced lymphomas, as a consequence of immunosuppression, were seen in recipients of renal, heart, liver, bone marrow, and thymic epithelial transplants [105]. The lymphoproliferations can be mono-, oligo-, and polyclonal and are predominantly located in lymph nodes, but extranodal manifestations are frequent in the CNS. Immunohistochemical analysis of the tumor cells from immunocomporomised patients with EBV lymphoproliferative disease demonstrated the presence of LMP, EBNA-2, CD23, LFA-3, and ICAM, antigens that had previously been found to be expressed on EBV infected cells in culture [106].

Cyclosporin inhibits the activation of T cells and the production of IL-2. The resulting defect in immunocompetence is probably a major factor in lymphomagenesis. Recently it was found that, in contrast to the inhibition of IL-2 production, cyclosporin-A does not inferfere with the production of IL-6 and may even stimulate IL-6 gene transcription [107]. Since IL-6 augments the proliferation of EBV infected B cells, the superinduction of the IL-6 gene by cyclosporine may support the emergence of lymphomas.

Withdrawal of the immunosuppressive therapy results in regression of the lymphomas and this further supports the importance of immune surveillance in controlling latent EBV infection [108].

Congenital Immunodeficiencies
Primary immunodeficiencies are associated with an increased incidence of malignancies. Lymphomas represent a large portion of these tumors and the highest frequencies are observed in the Wiskott-Aldrich syndrome, ataxiatelangiectasia, and common variable immunodeficiency [105].

A strong association between EBV and lymphomas has also been documented for the X-linked lymphoproliferative syndrome or Duncan's syndrome [109]. Prior to EBV infection, these patients appear to have normal cellular and humoral immune function. Upon infection, they develop fulminant IM with excessive proliferation of CTL. Approximately 25% of the patients develop malignant lymphoma. The tumor cells are EBV-positive lymphoblasts with infiltration of the intestine, liver, and CNS.

HIV Infection
HIV infection is associated with signs of reactivation of EBV infection and a significant proportion of non-Hodgkin's lymphomas that develop in AIDS patients are EBV-positive [111]. Peripheral blood of AIDS patients contains an elevated number of EBV infected cells [112]. Together with defective cellular immunity to EBV [112], this provides a possible basis for the generation of immortalized B cells which are not yet completely transformed. BL in AIDS show the same chromosomal abnormalities that are found in endemic Burkitts patients and include translocation of the cellular oncogene *myc* [113]. Expression of the *myc* gene in EBV-positive lymphoblasts resulted in fully transformed B cells. Although EBV can stimulate B cells, its role in the development of EBV-positive lymphomas is probably indirect and relates to the

destruction of cellular immunity by HIV. In this context the scenario in HIV infection is reminiscent of the events in transplant recipients that are therapeutically immunosuppressed. However, it has also been documented that a significant number of lymphomas in AIDS patients are EBV-negative. It is of interest that these also showed translocation of c-*myc* [114], suggesting that rearrangement of this locus, together with either the presence of EBV or a second as yet undefined factor, results in tumor development.

EBV and RA

For the past 15 years EBV has been the subject of active research to define its role in the pathogenesis of RA. Different facets of a potential role of the virus in this disease have been examined, and, with advances in the understanding of the virus and the immune responses against it, new approaches and potential mechanisms have continued to emerge.

RA Nuclear Antigen and its Relation to EBNA

Research into the role of EBV in RA began in 1976 when Alspaugh and Tan reported that sera from RA patients contained increased titers of precipitating antibody against a nuclear antigen that was present in EBV infected, but not in noninfected cells [15]. This antigen was termed the RA nuclear antigen (RANA). Initially, identification of the nature of this antigen proved difficult since EBV encoded proteins that are expressed in infected cells had not yet been characterized. It became clear later that RANA and EBNA-1 are the same molecule [116, 117]. Since EBNA-1 has been shown to cross-react with human cellular proteins [81], the importance of the immune response against RANA/EBNA-1 will be better appreciated after the cross-reactive cellular proteins have been characterized.

Control of Outgrowth of EBV Infected B Cells

Slaughter et al. observed that, in cultures of PBMC from RA patients, spontaneous outgrowth of permanently transformed lymphoblastoid cell lines occurred at a higher frequency than in healthy controls [118]. In addition, after in vitro infection with EBV, lymphoblasts developed more rapidly in cells from RA patients. Based on these findings studies were initiated to examine the cellular immune response to EBV in RA.

One of the earliest assays to quantify anti-EBV immune responses was inhibition of EBV induced B cell outgrowth. In this assay, the number of T cells required to inhibit outgrowth of a constant number of infected cells is determined. A higher number of RA T cells is needed to obtain a level of outgrowth inhibition identical to that obtained with cells from normal controls [119, 120]. Tosato et al. then showed that T cells from RA patients are defective in suppressing EBV induced Ig synthesis of autologous B cells [121]. This suggested a qualitative defect in the cellular control of EBV infection, and subsequent studies analyzed mechanisms responsible for this. After class I and class II IFN had been shown to mediate cellular control of EBV infection, Hasler et al. studied the production of IFNγ by cells from RA patients [122]. PBMC were activated by an autologous mixed lymphocyte reaction and the conditioned media from these cultures were found to contain lower levels of IFNγ as compared to cells from healthy controls. This decrease in IFNγ production was thought to be related to an increased sensitivity of RA T cells to prostaglandin [123]. We developed a system to directly test the production of IFNs after in vitro infection of RA blood mononuclear cells with EBV. Cells from RA patients released slightly higher levels of IFNα than cells from normal donors [124]. This production of IFNα occurs within 24 h after infection and represents a response of B cells and NK cells to the infection. IFNγ production is maximal between 3–5 days after infection; in RA culture levels of IFNγ were significantly lower than in controls. IFNγ production is a T cell function and depends on the prior release of IL-1 and IL-2. Analysis of IL-1 and IL-2 also showed lower levels in RA. The addition of IL-1 and IL-2 to RA PBMC restored the defect in IFNγ production. Since removal of monocytes from RA PBMC cultures resulted in normal IFNγ production, a monocyte dependent suppressive mechanism seemed responsible. It was found that RA monocytes released a factor that inhibited the biological activity of IL-1 in the lymphocyte activating factor assay. This activity, referred to as IL-1 inhibitor, also reduced the production of IFNγ in normal PBMC cultures. The identity of this functionally defined factor is not yet established but TGF-β and a recently described IL-1 receptor antagonist [125] are able to express similar biological activities. IL-10 [99], also inhibits IFNγ production and it will therefore be of interest to study its production in RA.

To understand the significance of defective cytokine release after EBV infection for RA pathogenesis, we determined the disease specificity of this finding. Analysis of PBMC from patients with multiple sclerosis, myasthenia gravis, or AIDS showed that patients with these conditions can also have impaired responses to EBV infection in vitro [126, 127, 128]. Consistent with this, other investigators have also demonstrated defects in cellular immunity against EBV in seronegative arthritis, multiple sclerosis, and myasthenia gravis [128, 129]. In any of these conditions, including RA, it is not clear whether the observed defects are present early in the disease or whether they are the result of chronic inflammation, in which immune defects may be a result of adaptive host mechanisms to down-regulate immune and inflammatory activation. The lack of disease specificity of the defects in T cell control of EBV infection indicates that a potential role of EBV in RA depends on additional factors.

Frequency of EBV Infected B Cells

As a manifestation of the T cell defects in control of EBV infection, increased numbers of infected cells might be expected to be present in tissues from RA patients. Peripheral blood from RA patients contains more infected B cells than blood from normal controls [130]. The techniques used to enumerate infected cells depend on outgrowth of B lymphoblasts under limiting dilution conditions and are very sensitive.

Attemps to detect infectious virus or EBV DNA in RA synovial tissues, however, have been negative [131]. With the use of more sensitive techniques it might be possible to detect extremely small numbers of infected cells or copies of viral DNA, but it appears that RA synovium is not a site of active EBV replication nor a tissue that contains significant numbers of latently infected cells.

HLA-DR4, EBV Infection, and RA

RA is associated with the HLA antigen HLA-Dw4 [132]. Disease susceptibility maps to the amino acid sequence QKRAA located in the third hypervariable region of the DR1 chain of the HLA-Dw4 molecule. The EBV glycoprotein gp110, which is encoded by the BALF4 ORF, contains the sequence QKRAA [89]. Healthy, non-HLA-Dw4 humans with past EBV infection have serum antibodies to gp110 and peripheral blood T cells that recognize peptides from gp110 and HLA-Dw4 encompassing the QKRAA determinant [90]. In HLA-Dw4-positive individuals, tolerance of self HLA antigens might delete T cells specific for the QKRAA determinant on gp110 and modify the course of EBV infection. Conversely, if QKRAA reactive T cells are not deleted completely, EBV infection may amplify HLA-Dw4 reactive T cells in some HLA-Dw4 individuals and thus propagate autoreactive T cells. Our preliminary results in the mouse suggest that self MHC peptides are tolerated in normal animals. In certain strains, however, animals may develop T cells reactive to self MHC peptides when immunized with cross-reactive antigens (Roudier, unpublished).

Thus, HLA-Dw4 and EBV gp110 share a T cell epitope to which susceptibility to RA maps [133]. Analysis of T cell responses to this epitope in HLA-Dw4 normals and RA patients and testing of the immune response to gp110 in the control of EBV infection will be needed to evaluate the importance of this finding.

Conclusion

EBV is an ancient and a lifelong host of the human species. As such, it has developed efficient adaptation mechanisms to escape the antiviral immune response. Analysis of these mechanisms and of their consequences will be needed to determine whether EBV can trigger autoimmune disease.

Specifically, it has to be evaluated which antigens are the main effective targets and which epitopes on these antigens are dominant. In this respect, it will be important to define the functional significance of T cell responses against the EBV antigens that mimic human tissue antigens, in particular, human HLA antigens. For instance, gp110 is the EBV equivalent of the gB proteins of herpes and cytomegalovirus (CMV). The gB proteins are major targets in the control of herpes and CMV infections [134]. EBV gp110 is a target for B cells and T cells in human infection by EBV. However, it is not known whether it is a necessary target and which epitopes on gp110 are dominant. These elements are needed to understand the significance of a modified pattern of T cell recognition of gp110 induced by self tolerance in HLA-Dw4 individuals.

Examples of mimicry in antibody responses have been observed. The identification of the cellular proteins that cross-react with EBNA-1 will help in understanding the humoral aspects of EBV induced autoimmunity.

Acknowledgements. Supported by NIH grant AR39799, Arthritis Foundation, INSERM, Association pour la Recherche sur la Polyarthrite, and Fondation pour la Recherche Medical.

References

1. Epstein MA, Achong BG (1979) The Epstein-Barr virus. Springer, Berlin Heidelberg New York
2. McGeoch DJ (1989) The genomes of the human herpesviruses. Ann Rev Microbiol 43:235–265
3. Liebowitz D, Kieff E, Sample J, Birkenbach M, Wang F (1990) Epstein-Barr virus transformation of B lymphocytes: molecular pathogenesis. In: Ablashi D (ed) EBV and human diseases II. Humana Press, Clifton, New Jersey, pp 3–15
4. Miller G (1980) Biology of Epstein-Barr virus. In: Klein G (ed) Advances in viral oncology. Raven Press, New York, pp 713–719
5. Blazar BA, Murphy AM (1990) Induction of B cell responsiveness to growth factors by Epstein-Barr virus conversion: comparison of endogenous factors and interleukin-1. Clin Exp Immunol 80:62–68
6. Tosato G, Tanner J, Jones KD, Revel M, Pike SE (1990) Identification of interleukin-6 as an autocrine growth factor for Epstein-Barr virus-immortalized B cells. J Virol 64:3033–3041
7. Reisbach G, Sindermann J, Kremer JP, HültnerL, Wolf H, Dörner P (1989) Macrophage colony-stimulating factor (CSF-1) is expressed by spontaneously out-growth EBV-B cell lines and activated normal B lymphocytes. Blood 74:959–964
8. Wang D, Liebowitz D, Wang F, Gregory C, Rickinson A, Larson R, Springer T, Kieff E (1988) Epstein-Barr virus latent infection membrane protein alters the human B-lymphocyte phenotype: deletion of the amino terminus abolishes activity. J Virol 62:4173–4184
9. Cordier M, Calender A, Bilaud M, Zimber U, Rousselet G, Pavlish O, Banchereau J, Tursz T, Bornkamm G, Lenoir GM (1990) Stable transfection of Epstein-Barr virus

(EBV) nuclear antigen 2 in lymphoma cells containing the EBV P3HR1 genome induces expression of B-cell activation molecules CD21 and CD23. J Virol 64:1002–1013

10. Wang F, Gregory C, Sample, Rowe M, Liebowitz D, Murray R, Rickinson A, Kieff E (1990) Epstein-Barr virus latent membrane protein (LMP1) and nuclear proteins 2 and 3C are effectors of phenotypic changes in B lymphocytes: EBNA-2 and LMP1 cooperatively induce CD23. J Virol 64:2309–2318

11. Slaughter L, Carson DA, Jensen FC, Holbrook TL, Vaughan JH (1978) In vitro effects of Epstein-Barr virus on peripheral blood mononuclear cells from patients with rheumatoid arthritis and normal subjects. J Exp Med 148:1429–1434

12. Pearson GR, Vroman B, Chase B, Sculley T, Hummel M, Kieff E (1983) Identification of polypeptide components of the Epstein-Barr virus early antigen complex with monoclonal antibodies. J Virol 47:193–201

13. Allday MJ, Crawford DH, Griffin BE (1989) Epstein-Barr virus latent gene expression during the initiation of B cell immortalization. Gen Virol 70:1755–1764

14. Longnecker RE, Kieff E (1990) A second Epstein-Barr virus membrane protein (LMP2) is expressed in latent infection and colonizes with LMP1. J Virol 64:2319–2326

15. Rowe DT, Hall L, Joab I, Laux G (1990) Identification of the Epstein-Barr virus terminal protein gene products in latenly infected cells. J Virol 64:2866–2875

16. Frech B, Zimber Strobl U, Suentzenich KO, Pavlish O, Lenoir GM, Bornkamm GW, Mueller Lantzsch N (1990) Identification of Epstein-Barr virus terminal protein 1 (TP1) in extracts of four lymphoid cell lines, expression in insect cells, and detection of antibodies in human sera. J Virol 64:2759–2767

17. Tomei LD, Noyes I, Blocker D, Holliday J, Glaser R (1987) Phorbol ester and Epstein-Barr virus dependent transformation of normal primary human skin epithelial cells. Nature 329:73–75

18. Sixbey JW, Vesterinen EH, Nedrud JG, Raab-Traub N, Walton LA, Pagano JS (1983) Replication of Epstein-Barr virus in human epithelial cells infected in vitro. Nature 306:480–483

19. Dawson CW, Rickinson AD, Young LS (1990) Epstein-Barr virus latent membrane protein inhibits human epithelial cell differentiation. Nature 344:777–780

20. Sauvageau G, Stocco R, Kasparian S, Menezes J (1990) Epstein-Barr virus receptor on human $CD8^+$ (cytotoxic/suppressor) T lymphocytes. J Gen Virol 71:379–386

20a. Watry D, Hedrick JA, Siervo S, Rhodes G, Lamberti JJ, Lambris JD, Tsoukas CD (1991) Infection of human thymocytes by Epstein-Barr Virus. J Exp Med 173:971–980

21. Fingeroth JD, Weis JJ, Tedder TF, Strominger JL, Bird PA, Fearon DT (1984) Epstein-Barr virus receptor of human B lymphocytes is the C3d receptor CR2. Proc Natl Acad Sci USA 81:4510–4516

22. Nemerow GR, Moore MD, Cooper NR (1990) Structure and function of the B-lymphocyte Epstein-Barr virus/C3d receptor. Adv Cancer Res 54:273–300

23. Nemerow GR, Houghton RA, Moore MD, Cooper NR (1989) Identification of an epitope in the major envelope protein of Epstein-Barr virus that mediates viral binding to the B lymphocyte EBV receptor (CR2). Cell 56:369–377

24. Nemerow GR, Wolfert R, McNaughton ME, Cooper NR (1985) Identification and characterization of the Epstein-Barr virus receptor on human B lymphocytes and its relationship to the C3d complement receptor. J Virol 55:347–351

25. Nemerow GR, Mullen JJ, Dickson PW, Cooper NR (1990) Soluble recombinant CR2 (CD21) inhibits Epstein-Barr virus infection. J Virol 64:1348–1352

26. Tanner J, Whang Y, Sample J, Sears A, Kieff E (1988) Soluble gp50/220 and deletion mutant glycoproteins block Epstein-Barr virus adsorption to lymphocytes. J Virol 62:4452–4464

27. Ahern JM, Fearon DT (1989) Structure and function of the complement receptors, CR1 (CD35) and CR2 (CD21). Adv Immunol 46:183–219

28. Gordon J, Walker L, Guy GR, Brown G, Rickinson A, Rowe M (1986) Control of human B-lymphocyte replication II. Transforming Epstein-Barr virus exploits three distinct signals to undermine three separate control points. Immunology 58:591–595

29. Guy GR, Gordon J (1989) Epstein-Barr virus and tumor-promoting phorbol ester use similar mechanisms in the stimulation of human B-cell proliferation. Int J Cancer 43:703–708

30. Young LS, Sixbey JW, Rickinson AD (1986) Epstein-Barr virus receptors on human pharyngeal epithelia. Lancet I:240–242

31. Young LS, Dawson CW, Brown KW, Rickinson AB (1989) Identification of a human epithelial cell surface protein sharing an epitope with the C3d/Epstein-Barr virus receptor molecule of B lymphocytes. Int J Cancer 43:786–794

32. Shapiro IM, Volsky DJ, Seamundson A, Anisimova E, Klein G (1982) Infection of the human T cell derived leukemia line Molt-4 by Epstein-Barr virus (EBV): induction of EBV determined antigen and virus production. Virology 120:171–181

33. Stevenson M, Volsky B, Hedenskog M, Volsky D (1986) Immortalization of human T lymphocytes after transfection of Epstein-Barr virus DNA. Science 223:980–984

34. Kikuta H, Taguchi Y, Tomizawa K, Kojima K, Kawamura N, Ishizaka A, Sakiyama Y, Matsumoto S, Imai S, Kinoshita T, Koizumi S, Osato T, Kobayashi I, Hamada I, Hirai K (1988) Epstein-Barr virus genome-positive T lymphocytes in a boy with chronic active EBV infection associated with Kawasaki-like disease. Nature 333:455–457

35. Jones JF, Shurin S, Abramowski C, Tubbs RR, Sciotto CG, Wahl R, Sands J, Gottman D, Katz BZ, Sklar J (1988) T cell lymphomas containing Epstein-Barr viral DNA in patients with chronic Epstein-Barr virus infections. N Engl J Med 318:733–741

36. Fearon DT (1984) Cellular receptors for fragments of the third component of complement. Immunol Today 5:105–110

37. Inada S, Brown EJ, Gaither TA, Hammer CH, Takahashi T, Frank MM (1983) C3d receptors are expressed on human monocytes after in vitro cultivation. Proc Natl Acad Sci USA 80:2351–2355

38. Fujisaku A, Harley JB, Frank MB, Gruner BA, Frazier B, Holers VM (1989) Genomic organization and polymorphism of the human C3d/Epstein-Barr virus receptor. J Biol Chem 264:2118–2125

39. Toothaker LE, Henjes AJ, Weis JJ (1989) Variability of CR2 gene products is due to alternative exon usage and different CR2 alleles. J Immunol 142:3668–3675

40. Hurley E, Thorley-Lawson DA (1988) B cell activation and the establishment of Epstein-Barr virus latency. J Exp Med 168:2059–2075

41. Abbot SD, Rowe M, Cadwallader K, Ricksten A, Gordon J, Wang F, Rymo L, Rickinson AB (1990) Epstein-Barr virus nuclear antigen 2 induces expression of the virus-encoded latent membrane protein. J Virol 64:2126–2134

42. Miller G, Robinson J, Heston L, Lipman M (1974) Differences between laboratory strains of Epstein-Barr virus based on immortalization, abortive infection and interference. Proc Natl Acad Sci USA 71:4006–4010

43. Rabson M, Gradoville L, Heston L, Miller G (1982) Non-immortalizing P3J-HR-1 Epstein-Barr virus: a deletion mutant of its transforming parent, Jijoye. J Virol 44:834–844

44. Wang F, Gregory CD, Rowe M, Rickinson AD, Wang D, Birkenbach M, Kikutani H, Kishimoto T, Kieff E (1987) Epstein-Barr virus nuclear antigen 2 specifically induces expression of the B cell activation antigen CD23. Proc Natl Acad Sci USA 84:3452–3456

45. Thorley-Lawson DA, Mann KP (1985) Early events in Epstein-Barr virus infection provide a model for B cell activation. J Exp Med 162:45–59

46. Straub C, Zubler RH (1989) Immortalization of EBV-infected B cells is not influenced by exogenous signals acting on B cell proliferation. J Immunol 142:87–93

47. Tosato G, Blaese RM, Yarchoan R (1985) Relationship between immunglobulin production and immortalization by Epstein-Barr virus. J Immunol 135:959–964

48. Scala G, Morrone G, Tamburrini M, Alfinito F, Pastore CI, D'Alessio G, Venuta S (1987) Autocrine growth function of human interleukin 1 molecules on ROHA-9, an EBV-transformed human B cell line. J Immunl 138:2527–2534

49. Tosato G, Seamon KB, Goldman ND, Sehgal PB, May LT, Whashington GC, Jones KD, Pike SE (1988) Identification of a monocyte-derived human B cell growth factor as interferon-2 (BSF-2; IL-6). Science 239:502–504

50. Scala G, Quinti I, Ruocco MR, Arcucci A, Mallardo M, Caretto P, Forni G, Venuta S (1990) Expression of an exogenous interleukin 6 gene in human Epstein Barr virus B cells confers growth advantage and in vivo tumorigenicity. J Exp Med 172:61–68

51. Breen EC, Rezai AR, Nakajima K, Beall GN, Mitsuyasu RT, Hirano T, Kishimoto T, Martinez-Maza O (1990) Infection with HIV is associated with elevated IL-6 levels and production. J Immunol 144:480–484

52. Van Oers MHJ, Van der Heyden AAPAM, Aarden LA (1988) Interleukin 6 (IL-6) in serum and urine of renal transplant recipients. Clin Exp Immunol 71:314–319

53. Swendeman S, Thorley-Lawson DA (1987) The activation antigen BLAST-2, when shed, is an autocrine BCGF for normal and transformed B cells. EMBO J 6:1637–1642

54. Cairns JA, Gordon J (1990) Intact, 45-kDa (membrane) from CD23 is consistently mitogenic for normal and transformed B lymphoblasts. Eur J Immunol 20:539–543

55. Paul CC, Baumann MA (1990) Modulation of spontaneous outgrowth of Epstein-Barr virus immortalized B-cell clones by granulocyte-macrophage colony-stimulating factor and interleukin-3. Blood 75:54–58

56. Jansson O, Kabelitz D (1988) Tumor necrosis factor selectively inhibits activation of human B cells by Epstein-Barr virus. J Immunol 140:125–130

57. Lotz M, Tsoukas CD, Fong S, Carson DA, Vaughan JH (1985) Regulation of Epstein-Barr virus infections by recombinant interferon. Selected sensitivity to interferon-gamma. Eur J Immunol 15:520–525

58. Knutson JC (1990) The level of c-*fgr* RNA is increased by EBNA-2, an Epstein-Barr virus gene required for B-cell immortalization. J Virol 64:2530–2536

59. Patel M, Leevers SJ, Brickell PM (1990) Regulation of c-*fgr* proto-oncogene expression in Epstein-Barr virus infected B-cell lines. Int J Cancer 45:342–346

60. Tsujimoto Y (1989) Overexpression of the human BCL-2 gene product results in growth enhancement in Epstein-Barr virus-immortalized B cells. Proc Natl Acad Sci USA 86:1958–1962

61. Lacy J, Summers WP, Summers WC (1989) Post-transcriptional mechanisms of deregulation of MYC following conversion of a human B cell line by Epstein-Barr virus. EMBO J 8:1973–1980

62. Lombardi L, Newcomb EW, Dalla-Favera R (1987) Pathogenesis of Burkitt lymphoma: expression of an activated c-*myc* oncogene causes the tumorigenic conversion of EBV-infected human B lymphoblasts. Cell 49:161–170

63. Seremetis S, Inghirami G, Ferrero D, Newcomb EW, Knowles DM, Dotto GP, Dalla-Favera R (1989) Transformation and plasmacytoid differentiation of EBV-infected human B lymphoblasts by *ras* oncogenes. Science 243:660–663

64. Aman P von Gabain A (1990) An Epstein-Barr virus immortalization associated gene segment interferes specifically with the IFN-induced anti-proliferative response in human B-lymphoid cell lines. EMBO J 9:147–152

65. Blomhoff HK, Smeland E, Mustafa AS, Godal T, Ohlsson R (1987) Epstein-Barr virus mediates a switch in responsiveness to transforming growth factor, type beta, in cells of the B cell lineage. Eur J Immunol 17:299–301

66. Kehrl JH, Roberts AB, Wakefiled Jakolew MB, Sporn MB, Fauci AS (1986) Transforming growth factor β is an important immunomodulatory protein for human B lymphocytes. J Immunol 137:3855–3860

67. Casali P, Burastero SE, Nakamura M, Inghirami G, Notkins AL (1987) Human lymphocytes making rheumatoid factor and antibody to ssDNA belong to Leu-1+ B-cell subset. Science 236:77–81

68. Fong S, Vaughan JH, Carson DA (1983) Two different rheumatoid factor-producing cell populations distinguished by the mouse erythrocyte receptor and responsiveness to polyclona B cell activators. J Immunol 130:162–164

69. Rickinson AB, Finerty S, Epstein MA (1982) Interaction of Epstein-Barr virus with leukemie B cells in vitro. I. Abortive infection and rare establishment from chronic lymphocytic leukemia cells. Clin Exp Immunol 50:347–354

70. Crain MJ, Sanders SK, Butler JL, Cooper MD (1989) Epstein-Barr virus preferentially induces proliferation of primed B cells. J Immunol 143:1543–1548

71. Aman P, Lewin N, Nordström, Klein G (1986) EBV-activation of human B-lymphocytes. Curr Top Microbiol Immunol 132:266–271

72. Hui MF, Lam P, Dosch HM (1989) Properties and heterogeneity of human fetal pre-B cells transformed by EBV. J Immunol 143:2470–2479

73. Lotz M, Tsoukas CD, Curd JG, Carson DA, Vaughan JH (1987) Effects of recombinant human interferons on rheumatoid arthritis B lymphocytes activated by Epstein-Barr virus. J Rheumatol 14:42–45

74. Thyphronitis G, Tsokos G, June CH, Levine AD, Finkelman FD (1989) IgE secretion by Epstein-Barr virus-infected purified human B lymphocytes is stimulated by interleukin 4 and suppressed by interferon. Proc Natl Acad Sci USA 86:5580–584

75. Rickinson AB (1989) Immune control mechanisms over EBV infection. In: Ablashi D (ed) EBV and Human Disease. Humana Press, Clifton, New Jersey, pp 171–178

76. Luka J, Chase RC, Person GR (1984) A sensitive enzyme-linked immunosorbent assay (ELISA) against the major EBV-associated antigens. I. Correlations between ELISA and immunofluorescence titers using purified antigens. J Immunol Methods 67:145-156

77. Hoffman GJ, Lazarowitz SG, Hayward SD (1980) Monoclonal antibody against a 250,000-dalton glycoprotein of Epstein-Barr virus identifies a membrane antigen and a neutralizing antigen. Proc Natl Acad Sci USA 77:2979–2983

78. Strnad BC, Schuster T, Klein R, Hopkins RF, Witmer T, Neubauer RH, Rabin H (1982) Production and characterization of monoclonal antibodies against the Epstein-Barr virus membrane antigen. J Virol 41:258–264

79. Rhodes G, Carson DA, Valbracht J, Houghten R, Vaughan JH (1985) Human immune responses to synthetic peptides from the Epstein-Barr nuclear antigen. J Immunol 134:211–216

80. Rhodes GH, Rumpold H, Smith RS, Horwitz CA, Vaughan JH (1987) Autoantibody generation during infectious mononucleosis. In: Levine PH, Ablashi DV, Nonoyama M, Pearson GR, Glaser R (eds) Epstein-Barr virus and human diseases. Humana Press, Clifton, New Jersey, pp 399–400

81. Rumpold H, Rhodes GH, Bloch PL, Carson DA, Vaughan JH (1987) The glycine-alanine repeating region is the major epitope of the Epstein-Barr nuclear antigen-1 (EBNA-1). J Immunol 138:593–599

82. Lam V, DeMars R, Chen BP, Hank JA, Kovats S, Fisch P, Sondel PM (1990) Human T cell receptor-gamma delta-expressing T-cell lines recognize MHC-controlled elements on autologous EBV-LCL that are not HLA-A, -B, -C, -DR, -DQ, or -DP. J Immunol 145:36–45

83. Murray RJ, Kurilla MG, Griffin HM, Brooks JM, Mackett M, Arrand JR, Rowe M, Burrows SR, Moss DJ, Kieff E, Rickinson AD (1990) Human cytotoxic T-cell responses against Epstein-Barr virus nuclear antigens demonstrated by using recombinant vaccinia viruses. Proc Natl Acad Sci USA 87:2906–2910

84. Burrows SR, Misko IS, Sculley TB, Schmidt C, Moss DH (1990) An Epstein-Barr virus-specific cytotoxic T-cell epitope present on A- and B-type transformants. J Virol 64:3974–3976

85. Burrows SR, Sculley TB, Misko IS, Schmidt C, Moss DJ (1990) An Epstein Barr virus-specific cytotoxic T cell epitope in EBV nuclear antigen 3 (EBNA 3). J Exp Med 171:345–349

86. Thorley-Lawson DA, Iraelsohn ES (1987) Generation of specific cytotoxic T cells with a fragment of the Epstein-Barr virus-encoded p63/latent membrane protein. Proc Natl Acad Sci USA 84:5384–5388

87. Petersen J, Rhodes G, Patrick K, Roudier J, Vaughan JH (1989) Human T cell responses to the Epstein-Barr nuclear antigen-1 (EBNA 1) as evaluated by synthetic peptide. Cell Immunol 123:325–333

88. Roudier J, Petersen J, Rhodes G, Carson DA (1989) T-cell response to peptides encompassing a 5 amino acid sequence shared by the EBV gp110 and the HLA DR4 beta1 chain. In: Ablashi D (ed) EBV and human disease II. Humana Press, Clifton, New Jersey

89. Roudier J, Rhodes G, Petersen J, Vaughan JH, Carson DA (1988) The Epstein-Barr virus glycoprotein gp110, a molecular link between HLA DR4, HLA DR1, and rheumatoid arthritis. Scand J Immunol 27:367–371

90. Roudier J, Petersen J, Rhodes GH, Luka J, Carson DA (1989) Susceptibility to rheumatoid arthritis maps to a T-cell epitope shared by the HLA Dw4 and DRβ-1 chain and the Epstein-Barr virus glycoprotein gp110. Proc Natl Acad Sci USA 86:5104–5108

91. Bejarano MT, Masucci GM, Morgan A, Morein B, Klein G, Klein E (1990) Epstein-Barr virus (EBV) antigens processed and presented by B cells, B blasts, and macrophages trigger T-cell-mediated inhibition of EBV-induced B-cell transformation. J Virol 64:1398–1401

92. Morgan AJ, Finerty S, Lovgren K, Scullion FT, Morein B (1988) Prevention of Epstein-Barr (EB) virus-induced lymphoma in cottontop tamarins by vaccination with the EB virus envelope glycoprotein gp340 incorporated into immunostimulating complexes. J Gen Virol 69:2093–2096

93. Lotz M, Tsoukas CD, Fong S, Dinarello CA, Carson DA, Vaughan JH (1986) Release of lymphokines following Epstein-Barr virus infection in vitro. I. The sources and kinetics of production of interferons and interleukins in normal humans. J Immunol 136:3636–3642

94. Thorley-Lawson DA, Chess L, Strominger JL (1977) Supression of in vitro Epstein-Barr virus infection. A new role for adult T lymphocytes. J Exp Med 146:495–508

95. Thorley-Lawson DA (1981) The transformation of adult but not newborn lymphocytes by Epstein-Barr virus and phytohaemagglutinin is inhibited by interferon: the early suppression by T cells of Epstein-Barr infection is mediated by interferon. J Immunol 126:829–833

96. Andersson U, Britton S, DeLey M, Bird G (1983) Evidence for the ontogenic precedence of suppressor T cell functions in the human neonate. Eur J Immunol 13:6–13

97. Delcayre AX, Salas F, Mathur S, Kovats K, Lotz M, Lernhardt W (1991) Epstein-Barr virus/Complement C3d receptor is an alpha interferon receptor. EMBO J 10:919–926

98. Uze G, Lutfalla G, Gesser I (1990) Genetic transfer of a functional human interferon α receptor into mouse cells: cloning and expression of its cDNA. Cell 60:225–234

99. Moore KW, Vieira P, Fiorentino DF, Trounstine ML, Khan TA, Mosmann TR (1990) Homology of cytokine synthesis inhibitory factor (IL-10) to the Epstein-Barr virus gene BCRFI. Science 248:1230–1234

99a. Hsu DH, De Waal Malefyt R, Fiorentino DF, Dang MN, Vieria P, De Vries J, Spits H, Mossman TR, Moore KW (1990) Expression of Interleukin-10 activity by Epstein Barr Virus protein BCRF-1. Science 250:830–831

99b. Roudier J, Sette A, Lamont A, Albani S, Karras J, Carson DA (1991) Tolerance to a self peptide from the third hypervariable region of the Eβs chain. Implications for molecular mimicry models of autoimmune disease. Submitted

100. Henle W, Henle G (1982) Immunology of Epstein-Barr virus. In: Rorzman B. The Herpesviruses, Vol 1. Plenum Press, New York, pp 204–252

101. Klein G, Purtillo D (1981) Summary: symposium on Epstein-Barr virus induced lymphoproliferative diseases in immunodeficient patients. Cancer Res 41:4302–4308

102. Klein G (1989) Epstein-Barr virus and its association with human disease: an overview: In: Ablashi D (ed) Epstein-Barr Virus and Human Disease II. Humana Press, Clifton, New Jersey, pp 17–27

103. Voltz R, Jilg W, Wolf H (1989) Modification of HLA expression as a possible factor in the pathogenesis of Burkitt's lymphoma. Hamatol Bluttransfus 32:289–292

104. Lu SJ, Day NE, Degos L, LepageV, Wang PJ, Chan SH, Simons M, McKnight B, Easton D, Zeng Y, de-The G (1990) Linkage of a nasopharyngeal carcinoma susceptibility locus to the HLA region. Nature 346:470–471

105. Brusamolino E, Pagnucco G, Bernasconi C (1989) Secondary lymphomas: a review on lymphoproliferative diseases arising in immunocompromised hosts: prevalence, clinical features and pathogenetic mechanisms. Hematologica 74:605–622

106. Young L, Alfieri C, Hennessy K, Evans H, O'Hara C, Anderson KC, Ritz J, Shapiro RS, Rickinson A, Kieff E, Cohen JI (1989) Expression of Epstein-Barr virus transformation-associated genes in tissues of patients with EBV lymphoproliferative disease. N Engl J Med 321:1080–1085

107. Walz G, Zanker B, Melton LB, Suthanthiran M, Storm TB (1990) Possible association of the immunosuppressive and B cell lymphoma-promoting properties of cyclosporine. Transplantation 49:191–194

108. Starzl TE, Porter KA, Iwatsuki S et al (1984) Reversibility of lymphomas and lymphoproliferative lesions developing under cyclosporin-steroid therapy. Lancet 1:583–587

109. Purtilo DT, Svedmyr E, Klein G et al (1980) Fatal infectious mononucleosis. N Engl J Med 303:159–160

110. Sullivan JL, Byron KS, Brewster FE, Baker SM, Ochs HD (1983) X-linked lymphoproliferative syndrome. Natural history of the immunodeficiency. J Clin Invest 71:1765–1778

111. Ziegler JL, Miner RC, Rosenbaum E, Lennette ET, Shillitoe E, Casavant C, Drew WL, Mintz L, Gershow J, Greenspan J, Beckstead J, Yamamoto K (1982) Outbreak of Burkitt's-like lymphoma in homosexual men. Lancet I:631–633

112. Birx DL, Redfield RR, Tosato G (1986) Defective regulation of Epstein-Barr virus infection in patients with acquired immunodeficiency syndrome (AIDS) or AIDS-related disorders. N Engl J Med 31:874–879

113. Whang-Peng J, Lee EC, Sievert H, Magrath IT (1984) Burkitt's lymphoma in AIDS: cytogenetic study. Blood 63:818–822

114. Subar M, Neri A, Inghirami G, Knowles DM, Dalla-Favera R (1988) Frequent c-*myc* oncogene activation and infrequent presence of Epstein-Barr virus genome in AIDS-associated lymphoma. Blood 72:677–671

115. Alspaugh MA, Tan EM (1976) Serum antibody in rheumatoid arthritis reactive with a cell-associated antigen. Arthritis Rheum 19:711–719

116. Billings PB, Hoch SO, Vaughan JH (1984) Polymorphism of the EBNA/RANA antigen in Epstein-Barr virus-positive cell lines. Arthritis Rheum 27:1423–1427

117. Billings PB, Hoch SO, White PJ, Carson DA, Vaughan JH (1983) Antibodies to the Epstein-Barr virus nuclear antigen and to rheumatoid arthritis nuclear antigen identify the same polypeptide. Proc Natl Acad Sci 80:7104–7108

118. Slaughter L, Carson DA, Jensen FC, Holbrook TL, Vaughan JH (1978) In vitro effects of Epstein-Barr virus on peripheral blood mononuclear cells from patients with rheumatoid arthritis and normal subjects. J Exp Med 148:1429–1434

119. Bardwick P, Bluestein H, Zvaifler NJ, Depper J, Seegmiller J (1980) Altered regulation of EBV induced lymphoblast proliferation in rheumatoid arthritis lymphoid cells. Arthritis Rheum 23:626–632

120. Depper JM, Bluestein HG, Zvaifler NJ (1981) Impaired regulation of Epstein-Barr virus-induced lymphocyte proliferation in rheumatoid arthritis is due to a T cell defect. J Immunol 127:1899–1902

121. Tosato G, Steinberg AD, Blaese RM (1981) Defective EBV-specific suppressor T-cell function and rheumatoid arthritis. N Engl J Med 305:1238–1243

122. Hasler F, Bluestein HG, Zvaifler NJ, Epstein LB (1983) Analysis of the defects responsible for the impaired regulation of Epstein-Barr virus-induced B cell proliferation by rheumatoid arthritis lymphocytes. I. Diminished gamma interferon production in response to autologous stimulation. J Exp Med 157:173–188

123. Hasler F, Bluestein HG, Zvaifler NJ, Epstein LB (1983) Analysis of the defects responsible for the impaired regulation of EBV-induced B cell proliferation by

       rheumatoid arthritis lymphocytes. II. Role of monocytes and the increased sensitivity
       of rheumatoid arthritis lymphocytes to prostaglandin E. J Immunol 131:768–772
124.   Lotz M, Tsoukas CD, Fong S, Dinarello CA, Carson DA, Vaughan JH (1986) Release
       of lymphokines after infection with Epstein-Barr virus in vitro. II. A monocyte-
       dependent inhibitor of interleukin-1 downregulates the production of interleukin-2
       and interferon-gamma in rheumatoid arthritis. J Immunol 136:3643–3648
125.   Arend WP, Joslin FG, Thompson RC, Hannum CH (1989) An IL-1 inhibitor from
       human monocytes. Production and characterization of biologic properties. J Immunol
       143:1851–1858
126.   Lotz M, Tsoukas CD, Hench PK, Carson DA, Vaughan JH (1986) Release of
       lymphokines following Epstein-Barr virus infection in vitro of blood lymphocyts from
       patients with autoimmune diseases. Trans Assoc Am Physicians 99:114–124
127.   Lotz M, Tsoukas CD, Carson DA, Vaughan JH (1987) Interleukins and interferons
       during EBV infection. In: Levine PH, Ablashi DV, Nonoyama M, Pearson GR (eds)
       Epstein-Barr virus and human diseases. Humana Press, Clifton, New Jersey, pp 349–
       353
128.   Gaston JSH, Rickinson AB, Yao QY, Epstein MA (1986) The abnormal cytotoxic T
       cell response to Epstein-Barr virus in rheumatoid arthritis is correlated with disease
       activity and occurs in other arthropathies. Clin Exp Immunol 45:932–936
129.   Shore A, Klock R, Lee P, Snow KM, Keystone EC (1989) Impaired late suppression of
       Epstein-Barr virus (EBV)-induced immunoglobulin synthesis: a common feature of
       autoimmune disease. J Clin Immunol 9:103–110
130.   Tosato G, Steinberg AD, Yarchoan R, Heliman CA, Pike SE, DeSeau V, Blaese RM
       (1984) Abnormally elevated frequency of Epstein-Barr virus-infected B cells in the
       blood of patients with rheumatoid arthritis. J Clin Invest 73:1789–1795
131.   Alspaugh MA, Shoji H, Nonoyama M (1983) A search for rheumatoid arthritis-
       associated nuclear antigen and Epstein-Barr virus specific antigens or genomes in
       tissues and cells from patients with rheumatoid arthritis. Arthritis Rheum 26:712–720
132.   Gregersen PK, Shen M, Song Q-L, Merryman P, Degar S, Seki T, Maccari J, Goldberg
       D, Murphy H, Schwenzer J, Wang CY, Winchester RJ, Nepom GT, Silver J (1986)
       Molecular diversity of HLA-DR4 haplotypes. Proc Natl Acad Sci USA 83:2642–2646
133.   Gregersen PK, Silver J, Winchester RJ (1987) The shared epitope hypothesis – an
       approach to understanding the molecular genetics of susceptibility to rheumatoid
       arthritis. Arthritis Rheum 30:1205–1213
134.   Gong M, Ooka T, Matsuo T, Kieff E (1987) Epstein-Barr virus glycoprotein
       homologous to Herpes Simplex Virus gB. J Virol 61:499–508

Antibodies to EBV-Encoded Proteins in Rheumatoid Arthritis

P. J. W. Venables

Senior lecturer in Rheumatology, Division of Clinical Immunology, Kennedy Institute, London W6 7DW, UK

Introduction

The Epstein-Barr virus has been considered a possible pathogen for RA because it is ubiquitous, has profound effects on the immune system [1] and is able to persist in two cell types, lymphoid cells [2] and the salivary gland epithelium [3]. Both of these could envisaged as possible sources for the pathogenic features of RA, either by causing polyclonal activation of B cells, a prominent feature of the disease, or by leading to salivary gland inflammation (as secondary Sjögren's syndrome). Evidence from cellular studies suggesting possible involvement in RA includes the ability of the virus to induce rheumatoid factor production in vitro and impaired T cell regulation of EBV-infected B cells (see Lotz and Roudier, this volume), and some in vivo studies which suggest increased virus load. A second body of evidence comes from serological studies which have shown increased titres of antibodies to a variety of EBV-encoded antigens. This has been interpreted as suggesting more active EBV infection in RA. However, the results of much of this work must be interpreted with caution, as many of the earlier assays for EBV antibodies were crude, semiquantitative, subject to a variety of artefacts and not always performed with age- and sex-matched controls.

The Serological Response to EBV

The Epstein-Barr virus is one of at least seven known herpesviruses, all of which are characterized as large DNA viruses with a lipid envelope and a capacity to persist in lymphoid cells as well as in other tissues. The EBV genome is 175 kilobases long and contains approximately 100 open reading frames. Its size and complexity are reflected in the large number of antigens which it encodes. The antigens can be divided into five groups: the membrane antigens (glycoproteins which are inserted into the envelope) the viral capsid antigens

Smolen, Kalden, Maini (Eds.)
Rheumatoid Arthritis
© Springer-Verlag Berlin Heidelberg 1992

(VCAs), the Epstein-Barr nuclear antigens (EBNAs), the early antigens and the latent membrane protein(s) [4]. The membrane antigens may be the most important in antibody-meditated control of EBV infection, as it is these – particularly the largest, gp 340 – which are thought to interact with the EBV receptor. The receptor is the CR2 receptor (CD 21) which is present on B cells and weakly expressed on some T cells. An antigen reactive with an anti-CR2 receptor antibody has also been described on epithelial cells [5], suggesting that a similar molecule, though not necessarily the receptor itself, may be present on non-lymphoid cells. This widespread distribution of CR2 receptor, or CR2 receptor-like molecules, could explain the varied topism of the virus, including the well-established infectibility of B cells, of the epithelium in salivary gland and possibly the genital tract, through to the most recent identification of the virus in T cell leukaemias. Even though the serological response to gp 340 may be the neutralizing antibody, and therefore a most important protection against EBV infection, it has received little attention in RA, partly because of difficulties in measuring antibodies to this group of antigens, though one study using immunoblotting [6] did find elevated titres of antibodies to gP 340 in both RA and SLE. There are no reports of the immune response to the latent membrane proteins in RA. It is possible that the immune response to this group is restricted to cytotoxic T cells. Studies of the serological responses in RA have therefore concentrated largely on the VCAs, the early antigens and the EBNAs.

Antibodies to the Viral Capsid Antigen

The viral capsid antigen complex represents a series of proteins surrounding the nucleic acid core of the virus and can be detected as a granular cytoplasmic staining pattern in productively infected lymphoblastoid cells (Fig. 1d). Because an immune response to VCA is virtually universal in EBV-infected individuals, the antibody is frequently used as the basis of seroepidemiological studies of the virus. In RA, antibodies to EBVCA have been used to examine two aspects of infection by the virus: (a) for prevalence studies and (b) for analyzing the immune response to the virus. Studies of the prevalence of EBV infection have been complicated by the fact that EBV is one of the most ubiquitous of all pathogens infecting man. In European populations the rate of seroconversion gradually increases with age, so that over 90% of 25-year-olds are seropositive [7]. In RA the few attempts at analyzing the prevalence of EBV infection have shown it to be normal. In our study of 100 RA patients [8], 94 were EBVCA seropositive, similar to the number which would bve expected from the frequency in the local population (92%) and slightly lower than that found in our adult controls (97%). Ferrel et al. [9] found a slightly higher prevalence in RA patients (97%) than controls (91%), though the difference was not statistically significant. It a study by Elson et al. in Bristol, the prevalence in RA patients was 83% [10], a number which corresponded to the lower

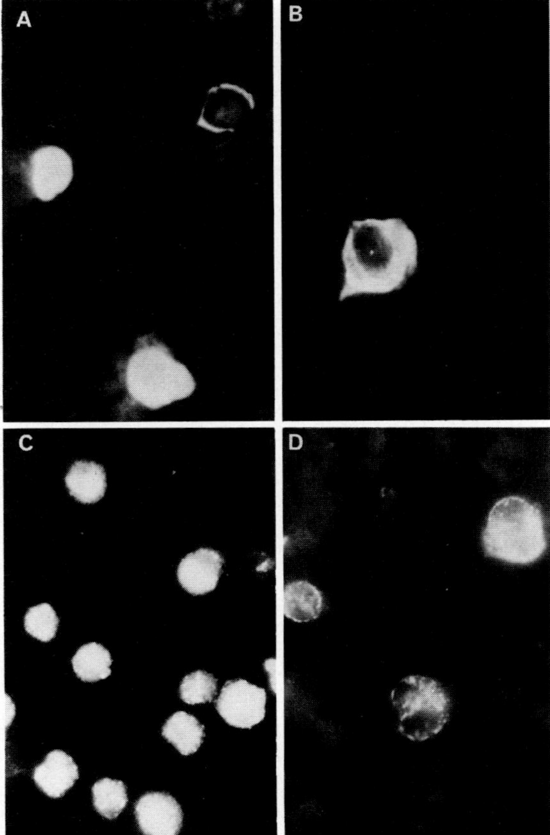

Fig. 1 a–d. Cellular distribution of EBV-encoded antigens demonstrated by indirect immunofluorescence with anti-EBV monoclonal antibodies or (in *c*) a human reference serum.
(a) Early antigen (diffuse);
(b) early antigen (restricted);
(c) Epstein-Barr nuclear antigen; **(d)** viral capsid antigen

frequency of EBV infection in the west of England. In an attempt to circumvent the problems associated with the very high prevalence of EBV in London, we examined sera from children with juvenile chronic arthritis in whom the expected frequency of EBV infection was lower. In the subgroup with juvenile RA (erosive joint disease and rheumatoid factor positive) the frequency was 60%, again corresponding to the frequency of 43%–70% which was reported for their age-group [11]. The two studies which included the largest number of EBV-seronegative subjects [8, 10] also pointed out that these patients, apparently free of EBV infection, did not show any clinical or serological differences from the EBV-positive patients with RA, implying that the virus was not an essential aetiological agent for all patients with the disease.

Some studies have examined titres of antibodies to EBVCA in RA, on the grounds that elevated titres may reflect an abnormal response to the virus or an increase in infection load. The results are conflicting: some studies have reported an approximately twofold increase in titre in RA, and some have found no difference between RA patients and normal controls (Table 1).

Table 1. Titres of antibodies to EBVCA in RA and controls

Reference	Geometric mean titre of anti-EBVCA	
	RA	Controls
Catalano et al. [12]	160	160
Bardwick et al. [13]	320	320
Alspaugh et al. [14]	226*	104
Ferrel et al. [9]	133*	58
Tosato et al. [15]	234*	87
Gaston et al. [16]	416	380
Venables et al. [17]	216	160
Yao et al. [18]	1,498*	627

* Titres reported as being significantly increased above normal

The finding of elevated levels of anti-EBVCA antibodies in RA has often been interpreted as indicating "hyper-responsiveness" of RA patients to the virus or impaired control of EBV infection.

However, it is important to remember that not all studies agree on the finding of high anti-VCA titres in RA. In addition, similar elevations in titre have been reported in multiple sclerosis [19], systemic lupus erythematosus [14], Sjögren's syndrome [20] and scleroderma [14]. If the response to EBV is abnormal in RA, the studies of anti-VCA antibodies to date have revealed little about pathogenic mechanisms which show any specificity for the virus or for the disease.

Antibodies to Early Antigens

The early antigen complex, which comprises the restricted (EA-R) and the diffuse components (EA-D), is expressed during lytic infection by EBV. EA-R is so called because its expression is restricted to the cytoplasm of EBV-infected cells (Fig. 1b), whereas EA-D is found in both cytoplasm and nucleus (Fig. 1a). High titres of antibodies to both components are found in patients with infectious mononucleosis (IM) and nasopharyngeal carcinoma, reflecting an immune response to the antigens in productively infected cells. Several studies have reported an increased frequency or titre of antibodies to early antigens in RA, though there has been disagreement as to whether the predominant target has been the diffuse or the restricted component (Table 2).

In an attempt to quantitative any differences in anti-EA-D antibodies between RA patients and healthy subjects, we used a synthetic peptide termed k7b, which represents an important epitope on EA-D in an ELISA system. No

Table 2. Percent frequency or geometric mean titres (GMT) of antibodies to EA-D and EA-R in RA patients and controls

Reference	RA	Controls	Specificity
Alspaugh et al. [14]	38*	9.8	EA-R
	4	1.2	EA-D
Ferrel et al. [9]	53*	19	EA-D
Tosato et al. [15]	75*	25	EA-R
	75*	15	EA-D
Gaston et al. [16] (GMT)	10.3	8.7	–
Yao et al. [18] (GMT)	30*	9	–

* Frequency or titres reported as significantly increased above normal
–, Not stated whether EA-D or EA-R

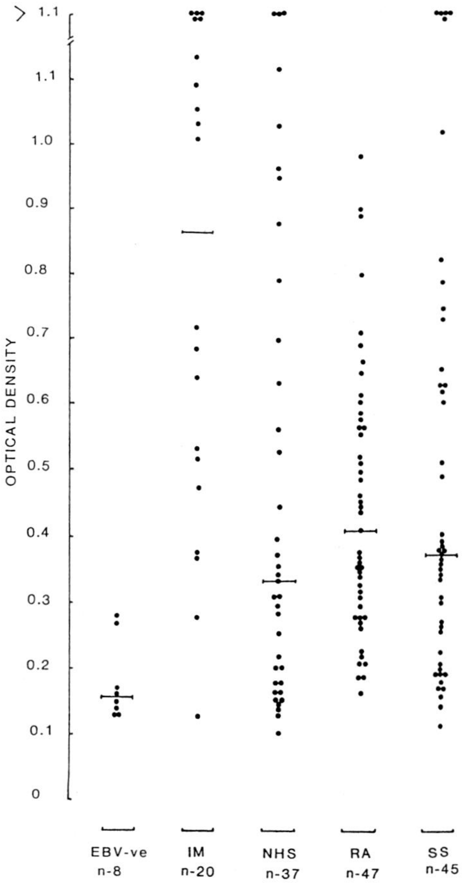

Fig. 2. Antibody levels by ELISA to K7B, a synthetic peptide representing an epitope on early antigen (diffuse) measured in healthy subjects with no serological evidence of EBV infection *(EBV-ve)*, infectious mononucleosis *(IM)*, normal human sera *(NHS)*, rheumatoid arthritis *(RA)*, Sjögren's syndrome *(SS)*

difference was found between RA and normal subjects (Fig. 2). However, we did find elevated IgG antibodies to the peptide in infectious mononucleosis and low levels in EBV-negative subjects, providing evidence of the specificity of the assay.

Antibodies to Epstein-Barr Nuclear Antigens

The Epstein-Barr nuclear antigens (EBNAs) are now known to consist of at least five polypeptides with molecular weights between 68 and 150 kD which are traditionally detected by an anti-complementary immunofluorescent (ACIF) technique in the nucleus of EBV-infected cells (Fig. 1d). Because expression of the EBNAs is restricted to cells transformed by the virus, the EBNAs are thought to play a major role in oncogenesis. Detected by ACIF, anti-EBNA antibodies give a bright, slightly granular nuclear staining pattern in lymphoblastoid cells (Fig. 1d). In RA, titres of anti-EBNA antibodies detected by ACIF have been largely reported as normal, reduced or increased above controls (Table 3).

Antibodies to RANA

The strongest serological evidence of a link between EBV was suggested by the description of an apparently distinct antigen, rheumatoid arthritis nuclear antigen (RANA), which was present in EBV-transformed cells. The antigen was first detected by immunodiffusion using homogenized lymphoblastoid cells as a source of antigen [22]. Subsequently, it was shown [23] that sera containing high

Table 3. Titres of antibodies to EBNA in RA patients and controls

Reference	Geometric mean titre of anti-EBNA	
	RA	Controls
Catalano et al. [12]	40*	11
Alspaugh et al. [14]	32	39
Ferrel et al. [9]	119	112
Tosato et al. [15]	56*	26
Gaston et al. [16]	19.9	51.5
Rhodes et al. [21]	84	73

* Titres reported as significantly increased above normal

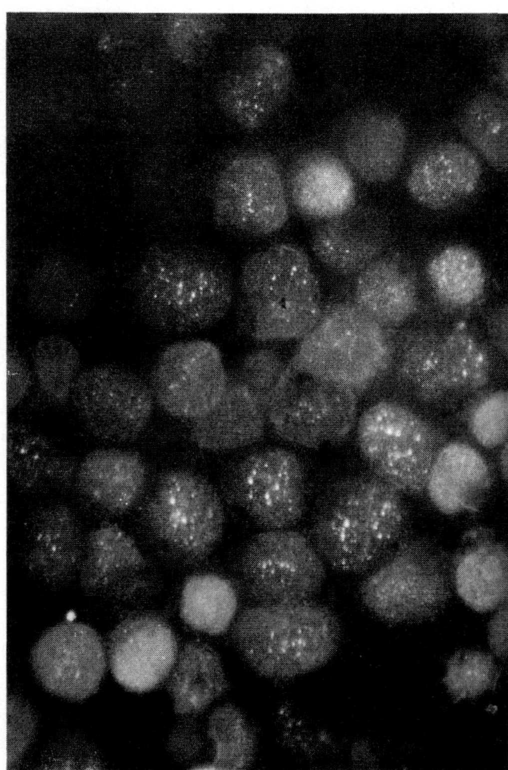

Fig. 3. Indirect immunofluorescence on an air-fixed, cytocentrifuged preparation of WI-L2 cells with an anti-RANA reference serum. The antigen appears as fine, discrete nuclear speckles

Table 4. Prevalence of antibodies to RANA in RA patients and controls

Reference	RA	Controls
Alspaugh and Tan [22]	67*	8
Catalano et al. [12]	94*	26
Ng et al. [24]	94*	16
Alspaugh et al. [14]	90*	6
Ferrel et al. [9]	71*	6
Venables et al. [8]	86*	54
Male et al. [25]	94*	41
Le Clerq and Davis [26]	71*	41
Hazelton et al. [27]	80*	26

* Prevalence or titres reported as significantly increased above normal

titres of precipitating antibodies also reacted with air-fixed lymphoblastoid cells on immunofluorescence with a characteristic fine, speckled nuclear staining pattern (Fig. 3). In contrast to antibodies to other EBV-encoded antigens, antibodies to RANA have been universally reported as significantly increased in

RA, suggesting that RANA is a selective target for antibodies in this disease (Table 4).

Some of the earliest reports found such a difference between the frequencies of anti-RANA in RA and controls that it was suggested that the antibodies were of diagnostic significance, with one study even claiming that they were "marker antibodies" [24]. The finding of anti-RANA in 40%–50% of healthy controls has challenged this claim to the extent that no one would recommend an "anti-RANA test" as diagnostically useful to the rheumatologist [8, 25, 28, 29]. Nevertheless, in spite of variability of the reports of anti-RANA antibody prevalence, there is general agreement that it is significantly increased in RA with about a fourfold increase above normal in anti-RANA titres. This represents the strongest serological evidence linking EBV to the disease.

The Identity of RANA

Anti-RANA antibodies were initially thought to be distinct from anti-EBNA because of differences in the properties of the two antigens and a striking dissociation of the antibody response (reviewed in [29]). A possible indentity for RANA was found by Sculley et al. [30], who suggested on the basis of correlative studies that RANA was EBNA-2. However, a previous study suggested that the target for anti-RANA antibodies was the EBNA-1 polypep-

```
  1    MSDEGPGTGP  GNGLGEKGDT  SGPEGSGGSG
 31    PQRRGGDNHG  RGRGRGRGRG  GGRPGAPGGS
 61    GSGPRHRDGV  RRPQKRPSCI  GCKGTHGGTG
 91    AGAGAGGAGA  GGAGAGGGAG  AGGGAGGAGG
121    AGGAGAGGGA  GAGGGAGGAG  GAGAGGGAGA
151    GGGAGGAGAG  GGAGGAGGAG  AGGGAGAGGG
181    AGGAGAGGGA  GGAGGAGAGG  GAGAGGAGGA
211    GGAGAGGAGA  GGGAGGAGGA  GAGGAGAGGA
241    GAGGAGAGGA  GGAGAGGAGG  AGAGGAGGAG
271    AGGGAGGAGA  GGGAGGAGAG  GAGGAGAGGA
301    GGAGAGGAGG  AGAGGGAGAG  GAGAGGGGRG
331    RGGSGGRGRG  GSGGRGRGCS  GGRRGRGRER
361    ARGGSRERAR  GRGRGRGEKR  PRSPSSQSSS
391    SGSPPRRPPP  GRRPFFHPVG  EADYFEYHQE
421    GGPDGEPDVP  PGAIEQGPAD  DPGEGPSTGP
451    RCQGDGGRRK  KGGWFGKHRG  QGGSNPKFEN
481    IAEGLRALLA  RSHVERTTDE  GTWVAGVFVY
511    GGSKTSLYNL  RRGTALAIPQ  CRLTPLSRLP
541    FGMAPGPGPQ  PGPLRESIVC  YFMVFLQTHI
571    FAEVLKDAIK  DLVMTKPAPT  CNIRVTVCSF
601    DDGVDLPPWF  PPMVEGAAAE  GDDGDDGDEG
631    GDGDEGEEGQ  E
```

Fig. 4. Amino acid sequence of EBNA-1 predicted from the DNA sequence of the *Bam*H1 K restriction fragment from B95-8. The sequences corresponding to p62 are *underlined*

tide by immunoblotting [31]. Furthermore, we showed that RANA was present in P3HR-1, a cell line which contains EBNA-1, but not EBNA-2 [32].

An explanation for the dissociation of anti-RANA and anti-EBNA antibodies may be found in the structure of EBNA-1. It is a highly polymorphic protein, varying in molecular weight between 68 and 90 kD in different cell lines; the variation is due to a sequence of approximately 20 kD, which consists entirely of the amino acids glycine and alanine arranged in a glycine-rich sequence (Fig. 4). By constructing synthetic peptides equivalent to a number of the potential epitopes on the molecule, Rhodes et al. [21] showed that the greatest difference in antibody levels between RA and normal sera was obtained with peptides from the repeat sequence, particularly P62, with the sequence AGAGGGAGGAGAGGGAGGAG. We confirmed their findings in a controlled study which showed that, like anti-RANA antibodies, anti-P62 antibodies increased approximately fourfold in RA [32]. Furthermore, we demonstrated conclusively that anti-RANA as detected by immunofluorescence was the same as anti-P62 by showing that affinity purified anti-P62 antibodies gave the characteristic fine speckled staining pattern on lymphoblastoid cells [32]. The purified antibodies did not react with RANA by immunodiffusion, suggesting that the precipitin reaction involved epitopes outside the sequence represented by P62.

The Selectivity of the Antibody Response
to the Glycine Alanine Repeat Sequence

The elevated titres of antibodies to RANA and P62 suggests that the glycine alanine (gly/ala) repeat sequence on EBNA-1 is a specific target for the antibody response to EBV in RA. It is difficult to explain this phenomenon merely by invoking a generalized hightened response to the virus because of the finding of normal antibody levels to other EBV-determined antigens in RA, including epitopes on EBNA-1 which do not include this sequence. The concept of generalized hyper-responsiveness in RA is also challenged by serological studies of nasopharyngeal carcinoma. In this disease, known to be associated with productive infection by virus in the tumour, antibodies to RANA or P62 are normal or only slightly increased, whereas antibody levels to VCA, to EBNA by ACIF, and to the carboxyl terminus of EBNA-1 are elevated fivefold [33]. This suggests that the repeat sequence of EBNA-1 has special properties in relation to the immune response in RA but not in other diseases that are known to be associated with active virus infection.

Cross-reactions Between the gly/ala Repeat and Host Proteins

A feature of the gly/ala repeat which could account for its targeting of the immune response in RA is its extensive homology with host proteins. This was first suggested by our findings that anti-RANA antibodies were depleted, but not abolished, by absorption of sera with Ramos, an EBV negative lymphoblastoid line [8]. Cross-reactions between the gly/ala repeat and host proteins were subsequently demonstrated with more precision by Rhodes et al., who showed that IgM antibodies to P62 in infectious mononucleosis reacted with a number of polypeptides in uninfected cells on immunblotting [34]. Recent studies have demonstrated similar cross-reactions of IgG antibodies in RA, as well as sequence homologies between P62, cyokeratins and collagens [33, 35, 36]. We showed that affinity-purified anti-P62 antibodies reacted with epidermis and cytoskeletal antigens in HEp-2 cells by immunofluorescence, and with a 60-kD polypeptide in keratinocytes and other tissues by immunoblotting [33]. Birkenfeld et al. showed cross-reactions of antibodies between the same peptide (which they termed p107) and collagen and keratin using both inhibition and purified antibodies [35]. More recently we have confirmed extensive cross-reactons of anti-p62 antibodies purified from four of 12 RA sera (Fig. 5). The anti-p62 antibodies reacted with human epidermal cytokeratin, denatured collagen type II and actin, but not with influenza haemaglutinin (a control antigen).

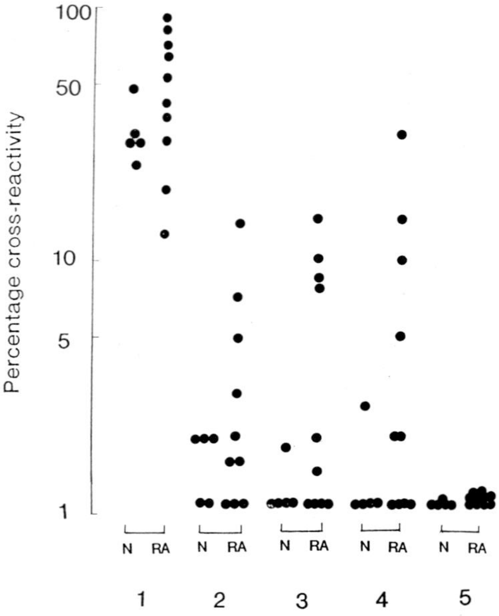

Fig. 5. Percentage recovery of purified antibodies to p62 (1) and their cross-reaction with denatured collagen (2), human epidermal keratin (3), actin (4), and influenza A (5) from P62 affinity purification columns. The percentage represents the proportion of the antibody of each specificity which bound to the P62 column (i.e. the proportion cross-reactive with P62). The antibodies were purified from sera from patients with RA and normal healthy individuals (N)

Cross-reactions between the gly/ala repeat and host proteins have also been demonstrated with monoclonal antibodies. Fox et al. [37] showed reactivity with a 60-kD protein in synovial membrane using a monoclonal antibody to p62. This is likely to be different from the cross-reactive 60-kD polypeptide which we have characterized, because our experiments suggested that it was cytokeratin and present in several tissues, whereas Fox et al. found the antigen was restricted to synovial membrane and did not react with a panel of anti-cytokeratin antibodies. Furthermore, repeated experiments with our purified anti-p62 antibodies have failed to demonstrate reactivity with synovial membrane by immunofluorescence (unpublished data). This suggests that the cross-reaction observed by Fox et al. may reflect a peculiar property of the monoclonal antibody they used. Nevertheless, a cross-reaction suggesting molecular mimicry between a synovial antigen and a major epitope on EBV is an important finding which certainly merits further study. A monoclonal antibody to EBNA produced by Garzelli et al. [38] cross-reacted with cytoskeletal antigens and smooth muscle. Although this antibody was derived from a patient with acute infectious mononucleosis, was of IgM class, and may have indicated more about autoimmunity in IM than RA, it again emphasized the extensive cross-reactions which have been demonstrated between EBNA-1 and host proteins.

Other Cross-reactive EBV-encoded Antigens

Although homologies between the repeat sequence of EBNA-1 and host proteins are the best studied, other cross-reactions or potential reactions (indicated by sequence homologies) have also been described. These include the chance finding of a cross-reaction between the Fc portion of IgG and EBVCA [39] and sequence homologies between EBNA-2 and the collagens which could relate to the higher levels of antibodies to EBNA-2 in RA, as judged by the intensity of bands on immunoblotting [30]. Another intriguing homology was described by Roudier et al. [40], who found that a five-amino-acid sequence (QKRAA) on the third hypervariable region of the HLA haplotypes that determine susceptibility to RA (HLA DR1, Dw4 and Dw14) was identical to a sequence on Gp 10 in the VCA complex. Studies by the same group indicated that this sequence acted predominantly as a T cell rather than a B cell epitope.

Implications for Pathogenesis

Elevated levels of antibodies to the glycine alanine repeat sequence, the major epitope on RNA, thus represent the only consistent serological finding linking

EBV infection to RA. Although it is not generally believed the EBV is the cause of the disease, it is a finding that warrants explanation and, it may indicate a contribution of the virus to pathogenesis. Four possible mechanisms are proposed.

1. The simplest explanation is based on the cross-reactions between the gly/ala repeat and collagens and cytokeratins. Antibodies to both groups of proteins have been described as elevated in RA (see by Holmdahl and by Hoet and van Venrooij, this volume), and it is possible that these autoantibodies also react with the gly/ala repeat and cause an apparent elevation of the anti-RANA/anti-P62 titre. If this were the case, it would be possible to explain these elevated antibody titres without invoking an abnormal serological response to EBV or indeed any pathogenic role for the virus in the disease.

2. A second possible explanation invokes a breakdown in tolerance due to the cross-reactions. Molecular mimicry between collagen and a virally encoded protein (EBNA) leads to breakdown of tolerance to denatured collagen. Continued exposure to what is now an immunogenic autoantigen within the joint results in local production of autoantibodies, the perpetuation of inflammation and immune-mediated damage to cartilage and bone. Some evidence in favour of this hypothesis may be found in the threefold specific concentration of anti-collagen antibodies in synovial fluid, suggesting local secretion of anti-collagen antibodies [41] and the demonstration of collagen antibody-secreting plasma cells in the synovial membrane [42].

3. One of the more popular ideas linking EBV to the pathogenesis of RA is based on the concept that impaired regulation of EBV infection by RA T cells (reviewed in Lotz and Roudier, this volume) results in increased viral load and a corresponding exaggeration of the humoral immune response to the virus. This explains those studies which have showed elevated titres of antibodies to virtually all of the EB virally encoded antigens but not those which suggest that the hyper-responsiveness is selective for the gly/ala repeat sequence. If the immune response does prove to be selective, it is possible that the gly/ala repeat is preferentially expressed in some infected cell types (such as B cells), possibly along with early antigens, whose antibodies are also elevated in most serological studies of RA (Table 2). One relatively specific mechanism for the increased viral load is suggested by the sequence homologies between an epitope on the VCA and the QKRAA sequence on the DRβ chain which predisposes to RA [40]. It could be proposed that tolerance to this sequence on VCA in patients who carry the appropriate haplotype (i.e. 80% of RA patients) results in impaired T-cell-mediated killing of cells productively infected with the virus. This would result in increased virus load and in serological hyper-responsiveness to many of the EBV-determined antigens, with the exception of VCA. This again would be concordant with the findings of many of the published studies.

4. The final, and least investigated possibility depends on the observation that the response to the gly/ala repeat is mediated by CD5 +ve B cells. It is almost universally agreed that such B cells are increased in number in the blood of RA patients and are responsible for the secretion of "natural antibodies". These immunoglobulins, predominantly IgM but often also of IgG class, are

thought to be derived from unmutated germline genes and to cross-react with a number of different antigens, amongst which cytoskeletal antigens figure prominently (see Plater-Zyberk et al., this volume). It is possible that a proportion of the anti-P62 antibodies found in RA are derived from such cells, though there is no experimental evidence to date in support of this.

Conclusion

Over the past 20 years there have been a number of serological phenomena described which could be interpreted as providing evidence of a link between EBV and RA. So far, nothing has suggested a primary causative role for the virus; indeed, all of the serological abnormalities can be explained by alteration of the immune response by the disease, without the virus necessarily making any contribution to its pathogenesis. However, there have been several hints at mechanisms by which EBV could exacerbate the disease by amplifying the immune response, in which case EBV could be one of the several factors contributing to disease severity. This latter possibility still merits investigation, not only because it could provide insight into disease mechanisms in RA, but also because it could lead to treatments aimed at modifying, if not curing, the disease.

References

1. Tosato G, Blaese RM (1985) Epstein-Barr virus infection and immunoregulation in man. Adv Immunol 37:99–149
2. Jondal J, Klein G (1973) Surface markers on human B and T lymphocytes. II. Presence of Epstein-Barr virus receptors on B lymphocytes. J Exp Med 138:1365–1378
3. Wolf H, Haus M, Wilmes E (1984) Persistence of Epstein-Barr virus in the parotid gland. J Virol 51:795–798
4. Pearson GR (1985) Advances in the identification of EBV-specific proteins. In: Levine et al. (eds) Epstein-Barr virus and associated diseases. Nijhoff, Boston
5. Young LS, Clark D, Sixbey JW, Rickinson AB (1986) Epstein-Barr virus receptors on human pharyngeal cells. Lancet 1:240–242
6. Yokochi T, Yanagawa A, Kimura Y, Mizushima Y (1989) High titre of antibody to Epstein-Barr virus membrane antigen in sera from patients with rheumatoid arthritis and systemic lupus erythematosus. J Rheumatol 16:1029–1032
7. Edwards JMB, Woodroof M (1979) EB virus-specific IgA in serum of patients with infectious mononucleosis and of healthy people of different ages. J Clin Pathol 32:1036–1041
8. Venables PJW, Roffe LM, Erhardt CC, Maini RN, Edwards JMB, Porter AD (1981) Titers of antibodies to RANA in rheumatoid arthritis and normal sera. Arthritis Rheum 24:1459–1464
9. Ferrel PB, Aitcheson CT, Pearson GR, Tan EM (1981) Seroepidemiological study of relationships between EBV and rheumatoid arthritis. J Clin Invest 67:681–687

10. Elson CJ, Crawford DM, Bucknall RC, Allen C, Thomson JL, Hall ND, Bacon PA, Epstein MA (1979) Infection with Epstein-Barr virus and rheumatoid arthritis. Lancet 1:105

11. Gear AJ, Venables PJW, Edwards JMB, Maini RN, Ansell BM (1986) Rheumatoid arthritis, juvenile arthritis, iridocyclitis and the Epstein-Bar virus. Ann Rheum Dis 45:6–8

12. Catalano MA, Carson DA, Nierderman JC, Feorino P, Vaughan JH (1980) Antibody to rheumatoid arthritis nuclear antigen: its relationship to in vivo Epstein-Barr virus infection. J Clin Invest 65:1238–1242

13. Bardwick PA, Bluestein HG, Zwaifler NG, Depper JM, Seegmiller JE (1980) Altered regulation of EBV-induced lymphoblast proliferation on rheumatoid arthritis lymphoid cells. Arthritis Rheum 23:626–632

14. Alspaugh MA, Henle G, Lennette FT, Henle W (1981) Elevated levels of antibodies to EBV antigens in sera and synovial fluid of patients with rheumatoid arthritis. J Clin Invest 67:1134–1140

15. Tosato G, Steinberg AD, Blaese RM (1981) Defective Epstein-Barr-specific suppressor T cell function in rheumatoid arthritis. N Engl J Med 305:1238–1243

16. Gaston JSH, Richinson AB, Epstein MA (1982) Epstein-Barr virus-specific cytotoxic T cell responses in rheumatoid arthritis patients. Rheumatol Int 2:155–159

17. Venables PJW, Ross MGR, Charles PJ, Melsom RD, Griffiths PD, Maini RN (1985) A seroepidemiological study of cytomegalovirus and Epstein-Barr virus in rheumatoid arthritis and sicca syndrome. Ann Rheum Dis 44:742–746

18. Yao QY, Rickinson AB, Gaston JSH, Epstein MA (1986) Disturbance of Epstein-Barr virus host balance in rheumatoid arthritis patients: a quantitative study. Clin Exp Immunol 64:302–310

19. Larsen PD, Bloomer LC, Bray PF (1985) Epstein-Barr nuclear antigen and viral capsid antigen antibody titres in multiple sclerosis. Neurology 35:435–438

20. Yamaoka K, Miyasaka N, Yamamoto K (1988) Possible involvement of Epstein-Barr virus in polyclonal B cell activation in Sjögren's syndrome. Arthritis Rheum 31:1014–1021

21. Rhodes G, Carson DA, Valbract J, Houghten R, Vaughan JH (1985) Human immune responses to synthetic peptides from the Epstein-Barr nuclear antigen. J Immunol 134:211–216

22. Alspaugh MA, Tan EM (1976) Serum antibody in rheumatoid arthritis reactive with a cell-associated antigen. Arthritis Rheum 19:711–719

23. Alspaugh MA, Jensen FC, Rabin H, Tan EM (1978) Lymphocyts transformed by Epstein-Barr virus: induction of nuclear antigen reactive with serum antibody in rheumatoid arthritis. J Exp Med 147:1018–1027

24. Ng KC, Brown KA, Perry JA, Holborow EJ (1980) Anti-RANA antibody: a marker for seronegative and seropositive rheumatoid arthritis. Lancet 1:447–449

25. Male D, Young A, Pilkinton C, Sutherland S, Roitt IN (1982) Antibodies to EB virus- and cytomegalovirus-induced antigens in early rheumatoid disease. Clin Exp Immunol 50:341–346

26. Le Clerk SA, Davis P (1982) Anti-RANA antibody in rheumatoid arthritis, seronegative polyarthritis and normal controls. Rheum Int 1:177–180

27. Hazelton RA, Cross SM, Robert G, Strachan N (1986) A family study of the prevalence of antibodies to the rheumatoid arthritis nuclear antigen (RANA). Br J Rheumatol 25:349–352

28. Lydyard PM, Irving WV (1988) Is there a role for Epstein-Barr virus in the aetiology of rheumatoid arthritis? Br J Rheumatol 27 [Suppl] 120–127

29. Venables PJW (1988) Leading article: Epstein-Barr virus and autoimmunity in rheumatoid arthritis. Ann Rheum Dis 47:265–269

30. Sculley TB, Pope JH, Hazelton RA (1986) Comparison between the presence of antibodies to Epstein-Barr virus nuclear antigen 2 and the rheumatoid arthritis nuclear antigen in rheumatoid arthritis patients. Arthritis Rheum 29:964–970

31. Billings PB, Hoch SO, White PJ, Carson DA, Vaughan JH (1983) Antibodies to the Epstein-Barr nuclear antigen and to the rheumatoid arthritis nuclear antigen identify the same polypeptide. Proc Natl Acad Sci USA 80:7104–7108

32. Venables PJW, Pawlowski T, Mumford PA, Brown C, Crawford DH, Maini RN (1988) Reaction of antibodies to rheumatoid arthritis nuclear antigen with a synthetic peptide corresponding to part of Epstein-Barr nuclear antigen-1. Ann Rheum Dis 47:270–279
33. Baboonian C, Halliday D, Venables PJW, Pawlowski T, Millman G, Maini RN (1989) Antibodies in rheumatoid arthritis react specifically with the glycine alanine repeat sequence of Epstein-Barr nuclear antigen-1. Rheumatol Int 9:161–166
34. Rhodes G, Rumpold R, Kurki P, Patrick KM, Carson DA, Vaughan JH (1987) Autoantibodies in infectious mononucleosis have specificity for the glycine alanine repeating region of the Epstein-Barr nuclear antigen. J Exp Med 165:1026–1042
35. Birkenfeld P, Haratz N, Klein G (1990) Cross-reactivity between the EBNA-1 p107 peptide, collagen and keratin: implications for the pathogenesis of rheumatoid arthritis. Clin Immunol Immunopathol 54:14–25
36. Venables PJW (1989) Infection and rheumatoid arthritis. Curr Opinion Rheumatol 1:15–20
37. Fox R, Sportsman R, Rhodes G, Luka J, Pearson G, Vaughan JH (1986) Rheumatoid arthritis synovial membrane contains a 62000 molecular wt. protein that shares an antigenic epitope with the Epstein-Barr virus-encoded nuclear antigen. J Clin Invest 77:1539–1547
38. Garzelli C, Pacciardi A, Carmignani M, Conaldi PG, Basolo F, Falcone G (1989) A human monoclonal antibody isolated from a patient with infectious mononucleosis reactive with both self-antigens and Epstein-Barr nuclear antigen (EBNA). Immunol Lett 22:211
39. Inman RD, Chiu B, Hamilton NC (1987) Analysis of immune complexes in rheumatoid arthritis reveals cross-reactivity of viral capsid antigen and human IgG. J Immunol 138:407–412
40. Roudier J, Rhodes G, Petersen J, Vaughan JH, Carson DA (1988) The Epstein-Barr virus glycoprotein gp110, a molecular link between HLA DR4, HLA DR-1 and rheumatoid arthritis. Scand J Immunol 27:367–372
41. Rowley MJ, Williamson J, Mackay IR (1987) Evidence for local synthesis of antibodies to denatured collagen in the synovium in rheumatoid arthritis. Arthritis Rheum 12:1420–1426
42. Tarkowski A, Klareskog L, Carlsten H, Herberts P, Koopman W (1989) secretion of antibodies to types I and II by synovial tissue cells in patients with rheumatoid arthritis. Arthritis Rheum 2:1087–1092

Autoantibodies and Markers of Disease Activity

The Antiperinuclear Factor (APF)
and Antikeratin Antibodies (AKA)
in Rheumatoid Arthritis*

R. M. Hoet and W. J. van Venrooij

Department of Biochemistry, University of Nijmegen, P.O. Box 9101, NL 6500 HB Nijmegen, The Netherlands

Introduction

The diagnosis of rheumatoid arthritis (RA) is first of all based on clinical manifestations. Serological support for such a diagnosis is not very well established and it is based mainly on the presence of rheumatoid factors (RF). A positive RF test has a predictive value [1] and is related to disease with a more severe outcome [2]. However, RF is also present in other (autoimmune) diseases and in control sera from healthy persons [3]. Therefore, testing for a second RA-specific antibody would be very useful, and might even be necessary for the management of seronegative RA patients.

Three other antibody activities have been described as being specific for RA, all three directed against components of epithelial cells, namely: antibodies against the perinuclear factor in human buccal mucosa cells (APF), antibodies against keratin-like components in rat esophageal epithelium (AKA), and antibodies against intermediate filaments in cultured cells (AIFA). These three specificities are detectable only by the (indirect) immunofluorescence technique.

The antiperinuclear factor (APF) was originally described by Nienhuis and Mandema [4], who demonstrated its high specificity for RA. The antibodies, mostly of the IgG type, are directed against a protein component present in the 0.5–4 µm spherical keratohyalin granules [4–6] in the cytoplasm of human buccal mucosa cells and are found in 49%–91% of sera from RA patients [4–17]. A typical immunofluorescence staining pattern of a buccal mucosa cell from an APF-positive RA serum is shown in Fig. 1.

The so-called antikeratin antibodies (AKA) were first described by Young et al. [18] and can be found in 36%–59% of sera from RA patients. This antibody specificity also has been found to be specific for RA [6, 11, 14, 18–27]. A typical

* Part of the work described in this review was supported financially by "Het Nationaal Reumafonds" of The Netherlands.

Smolen, Kalden, Maini (Eds.)
Rheumatoid Arthritis
© Springer-Verlag Berlin Heidelberg 1992

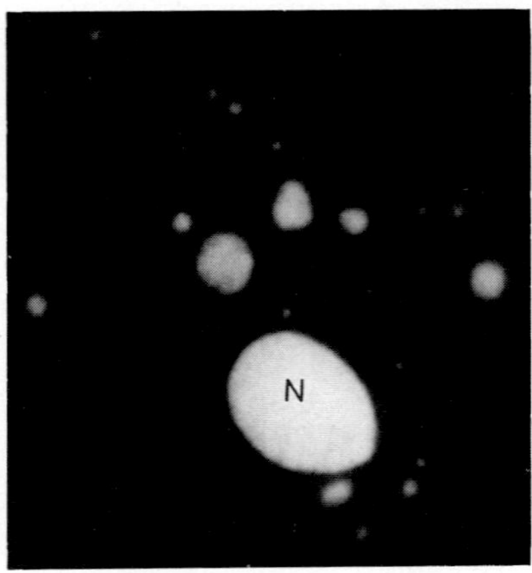

Fig. 1. Typical immunofluorescence staining pattern of a buccal mucosa cell with an APF-positive RA serum. The nucleus (*N*) is counter-stained with ethidium bromide

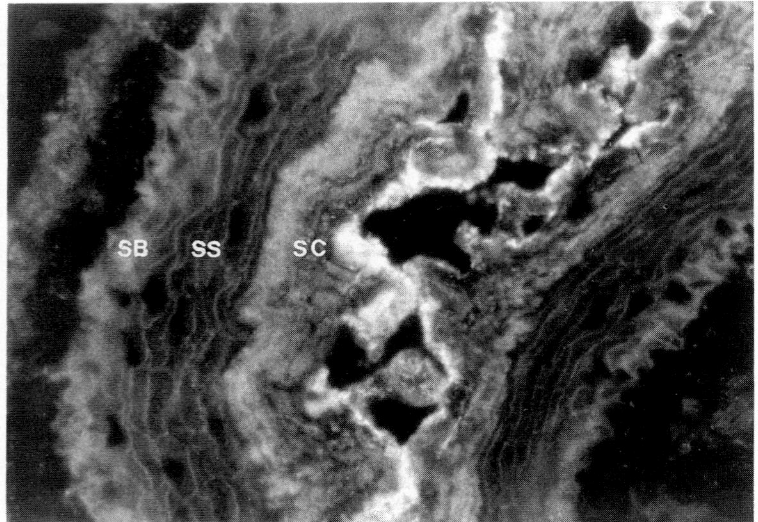

Fig. 2. Typical immunofluorescence staining pattern of an AKA-positive serum on a rat esophagus cryostat section. The laminar staining of the stratum corneum (*SC*) of rat esophagus is specific for RA. *SS*, stratum spinosum; *SB*, stratum basale; *SC*, stratum corneum

immunofluorescence staining pattern of AKA on a rat esophagus section is shown in Fig. 2.

AIFA in RA sera are believed to recognize the intermediate filament proteins vimentin and/or cytokeratin in cultured cells and are mostly of the IgM class [14, 28, 29]. Indeed, in 50%–80% of RA patients antibodies against vimentin [14, 27–31] and in 30%–40% anti-cytokeratin antibodies [14, 27, 28] have been found. Unfortunately, AIFA do not seem very specific for RA since they are also detectable after viral infections (65% of patients) [32] and in patients with infectious mononucleosis (92.5%) [14], systemic lupus erythematosus (30%–53%) [28, 33], Sjögren's syndrome (64%) [28], chronic active hepatitis (88%), primary biliary cirrhosis (93%), and alcoholic liver disease (50%–69%) [28], and even can be found in 14%–63% of sera from healthy individuals [14, 28, 34, 35].

Because of its low specificity, AIFA will not be discussed in this review further. Rather, we want to focus on APF and AKA, because these specificities are found only in very low incidence in normal human sera. Although they do not show an absolute specificity for RA (see below), their presence in RA sera is so frequent that one can use them as an additional serological marker for RA, especially when tests for RF are negative.

In the following paragraphs we will deal critically with the methods employed for the detection of APF and AKA and review the data on their specificity and sensitivity. We will discuss what is known about the biochemical characteristics of the antigens and their possible interrelationship.

The Antiperinuclear Factor

Detection of the APF

The Substrate

As substrate for the APF test buccal mucosa cells from so-called positive donors are used. Although the proportion of antigen-positive donors in a normal population is high (at least 70%–80%) [6, 36], most authors report that only a small percentage of the donors have sufficient antigen present in their buccal mucosa cells to allow easy detection of the APF. A low contamination with mouth flora is another consideration for the selection of a good donor [10–13, 16, 36].

Also the number of cells that carry the substrate for APF differs substantially among donors. The maximum number of positive cells one can find in a good donor cell preparation is about 60% (our unpublished data). The variations between donors are probably related to the site at which the antigenic granules are present in the buccal mucosa. The keratohyalin granules appear in the mucosa cells during the final stages of keratinization, i.e., in dying cells that are being degraded. In some individuals this site lies deep in the mucosa, in others it is more superficial (T. E. W. Feltkamp, personal communication), so it is quite possible that some people lose the epithelial cells containing the antigen more quickly than others.

Qualitative differences in antigen composition between donors have not been studied in depth, and the results obtained so far are somewhat contradictory. In our laboratory we tested buccal mucosa cells from seven donors using ten sera with different APF titers and found no evidence for more than one antigen. Sera that reacted strongly with cells from one donor reacted similarly with cells from other donors. Even so, sera that gave weak fluorescence with cells of one donor did the same with those of other donors. However, similar experiments were performed by others (F. de Keyser, E. M. Veys, P. Youinou and co-workers, unpublished data) who obtained opposite results; i.e., some sera reacted with the perinuclear factor from one donor but not with the granules from another donor and vice versa. It is clear that the possibility that more than one antigen is involved cannot be ruled out, and that the question of the complexity of the perinuclear factor can be solved only after isolation and biochemical characterization of the antigen.

The fact that the APF method is not widely used as a serological test for RA certainly has to do with the difficulty in obtaining good antigen preparations. Research efforts should therefore be directed at finding a more easily obtainable substrate. Although other substrates have been tested – e.g., human vaginal epithelial cells, human esophageal mucosa, and rabbit oral or esophageal mucosa – they were found to be less sensitive or less specific than the human buccal mucosa cells [5]. Other sources such as rat, cow, or pig oral mucosa did not contain the antigen [5].

Preparation of Buccal Mucosa Cells for Immunofluorescence

Buccal mucosa cells can be removed from the cheek of the donor with a small piece of foam plastic sponge (not too rigid and not too soft) after the teeth have been brushed and the mouth rinsed with water. The sponge is then squeezed and the cells are washed several times in a physiological buffer solution. Generally, about 10 µl cell suspension (about 1000 cells) is then spotted on a microscopic slide and air-dried. The cells are used without fixation because both acetone and methanol have a traumatic effect on the antigenicity of the perinuclear factor [4, 6]. Treatment of the buccal mucosa cells with 0.5% Triton-X100 increases the sensitivity of the APF test, probably because this treatment renders the cells more permeable to the antibodies and because it helps in reducing background staining by removing most soluble cellular proteins and residual bacterial contamination [6].

Serum Dilution and Second Antibody

Serum dilution seems a critical variable in the test protocol. In earlier studies undiluted sera were used [4], but at present mostly 1:5 diluted sera are used because of the higher sensitivity obtained [10, 11, 16]. Westgeest and co-workers [36, 37] found a positive APF result in 6% of 123 control blood donors and in 41% of 123 RA patients when undiluted sera were used. When the same sera were tested in a 1:10 dilution, 12% of the controls and 70% of RA patients showed a positive result. There was no difference in sensitivity between 1:10 or 1:5 diluted sera (A. M. Th. Boerbooms, personal communication). The sensitivity of the test thus increases and the specificity decreases when the serum is diluted. These findings are in accord with data in the literature (see Table 1), in that studies showing the lowest sensitivity used undiluted sera. The reasons why serum dilution is so critical are not well understood. A pH effect could be implicated, but another explanation could be that the high protein concentration in undiluted serum hampers the antibody-antigen recognition (prozone effect). The incubation time of the cells with the serum is usually 90 min at room temperature.

APF is mostly of the IgG class. Kataaha et al. [14] found IgG-APF activity in all 16 sera tested, although in four sera there was additional IgM and in three additional IgA activity. In most studies a total anti-Ig conjugate preparation has been used.

Criteria for Positivity and Reproducibility of the Test

Most workers have their own criteria for defining a positive test result. In most cases one considers one or a few cells showing the typical perinuclear staining on different granules (see Fig. 1) to be sufficient for a positive score. Others [38] consider a serum positive when 10% of the cells are stained.

In an interlaboratory assay five sera from RA patients were independently tested using the WHO reference RA serum (100 IU/ml) and a reference anti-Ig conjugate as standards. The sera contained APF activity ranging between 0 (control serum) and 400 IU/ml. The results showed that although all five laboratories involved used their own donors and their own criteria for positivity, the APF concentrations obtained were very comparable [56].

Specificity and Sensitivity of the APF

In Table 1 we have collected most data described in the literature on the frequency of appearance of APF. As noted above, undiluted sera show a lower sensitivity but higher specificity than diluted sera. However, one should mention the fact that the specificities were calculated from rather inhomogeneous cohorts of "healthy persons and other rheumatic diseases," which varied considerably between the various studies. Nevertheless, it is obvious that APF is very common among RA patients and that most authors, except Roques [9], find the APF to be specific for RA. It might not be surprising that the APF has also been found in synovial fluids of RA patients [4, 17]. Notwithstanding the obvious relationship between APF and RA, increased frequencies of APF in other autoimmune diseases have been described. These are summarized in Table 2.

Most authors have found increased APF frequencies in Sjögren's syndrome, even when no diagnostic association with RA was observed. Some authors found increased frequencies in systemic lupus erythematosus (SLE), systemic sclerosis (SSc), psoriasis, juvenile chronic arthritis, and infectious mononucleosis (IM). A subset of autoimmune thyroiditis (primary myxedema) patients have been found to be APF positive as well. Interestingly, Youinou and coworkers [45] found APF in sera from 40 of 79 (50.6%) patients with primary and in 21 of 36 (58.3%) patients with metastatic lung cancer. The conclusion from these data must be that although the APF is preferentially present in sera from RA patients, it can also be detected, though less frequently, in other (autoimmune) diseases. Therefore, the APF should be used only as an

Table 1. Percentages of sera positive for APF in RA patients, healthy controls, and other patients with rheumatic diseases, summarized from the literature

Reference	Number of positive sera/total			Sensitivity (%)	Specificity (%)	Serum dilution
	RA	Healthy controls	Other rheumatic diseases			
Nienhuis and Mandema [4]	51/105	4/431	1/84	48.6	99.0	Undiluted
Smit et al. [5]	77/97	4/96	–	79.4	95.8	1:5
Hoet et al. [6]	51/63	3/51	28/153	81.0	84.8	1:5
Visconti et al. [7]	29/37	–	3/148	78.4	98.0	Undiluted
Marmont et al. [8]	51/100	0/50	3/91	51.0	97.0	Undiluted
Roques [9]	91/165	16/66	9/48	55.2	78.1	Undiluted
Sondag-Tschroots et al. [10]	80/103	4/111	33/405	77.7	92.8	1:5
Johnson et al. [11]	82/102	8/60	4/57	80.4	89.7	1:5
	93/102[a]	12/60[a]	9/57[a]	91.2[a]	82.1[a]	
Cassani et al. [12]	74/90	7/100	25/218	82.2	89.9	1:10
Youinou et al. [13]	121/178	6/67[b]	19/138	68.0	86.9	1:5
		12/78[c]				
Kataaha et al. [14]	53/72	3/93	–	73.6	96.8	1:5
Westgeest et al. [15]	69/132	1/54	–	52.3	98.1	Undiluted
Janssens et al. [16]	110/127	–	11/262	86.6	95.8	1:5
Vivino and Maul [17]	44/75	5/50	36/100	58.7	72.7	1:5
Youinou et al.[d] [38]	76/100	3/108	28/398	76.0	93.9	1:5

[a] Also included are weak positive sera.
[b] <60 year
[c] >60 year
[d] Considers a serum positive when 10% of the cells are stained
–, Not tested

Table 2. Frequency of APF in other autoimmune diseases

Disease	Reference number											
	[4]	[8]	[10]	[39–41]	[12]	[14]	[16]	[44]	[17]	[6]	[42]	[38][c]
Ankylosing spondylitis	0/42		2/36		3/16		0/17					3/52
Psoriatic arthritis	0/5	0/5		4/11 41/72[a]	1/5		0/17					5/34
SLE	1/12	1/28	8/94	3/24	4/12		0/11	3/39	24/50	7/33		4/47
SSc	0/10		0/17		1/2		3/6		13/50	11/42		2/26
Infectious mononucleosis						1/40		28/55				
Primary Sjögren's syndrome	0/3	1/1	5/16	9/29 3/22[b]	1/2		0/1			10/34		3/42
Juvenile chronic arthritis					0/7		3/13					
Autoimmune thyroiditis			6/30								6/20[1] 0/20[2] 0/22[3]	

[a] Psoriasis without arthritis
[b] Secondary Sjögren's syndrome
[c] Values obtained considering sera positive when 10% of the buccal mucosa cells were stained
[1] Primary myxedema
[2] Graves' thyrotoxicosis
[3] Hashimoto's thyroiditis
SSc, Systemic sclerosis; SLE, systemic lupus erythematosus
Note: Only diseases with increased APF frequencies mentioned by at least two research groups are included.

Table 3. Correlation between the APF and RF in RA

Reference	RA sera (n)	APF(+)/RF(−) (%)	p value (χ^2-test)
Nienhuis and Mandema [4]	248	14	= 0.10
Hoet et al. [6]	63	6	< 0.50
Marmont et al. [8]	100	4	< 0.001
Sondag-Tschroots et al. [10]	103	11	< 0.001
Johnson et al. [11]	83	–	= 0.70
Cassani et al. [12]	90	13	< 0.001
Youinou et al. [13]	178	18	< 0.02
Westgeest et al. [15]	132	11	< 0.05
Janssens et al. [16]	127	9	< 0.02

–, Not specified

additional serological marker in cases where clinical features support the suspicion of a diagnosis of RA. Most important, the APF can be used as a serological indicator for RA in RF-negative sera.

Correlation Between the APF and RF

Youinou and co-workers were the first to suggest a possible relationship between RF and APF [41]. They purified RF by means of affinity chromatography and showed that the purified preparation still contained some APF activity. The possibility that the purified RF was contaminated with IgG-APF, however, could not be excluded. In a second type of experiment they treated APF-positive sera with aggregated IgG and subsequently observed decreased titers of APF, suggesting that with the removal of RF, part of the APF activity was removed as well. These results should be interpreted with care because in a serum containing both RF and APF, RF possibly amplifies the APF fluorescence by binding to the IgG-APF antibodies. When the RFs are removed a drop in APF titer might be the result. Another argument in favor of a possible relationship between APF and RF could be the fact that most APF-positive sera are found in the same patient groups in which IgG-RF is found, namely RA, psoriasis, and primary Sjögren's syndrome [41]. The APF titers are also significantly higher in RA patients when IgG-RF is present [41]. However, all these arguments are not sufficient to make acceptable the idea that APF is a special class of RF. In fact, the data in Table 3 show that there are quite a few patients who are APF positive and RF negative (ranging between 4% and 18%).

Correlation Between APF and Clinical Parameters

The question of whether there is a relation between APF and severity of disease or special clinical symptoms is still unsolved. In the early studies of Nienhuis and Mandema [4] a positive correlation between the presence of APF and the presence of subcutaneous nodules was indicated. Marmont et al. [8] reported a relation between APF and the stage of disease (a scale from I to IV calculated via clinical and laboratory parameters), and Youinou and co-workers [46] reported a correlation ($r = 0.51$, $P < 0.001$) between the actual activity of the disease and the APF titer. All these studies tried to find a relation between APF and disease activity – in fact, a very momentary impression of the disease. Westgeest and co-workers [15], instead of measuring disease activity, scored for disease severity and found that RF(−) APF(+) patients have a worse outcome of the disease than RF(−) APF(−) patients.

Recently, HLA-typing was carried out in 132 patients with RA divided into four groups; APF(+)/RF(+), APF(+)/RF(−), APF(−)/RF(+) and APF(−)/RF(−) [47]. The prevalence of HLA-DR4 was in all groups significantly higher than in a healthy control group, but no significant differences were found between the seropositive and the seronegative groups. Interestingly, in seronegative RA the HLA-DR4 was preferentially associated with the APF(+) group [47].

Attempts to Characterize the Perinuclear Factor

When Nienhuis and Mandema reported in 1964 [4] that antibodies in sera from RA patients reacted with granules in buccal mucosa cells, virtually nothing was known about the biochemical identity of these granules. The granules stain basophilic but seem not to contain RNA or DNA [4–6]. However, a recent report showed that granules containing the perinuclear factor have ultrastructural characteristics of aggregated rough endoplasmatic reticulum and exhibit histological features of nucleoproteins [17]. The antigenicity of the perinuclear factor is sensitive to trypsin, indicating that it is a protein [4, 6]. Smit and coworkers [5] were the first to show that the perinuclear factor is located in the so-called keratohyalin granules. This has recently been confirmed by immunoelectron-microscopic localization of the perinuclear factor [6]. The antigen-containing keratohyalin granules, also referred to as "single granules," have a shape and composition different from that of keratohyalin granules present in the granular layer of keratinized epithelium [48]. Smit et al. [5] tested a number of comparable epithelia from various species and detected the perinuclear factor also in vaginal epithelial cells of newborn babies and in human esophageal mucosa. They also detected an immunological reaction on sections from rabbit esophageal mucosa. but with lowered sensitivity and specificity. No reaction was found with rat, cow, and pig oral mucosa, although in rat oral mucosa many basophilic granules are present. The abundantly present keratohyalin granules of human foreskin (keratinized epithelium) do not show a reaction with RA sera, either [6]. These results thus demonstrate that the perinuclear factor is not necessarily organ or species specific, but it seems to be present in a particular type of squamous epithelium. Chemical treatments of the buccal mucosa cells showed that the perinuclear factor is a rather insoluble protein whose antigenicity is very sensitive to fixation [6]. Routine procedures used to prepare cytoskeletons (treatment with 0.5% Triton-X100) do not solubilize the perinuclear factor but remove the majority of background staining. As a result, the sensitivity of the APF detection is enhanced [6].

All epithelial cells are known to contain intermediate (keratin) filaments composed of a specific subset of cytokeratins. Using specific monoclonal antibodies directed against a variety of cytokeratins, as well as polyclonal anti-keratin antibodies and antibodies against other types of intermediate filament proteins, it was shown that keratohyalin granules in buccal mucosa cells do not contain detectable amounts of either cytokeratin, vimentin, or lamin [6]. The keratohyalin granules were stained only by antibodies against profilaggrin, a large 1000-kD protein which is a precursor of the 37-kD protein filaggrin [49]. This latter polypeptide is a keratin-associated protein present in most, if not all, keratinized epithelia [49]. Poly- and monoclonal antibodies against (pro)filaggrin show an exact co-localization of this protein with the perinuclear factor [6]. However, subsequent experiments indicated that (pro)filaggrin is not identical with the perinuclear factor, although immunoblotting of a buccal mucosa cell extract showed that some sera from RA patients do contain antibody against filaggrin [6]. These findings suggest that the perinuclear factor might be associated with profilaggrin in the keratohyalin granules of buccal mucosa cells, and that the perinuclear factor would be involved in the keratinization process of these cells as well.

Recently, we succeeded in culturing human buccal mucosa cells. Interestingly, the induced keratohyalin granules in these cultured cells did contain (pro)filaggrin, but there was no evidence for the presence of the perinuclear factor [50]. This finding can be explained in several ways. First, it could be that the absence of the perinuclear factor is a culturing phenomenon. Either the factor could be lost during culturing of the cells or the differentiation process of the keratinocytes in vitro cannot proceed far enough to produce the perinuclear factor. Second, it is possible that the perinuclear factor might be a protein coming from the outside (mouth flora) or is induced via infection of the buccal mucosa cells by a common virus such as Epstein-Barr virus (EBV). Support for such a hypothesis lies in the finding that 51% of patients with a recent EBV infection contain APF in their serum [44] and in the fact that squamous epithelial cells in vivo can be infected by EBV [51]. If this possibility is correct, however, one would expect all perinuclear factor "cheek cell donors" to contain antibody against EBV. This was tested with sera from positive cheek cell donors and seemed not to be the case [44, 52]. Monoclonal antibodies against EBV viral capsid antigen and early antigen (diffuse component) did not react, either, with keratohyalin granules of buccal mucosa cells from positive donors [6]. So, at the present our conclusion must be that the precise biochemical nature and complexity of the perinuclear factor are still a mystery.

Antikeratin Antibodies

Detection of Antikeratin Antibodies (AKA)

The Substrate

The detection of AKA by immunofluorescence was first reported by Young and co-workers [18]. In this study, and most subsequent ones, unfixed rat esophagus cryostat sections [4–5 µm) were used. Johnson et al. [11] found that the specificity and sensitivity of the test depends on the part of the esophagus that is used to prepare the cryosections. Low esophagus provided the best discrimination between RA and controls, and cardia of the stomach gave the highest incidence of staining in all groups (RA, other autoimmune diseases, and healthy controls). Nevertheless, in most studies the middle third of the esophagus has been used as substrate for the AKA test.

Serum Dilution and Second Antibody

A serum dilution of 1:10 is routinely used. Most AKA are of the IgG type and, according to Vincent and co-workers [26], only these IgG-AKA are specific for RA. Therefore, the use of an IgG-specific second antibody is recommended.

Table 4. Frequency of AKA in RA, other rheumatic diseases, and healthy controls

Reference	Number of positive sera/total sera			Sensitivity (%)	Specificity (%)
	RA	Healthy controls	Other rheumatic diseases		
Hoet et al. [6]	26/47	1/47	2/47	55.3	96.8
Johnson et al. [11]	52/102	0/60	2/47	51.0	97.4
Kataaha et al. [14]	39/72	0/93	–	54.2	100.0
Young et al. [18]	75/129	0/105	1/52	58.1	99.4
Scott et al. [19]	36/99	0/50	8/16	36.4	87.9
Ordeig and Guardia [20]	71/131	0/100	7/266	54.2	97.9
Hajiroussou et al. [21]	121/204	–	6/100	59.3	94.0
Kirnstein and Mathiesen [23]	73/156	2/80	0/61	46.8	98.6
Youinou et al. [24]	156/421	6/247	5/91	37.1	96.3
Meyer et al. [25]	67/122	1/30	3/75	54.9	96.2
Vincent et al.[a] [26]*	100/178	–	16/350	56.2	95.4
[b]	85/178	–	7/350	47.8	98.0
[c]	77/178	–	3/350	43.3	99.1
Quismorio et al. [27]	46/80	2/47	7/84	57.5	93.1

*, Results were computed according to three fluorescence intensity thresholds: a, 1.5; b, 1.75; c, 2.0
–, Not tested
Note: Most data in this table were taken from Vincent et al. [26]

Table 5. Frequency of AKA in other autoimmune diseases

Disease	Reference number									
	[18]	[22]	[27]	[19]	[24]	[20]	[11]	[23]	[26]	[54]
Ankylosing spondylitis	0/8		3/12		2/35	0/7	0/16	0/10	1/44	
SSc	1/7		4/20	8/16	2/26	1/18		0/2		
SLE	0/10		0/20		1/30	1/69	2/11	0/9	1/28	
Psoriasis	0/9		0/10[a]		5/69	0/12[a]	0/8	0/9[a]	0/40	0/14
Sjögren's syndrome		9/10			1/52			0/2		
Fibrosing alveolitis		5/5				1/2				

SSc, Systemic sclerosis; SLE, systemic lupus erythematosus
[a] Psoriatic arthritis
Note: Only diseases with increased AKA frequencies mentioned by at least two research groups are included.

Criteria for Positivity of the AKA Test

Most authors [11, 14, 19, 21, 26, 27, 53] regard only the distinct laminar staining of the keratin layer as a positive reaction (see Fig. 2), while others [20, 23] also consider a speckled fluorescence labeling pattern positive. Vincent et al. [26] studied different labeling patterns on the rat esophagus epithelium and found only the intense, linear laminated labeling restricted to the stratum corneum to be highly specific for RA (Fig. 2), while the weak, diffuse labeling of the three epithelial compartments (stratum basale, stratum spinosum, and stratum corneum) was not specific.

Specificity and Sensitivity of AKA

The frequency of occurrence of AKA in RA and control sera is shown in Table 4. All authors except Scott et al., who used acetone-fixed sections [19], find AKA to be very specific for RA but the sensitivity of detection to be relatively low. Vincent and co-workers [26] used a semi-quantitative immuno-fluorescence test and found, by changing the threshold of the intensity of the immunofluorescence staining from 1.5 to 1.75 to 2.0, that increased specificity for RA is accompanied by a decreased sensitivity.

AKA is considered specific for RA because this type of antibody is found in only rather low percentage in healthy controls and in other (autoimmune) diseases (see Table 5). Only in SSc did most authors find increased frequencies of AKA, as was true for the APF. In patients with primary myxedema, AKA is also more frequently present [24]. As expected, AKA can also be found in the synovial fluid of about 50% of RA patients [24, 27].

Correlation Between AKA and RF

A number of workers investigated the possible relation between AKA and RF. The results, summarized in Table 6, show that AKA, as was the case for APF, quite often occur in RF-negative sera. All studies claim 5% level correlations between AKA and RF. Nevertheless, a number of RA patients (roughly 10%) are seronegative but AKA positive, indicating that AKA and RF are different antibody specificities. Furthermore, Young et al. [18] have demonstrated that when RF activity of an RA serum was abolished by absorption with aggregated gammaglobulin the AKA activity was retained, implicating that the antigen for AKA is not related to RF. Therefore, it can be used as an additional serological marker for RA, in particular with RF-negative patients.

Correlation Between AKA, Clinical Data and Serum Variables

A number of clinical and serological parameters have been included in studies of AKA. Correlations between AKA, clinical data, and serum variables are

Table 6. Correlation between the AKA and RF in RA

Reference	RA sera (*n*)	RF(−)/AKA(+) (%)	*P*-value (χ^2-test)
Johnson et al. [11]	83	13.3	< 0.02
Youinou et al. [13]	178	–	< 0.001
Young et al. [18]	129	6.2	< 0.02
Scott et al. [19]	99	14.1	< 0.05
Ordeig and Guardia [20]	131	7.6	< 0.02
Hajiroussou et al. [21]	204	2.5	< 0.001
Mallya et al. [22]	98	–	< 0.001
Kirnstein and Mathiesen [23]	156	10.9	< 0.02
Vincent et al. [26]	350	6.0	< 0.001
Miossec et al. [53]	96	13.5	< 0.001

–, Not specified

summarized in Table 7. AKA seems not to be associated with sex or age, but it can be correlated with increased erythrocyte sedimentation rate, increased levels of C-reactive protein, and levels of soluble immune complexes. The association of AKA with clinical data such as functional indexes and subcutaneous nodules suggests that IgG-AKA are probably associated with the most severe or active forms of RA. A similar association was found between APF and disease severity [15]. The frequency of AKA in RA patients both negative and positive for HLA-DR4 was about the same [27]. Disease duration is probably not related to the incidence of AKA. This may indicate that AKA appear at the beginning of, or may even precede, the disease and suggests a predictive character of AKA that might be useful for an early diagnosis of RA [20]. It is obvious that more longitudinal studies are needed to sustain such a conclusion.

Attempts to Characterize the Antigen

Since the report of Young et al. [18], antibodies associated with RA that react with rat esophagus stratum corneum have always been referred to as antikeratin antibodies, partly because of the typical immunofluorescence labeling pattern, but also because keratins are the major protein components in this epithelial compartment. AKA seems not to be restricted to rat esophagus tissue but can also be found in the keratogenous zone of human hair follicles and to a lesser extent in mouse and monkey esophageal epithelia and human skin [18]. According to Yound and co-workers [18], the antigen recognized by AKA is related to fully differentiated keratin but this claim has never been substantiated by sound experimental data. In fact, other investigators have showed convincingly that IgG and IgM antibodies directed against epidermal cytokeratin polypeptides are not specific for RA and, for example, can be detected in most

Table 7. Relation between AKA, clinical data, and serum variables in rheumatoid arthritis

	Reference number												
	[11]	[19]	[53]	[22]	[27]	[20]	[14]	[24]	[21]	[25]	[23]	[26]	[6]
Sex (% men)	–	–	–	–	–	NS	–	–	++	NS	NS	NS	–
Age	–	–	–	–	–	+	–	–	NS	+	NS	NS	–
Disease duration	–	–	NS	–	–	NS	–	–	NS	NS	NS	NS	–
Functional indexes	–	NS	–	+	–	+	–	–	++	++	–	–	–
Subcutaneous nodules	–	NS	–	+++	–	+	–	+	++	NS	NS	+	–
Erythrocyte sedimentation rate	–	NS	+	+++	–	–	–	–	–	+++	NS	+	–
C-reactive protein	–	NS	–	+++	–	–	–	–	+++	–	–	+++	–
IgM rheumatoid factor	+	+	+++	+++	–	++	–	–	+	+	+	+++	–
Antinuclear antibodies	–	NS	–	+	NS	+	–	–	+	NS	–	NS	–
Soluble immune complexes	+++	–	–	–	–	–	–	–	–	–	–	+++	–
Antiperinuclear factor	+	–	+	–	–	–	NS	–	–	–	–	–	+

Significance of the tests is given as +, $P < 0.05$; ++, $P < 0.01$; +++, $P < 0.001$; NS, non-significant; –, not tested.
Note: only variables studied by at least two research groups are included. Most data in this table were taken from Vincent et al. [26]

normal human sera [55]. Other arguments against keratin as being the antigen are the studies of Quismorio and co-workers [27] who showed that the reaction of AKA against the keratin layer of rat esophagus could not be blocked by rabbit antibody against human keratin, and of Youinou et al. [24] who reported that a rabbit antihuman keratin serum only bound to the basal layer of rat esophagus. Monoclonal antibodies directed against keratin 4 and 13 did show a similar staining pattern as AKA positive RA sera [6], but immunoblotting of rat esophagus extracts with AKA positive and negative RA sera could not confirm that these keratins are the antigen (our unpublished results). The stratum corneum of the squamous epithelium of rat esophagus, however, contains besides keratin polypeptides a wide variety of other potentially antigenic molecules. One of them is profilaggrin, which, as we have discussed above, co-localizes with the perinuclear factor. Immunofluorescence studies with rabbit polyclonal antibodies against profilaggrin on rat esophagus demonstrated only a reaction with the stratum spinosum, a less differentiated layer or rat esophagus (our unpublished results).

Considering all the data that are available one must conclude that the name "antikeratin antibodies" is a most unfortunate choice. Vincent and co-workers [26] suggested "anti-stratum corneum antibodies" instead, but also this name seems inappropriate because of the lack of a specific reactivity of RA sera with stratum corneum of most (keratinized) tissues. It might be best to choose a more "to the point" name for which we want to propose "anti-rat esophagus antibodies" ("AREA").

Correlation between APF and AKA

There are two arguments supporting the idea that APF and AKA could be directed to immunologically related antigen(s). First of all, the antigens are localized in similar types of squamous epithelium. Further evidence for this comes from Smit and coworkers [5] who also found an "APF-like" reaction with human and rabbit esophagus superficial cells. Secondly, in our experience most AKA positive sera are also APF positive [6]. The reverse is not true, because the APF test is more sensitive than the AKA test. The positive correlation between APF and AKA is further demonstrated by the data in Table 8.

Possible Pathogenic Role of APF and AKA

Not much is known about the possible pathogenic role of APF and AKA in RA. Kataaha et al. [14] speculate that an infectious agent with an epithelial portal of entry confers enhanced immunogenicity on certain components of these

Table 8. Correlation between APF and AKA in sera from RA patients

Reference	Patients (n)	P-value (χ^2-test)
Hoet et al. [6]	63	< 0.02
Johnson et al. [11]	83	< 0.02
Youinou et al. [13]	178	< 0.001
Kataaha et al. [14]	72	$= 0.086$
Miossec et al. [53]	96	< 0.001

epithelial cells, and that this in turn may lead to production of the triad of autoantibodies AIFA, APF, and AKA.

Westgeest et al. [44] suggested that APF in RA patients could be a consequence of recurrent exposure of these patients to EBV, and if the antibody is really virus elicited, it probably cross-reacts with epitopes of human cell constituents. Mallya et al. [22] speculate that the presence of AKA could be explained by an as yet unidentified structural alteration of keratin in RA and Quismorio et al. [27] see a role for AKA in forming soluble immune complexes that participate in the pathogenesis of synovial inflammation, much like the proposed role of RF. All these hypotheses are very interesting, but they obviously need experimental support, which at present is not available.

The Future of AKA and APF as Serological Indicators for RA

Both APF and AKA occur rather specifically in sera from patients with RA. From the data presented above it is clear that the more sensitive test (APF) is also less specific. However, there are rather strong arguments for the assumption that in both tests the antigens that are recognized might be immunologically related. The most commonly used serological test for RA is the detection of RF. The main reason for this probably is not its specificity, which is not better than that of APF or AKA, but the fact that the test is simple and commercially available. Biochemical identification and/or purification of both the antigen for the antiperinuclear factor and "antikeratin antibodies" (AKA or AREA) is therefore needed. Until then, however, buccal mucosa cells or esophageal cryosections for the detection of APF and AKA, respectively, are useful as an additional serological marker for rheumatoid arthritis, in particular in cases where the RF is absent.

Acknowledgements. Part of this material was collected during a workshop on the APF organized in June 1989 by Prof. E. M. Veys and Dr. F. De Keyser (Ghent, Belgium). We wish to thank our colleagues T. E. W. Feltkamp (Amsterdam), P. Youinou (Brest), E. M. Veys and F. De Keyser (Ghent), and A. M. Th. Boerbooms (Nijmegen) for their suggestions and critical comments.

References

1. Valkenburg HA, Ball J, Burch TA et al. (1966) Rheumatoid factors in a rural population. Ann Rheum Dis 25:497–508
2. Kellgren JH, O'Brien WH (1962) On the natural history of rheumatoid arthritis in relation to sheep cell agglutination test (SCAT). Arthritis Rheum 5:115
3. Waller MV, Toone EC, Vaughan E (1964) Study of rheumatoid factor in a normal population. Arthritis Rheum 7:513
4. Nienhuis RLF, Mandema E (1964) A new serum factor in patients with rheumatoid arthritis. The antiperinuclear factor. Ann Rheum Dis 23:302–305
5. Smit JW, Sondag-Tschroots IRJM, Aaij C, Feltkamp TEW, Feltkamp-Vroom TM (1980) The antiperinuclear factor. II. A light-microscopical and immunofluorescence study on the antigenic substrate. Ann Rheum Dis 39:381–386
6. Hoet RM, Arends M, Boerbooms AMTh, van Venrooij WJ (1991) The antiperinuclear factor, a marker autoantibody for rheumatoid arthritis. Co-localization of the perinuclear factor and profilaggrin. Ann Rheum Dis 50:611–619
7. Visconti A, Cava L, Fontana G (1964) Ricerca del fattore antiperinucleare (APF) nell'artrite reumatoide ed in altre malattie. Osp Magg 59:1357
8. Marmont AM, Damasio EE, Bertorello C, Rossi F (1967) Studies on the antiperinuclear factor. Arthritis Rheum 10:117–128
9. Roques MT (1969) Les anticorps dits périnucléaires. Thesis, Paris
10. Sondag-Tschroots IRJM, Aaij C, Smit JW, Feltkamp TEW (1979) The antiperinuclear factor. 1. The diagnostic significance of the antiperinuclear factor for rheumatoid arthritis. Ann Rheum Dis 38:248–251
11. Johnson GD, Carvalho A, Holborow EJ, Goddard DH, Russel G (1981) Antiperinuclear factor and antikeratin antibodies in rheumatoid arthritis. Ann Rheum Dis 40:263–266
12. Cassani F, Ferri S, Bianchi FB, Zauli D, Pisi E (1983) Antiperinuclear factor in an Italian series of patients with rheumatoid arthritis. Ric Clin Lab 13:347–352
13. Youinou P, Le Goff P, Miossec P (1983) Untersuchungen zur Beziehung zwischen antiperinucleären Faktoren, Anti-keratin-antikörpern und dem agglutinierenden und nicht agglutinierenden Rheumafactor bei der chronischen Polyarthritis. Z. Rheumatol 42:36–39
14. Kataaha PK, Mortazavi-Milani SM, Russel G, Holborow EJ (1985) Anti-intermediate filament antibodies, antikeratin antibody, and antiperinuclear factor in rheumatoid arthritis and infectious mononucleosis. Ann Rheum Dis 44:446–449
15. Westgeest AA, Boerbooms AMTh, Jongmans M, Vandenbroucke JP, Vierwinden G, van de Putte LBA (1987) Antiperinuclear factor: indicator of more severe disease in seronegative rheumatoid arthritis. J Rheumatol 14:893–897
16. Janssens X, Veys EM, Verbruggen G, Declercq L (1988) The diagnostic significance of the antiperinuclear factor for rheumatoid arthritis. J Rheumatol 15:1346–1350
17. Vivino FB, Maul GG (1990) Histologic and electron microscopic characterization of the antiperinuclear factor antigen. Arthritis Rheum 33:960–969
18. Young BJJ, Mallya RK, Leslie RDG, Clark CJM, Hamblin TJ (1979) Antikeratin antibodies in rheumatoid arthritis. Br Med J 2:97–99
19. Scott DL, Delamere JP, Jones LJ, Walton KW (1981) Significance of laminar antikeratin antibodies to rat oesophagus in rheumatoid arthritis. Ann Rheum Dis 40:267–271
20. Ordeig J, Guardia J (1984) Diagnostic value of antikeratin antibodies in rheumatoid arthritis. J Rheumatol 11:602–604
21. Hajiroussou VJ, Skingle J, Gillett AP, Webley M (1985) Significance of antikeratin antibodies in rheumatoid arthritis. J Rheumatol 12:57–59
22. Mallya RK, Young BJJ, Pepys MB, Hamblin TJ, Mace BEW, Hamilton EBD (1983) Antikeratin antibodies in rheumatoid arthritis: frequency and correlation with other features of the disease. Clin Exp Immunol 51:17–20
23. Kirnstein H, Mathiesen FK (1987) Antikeratin antibodies in rheumatoid arthritis. Scand J Rheumatology 16:331–337

24. Youinou P, Le Goff P, Colaco CB, Thivolet J, Tater D, Viac J, Shipley M (1985) Antikeratin antibodies in serum and synovial fluid show specificity for rheumatoid arthritis in a study of connective tissue diseases. Ann Rheum Dis 44:450–454
25. Meyer O, Fabregas D, Cyna L, Ryckewaert A (1986) Les anticorps antikératine. Un marqueur des polyarthrites rhumatoïdes évolutives. Rev Rhum Mal Osteoartic 53:601–605
26. Vincent C, Serre G, Lapeyre F, Fournié B, Ayrolles C, Fournié A, Soleilhavoup J-P (1989) High diagnostic value in rheumatoid arthritis of antibodies to the stratum corneum of rat oesophagus epithelium, so-called antikeratin antibodies. Ann Rheum Dis 48:712–722
27. Quismorio PF, Kaufman RL, Beardmore T, Mongan ES (1983) Reactivity of serum antibodies to the keratin layer of rat esophagus in patients with rheumatoid arthritis. Arthritis Rheum 4:494–499
28. Kurki P, Helve T, Virtanen I (1983) Antibodies to cytoplasmic intermediate filaments in rheumatic diseases. J Rheumatol 10:558–562
29. Senecal JL, Rothfield NF, Oliver JM (1982) Immunoglobulin M autoantibody to vimentin intermediate filaments. J Clin Invest 69:716–721
30. Kurki P, Virtanen I (1984) The detection of human antibodies against cytoskeletal components. J Immunol Methods 67:209–223
31. Osung OA, Chandra M, Holborow EJ (1982) Intermediate filaments in synovial lining cells in rheumatoid arthritis and other arthritides are of the vimentin type. Ann Rheum Dis 41:74–77
32. Toh BH, Sotelo YJ, Osung O, Holborow EJ, Kanakoudi F, Small JV (1979) Viral infections and IgM autoantibodies to cytoplasmic intermediate filaments. Clin Exp Immunol 37:76–82
33. Alcover A, Molano J, Renart J, Gil-Aguado A, Nieto A, Avila J (1984) Antibodies to vimentin intermediate filaments in sera from patients with systemic lupus erythematosus. Arthritis Rheum 8:922–928
34. Osung OA, Chandra M, Holborow EJ (1982) Antibody to intermediate filaments of the cytoskeleton in rheumatoid arthritis. Ann Rheum Dis 41:69–73
35. Senecal JL, Olivier JM, Rothfield N (1985) Anticytoskeletal autoantibodies in the connective tissue diseases. Arthritis Rheum 28:889–895
36. Westgeest AAA (1988) Autoantibodies in rheumatic diseases, Chap 7. Rheumatoid arthritis and autoantibodies: a review of the literature on antinuclear antibody and antiperinuclear factor. Thesis, University of Nijmegen
37. Westgeest AAA, Boerbooms AMTh, van de Putte LBA (1990) The influence of serum dilution on findings of antiperinuclear factor prevalence in rheumatoid arthritis. Arthritis Rheum 33:759–760
38. Youinou P, Le Goff P, Dumay A, Lelong A, Fauquert P, Jouquan J (1990) The antiperinuclear factor. I. Clinical and serologic associations. Clin Exp Rheum 8:1–6
39. Youinou P, Pennec P, Le Goff P (1984) Antiperinuclear factor in Sjögren's syndrome in the presence or absence of rheumatoid arthritis. Clin Exp Rheumatol 2:5–9
40. Youinou P, Massé R, Peu-Duvallon P, Le Roux P, Grulier A, Miossec P, Dorval J-C, Lizan G, Férec C, Le Goff P (1982) Anticorps antipérinucléaires dans le psoriasis. Ann Dermatol Venereol 109:359–364
41. Youinou P, Le Goff P, Casburn-Budd R, Ferec C, Pennec Y (1984) Evidence for relationships between antiperinuclear and IgG rheumatoid factor. Rheumatol Int 4:111–114
42. Scherbaum WA, Youinou P, Le Goff P, Bottazzo GF (1984) Anti-perinuclear and rheumatoid factor in different forms of autoimmune thyroid disease. Clin Exp Immunol 55:516–518
43. Youinou P, Le Goff P, Miossec P, L'Hostis D, Pennec Y, Schwarzberg C, Ferrec C (1983) Intérêt des anticorps anti-périnucléaires dans le diagnostic et le pronostic de la polyarthrite rhumatoïde. Rev Rhum Mal Osteoartic 50:441–446
44. Westgeest AAA, van Loon AM, van der Logt JTM, van de Putte LBA, Boerbooms AMTh (1989) Antiperinuclear factor, a rheumatoid arthritis specific autoantibody: its relation to Epstein-Barr virus. J Rheumatol 16:626–630

45. Youinou P, Zabba C, Eveillaud C, Dewitte JD, Kerbourc'h JF, Ferec C, Clavier J (1984) Antiperinuclear activity in lung carcinoma patients. Cancer Immunol Immunother 2:80–81
46. Youinou P, Miossec P, Pennec Y, Boles JM, Le Goff P, Le Menn G (1983) Anticorps anti-périnucléaires et anti-kératine au cours des maladies du foie. Sem Hop Paris 59:589–592
47. Boerbooms AMTh, Westgeest AAA, Reekers P, van de Putte LBA (1990) Immunogenetic heterogeneity of seronegative rheumatoid arthritis and the perinuclear factor. Ann Rheum Dis 49:15–17
48. Holbrook KA (1989) Biologic structure and function: perspectives on morphologic approaches to the study of the granular layer keratinocyte. J Invest Dermatol 4S:84S–104S
49. Dale BA, Holbrook KA, Kimball JR, Hoff M, Sun T-T (1985) Expression of epidermal keratins and filaggrin during fetal skin development. J Cell Biol 101:1257–1269
50. Hoet RM, Voorsmit R, van Venrooij WJ (1991) Keratohyalin granules of cultured buccal mucosa cells do not contain the perinuclear factor. Clin Exp Immul 84:59–65
51. Allday MJ, Crawford DH (1988) Role of epithelium in EBV persistence and pathogenesis of B-cell tumours. Lancet I:855–857
52. Youinou P, Seigneurin JM, Le Goff P, Dumay A, Vicariot M Lelong A (1990) The antiperinuclear factor. II. Variability of the perinuclear antigen. Clin Exp Rheumatol 8:1–5
53. Miossec P, Youinou P, Le Goff P, Moineau MP (1982) Clinical relevance of antikeratin antibodies in rheumatoid arthritis. Clin Rheumatol 1:185–189
54. Cooper C, Cotton DWK, Jones SK, Cawley MID, Young BJJ (1986) Antikeratin antibody in rheumatoid and psoriatic arthritis. Ann Rheum Dis 145:349–350
55. Serre G, Vincent C, Viraben R, Soleilhavoup J-P (1985) Autoantibodies to keratins in normal huma sera, systemic lupus erythematosus, rheumatoid arthritis and psoriasis. Eur J Clin Invest 115:A36
56. Feltkamp TEW, Boerbooms AMTh, De Keyser F, Dumais M, Hoet RM, van Venrooij WJ, Verbruggen G, Veys EM, Youinou P (1990) Antiperinuclear factor – standardization program. Clin Rheumatol 9:112–113

Anti-RA 33: A New Antinuclear Antibody in Rheumatoid Arthritis*

W. Hassfeld, G. Steiner, W. Graninger, and J. S. Smolen

Second Department of Medicine, Center for Rheumatic Diseases, Lainz Hospital, and L. Boltzmann Institute for Rheumatology and Balneology, Vienna, Austria

Introduction

Systemic rheumatic diseases are commonly associated with autoantibodies to cell components, especially to nuclear antigens (ANA) [1–3]. Subspecificities of these antibodies often constitute marker antibodies for particular disorders and are therefore useful for diagnostic purposes. Thus several disease-specific autoantibodies are known, such as anti-Scl70 in progressive systemic sclerosis or anti-Jo1 in polymyositis [1–5]. Moreover, antibodies to Sm, a nuclear ribonucleoprotein, which occur almost exclusively in patients with systemic lupus erythematosus (SLE), have even been included among the immunological abnormalities listed in the revised criteria for the classification of SLE [6]. In addition, several antibody subsets were known to be correlated with clinical features, e.g. anti-Jo1, which is commonly associated with pulmonary fibrosis in polymyositis, or anti-Ro/SSA, which is associated with the neonatal lupus syndrome [7–9].

The diagnosis of rheumatoid arthritis (RA), the most common inflammatory rheumatic condition, is based primarily upon clinical criteria [10, 11]. In early stages these criteria are often not fulfilled, and appropriate therapeutic measures are therefore not instituted. Current serologic testing may be of only limited value, even though the positivity of rheumatoid factor (RF) represents one of the classification criteria for RA [10–13]. However, RF is often negative in RA, particularly in early stages; furthermore, RF is not pathognomonic and can be found in patients with many other rheumatic disorders, especially SLE and primary Sjögren's syndrome, as well as in many chronic inflammatory conditions, and even in healthy individuals, particularly with increasing age [14, 15].

In order to counteract these problems, several attempts have been made to find new serologic parameters for RA with disease specificity similar to those

* This study was supported by grants from the Fonds zur Förderung der wissenschaftlichen Forschung and the Medizinisch-Wissenschaftlicher Fonds des Bürgermeisters der Bundeshauptstadt Wien.

Smolen, Kalden, Maini (Eds.)
Rheumatoid Arthritis
© Springer-Verlag Berlin Heidelberg 1992

found in the other systemic rheumatic diseases mentioned above. With this aim in mind, sera from patients with classic or definite RA were investigated for the occurrence of autoantibodies to potentially new antigens.

Demonstration of Anti-RA 33 by Immunoblot

Using soluble nuclear extracts from HeLa cells, immunoblot analysis revealed reactivities of RA sera with one band which was particularly prominent and common to many of the sera tested [16] (Fig. 1). This band corresponded to an antigen of 33 kD, which was shown to be resistant to repeated cycles of freezing and thawing, to heat treatment (5 min at 96°C, 30 min at 56°C), to acid and alkali treatment (pH 2–pH 9), and to DNase or RNase digestion. The only treatment that eliminated the reactivity was proteinase-K digestion. Thus, the 33-kD antigen appeared to be of proteinaceous nature.

To evaluate whether the 33-kD protein was related to other known nuclear antigens comparative immunoblot analyses were performed, using sera specific for particular ANA subsets.

Antibodies to the newly described antigen were not associated with antibodies against Sm, nRNP, Scl70, Ro/SSA, and La/SSB or other autoantibodies found in sera from patients with connective tissue diseases such as anti-Jo1, anti-Ku, anti-Pm/Scl, anti-PCNA, and anti-centromere [5, 17–20]. There was also no correlation with antibodies to collagen, perinuclear factor, and histones, which have frequently been found in RA sera [21–24]. As was evident from the lack of relationship to previously described antigens, the 33-kD protein appeared to be a new nuclear antigen and was therefore termed RA 33.

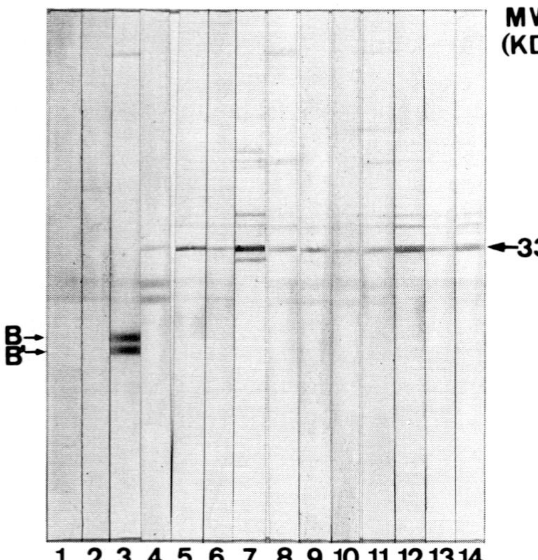

Fig. 1. Immunoblot analysis of a nuclear extract, using serum from a healthy control *(lane 1),* no serum (control; *lane 2*), anti-B/B'-positive serum from a patient with SLE *(lane 3),* and sera from patients with rheumatoid arthritis *(lanes 4–14).* A 33-kD band can be seen in lanes 4–14, which is not present in lanes 1–3. Autoantibodies were detected by the use of alkaline phosphatase-conjugated anti-human IgG (Fc)

Lack of Cross-reactivity with Other Autoantibodies Commonly Found in RA

Further studies showed that antibodies against RA 33 were not correlated with the presence or absence of rheumatoid factor. To exclude a possible cross-reactivity of RF with antigenic determinants in the nuclear extracts [24]. RF- and anti-RA 33-positive sera wee absorbed by passage over IgG affinity columns. Using immunoblot analysis the unbound, RF-depleted serum fraction retained the reactivity against RA 33, whereas the RF-containing fraction was anti-RA 33 negative (Fig. 2). In view of the commonly found reactivity of RA sera with EBV-encoded antigens, several anti-RA 33-positive and -negative sera were investigated for the presence of cross-reacting antibodies [25, 26]. Using both HeLa and Raji (EBV-infected cell line) nuclear extracts no discernable correlation (i.e., with antibodies to rheumatoid arthritis nuclear antigen) could be found. Moreover, sera from four patients with acute EBV infection drawn in the course of EBV infection were all anti-RA 33 negative.

Frequency of Anti-RA 33

As shown in Table 1, antibodies to RA 33 were detected in 51 of the 141 RA sera (36%) but in only two of various controls ($n = 311$), including sera from patients with connective tissue disorders and other joint diseases. The only non-RA sera

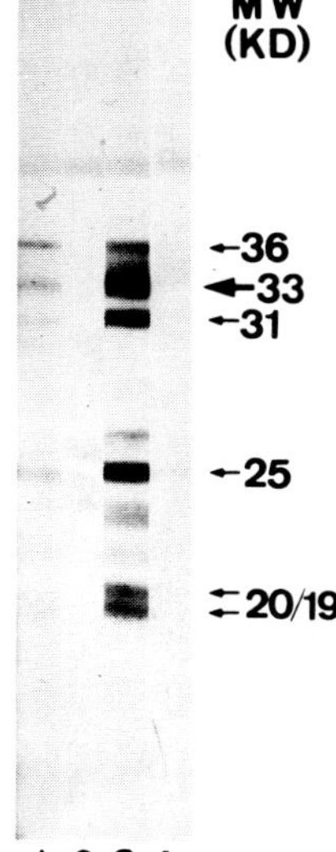

Fig. 2. Immunoblot demonstrating lack of reactivity of rheumatoid factor (RF) with RA 33. RF was absorbed by passing the sera over an IgG-affinity column; subsequently, bound RF was eluted with 0.2 *M* glycine-buffer, pH 2.5. *Lanes 1 and 3,* RF-depleted sera (unbound fraction); *lanes 2 and 4,* RF (-bound) fraction of the same sera. Note that in lane 1, and particularly in lane 3, a number of bands in addition to RA 33 are visible; these are described in greater detail in the text and in Fig. 3

Table 1. Frequencies of autoantibodies to RA 33 in sera of patients with rheumatoid arthritis and in various control sera

Patients	n	Anti-RA 33 positive
Rheumatoid arthritis	141	51 (36%)
Systemic lupus erythematosus	63	1
Other connective tissue diseases	38	0
Reactive arthritis	51	1
Ankylosing spondylitis	17	0
Psoriatic arthropathy	16	0
Osteoarthrosis	42	0
Liver cirrhosis	11	0
Crohn's disease	7	0
Allergy	14	0
EBV infections (4 patients, 12 sera)	12	0
Healthy controls	40	0
All controls	311	2

positive for anti-RA 33 were from a patient with SLE and another one with presumed reactive arthritis. Furthermore, anti-RA 33 was also found in patients with early RA.

To analyze whether anti-RA 33 could be demonstrated in synovial fluids, six paired samples of sera and synovial fluids were investigated by immunoblotting. Anti-RA 33 was found in three pairs of sera and synovial fluids. Furthermore, in both serum and synovial fluid anti-RA 33 was demonstrable not only when an anti-human IgG second antibody was used, but also when IgM was examined, demonstrating that anti-RA 33 was of both IgG and IgM isotype.

Correlation with Clinical Features

The presence of antibodies to RA 33 did not appear to be correlated with patient's age, with disease duration, or with disease stage, according to Steinbocker [27]; there was also no correlation between the occurrence of anti-RA 33 and remission-inducing drug therapy. However, the frequency of anti-RA 33 was found to be decreased in patients with long-term corticosteroid therapy (i.e., longer than 1 year and more than 6 mg methylprednisolone/day; Table 2, B). Furthermore, RA patients with vasculitis were observed to have a higher incidence of anti-RA 33 (Table 2).

Table 2. Correlation of anti-RA 33 in 95 patients with rheumatoid arthritis with (a) vasculitis and (b) long-term corticosteroid therapy

	A: Vasculitis		B: Long-term steroids	
	+	−	+	−
RA 33 +	8	26	1	33
RA 33 −	3	58	13	48
Chi square (Yates' corr.)	$p < 0.02$		$p < 0.05$	

Comparison of Nuclear Extracts

Further investigations revealed reasons for the detection of anti-RA 33 in this study but not in previous studies. Apparently, it was of major importance to use nuclear extracts prepared by other than by the commonly used methods. Thus, for example, nuclear extracts prepared according to Hartmuth and Barta [28] contained more protein in the molecular weight region between 30 and 40 kD, where RA 33 is located, than extracts prepared conventionally [29]. Although RA 33 could be detected in extracts prepared by other methods or even in several commercially available preparations, only a few sera with high anti-RA 33 titers were found to be reactive under such conditions.

Reactivity with RA 33 is Commonly Associated with Autoantibodies to Other New Nuclear Antigens

Further immunoblot studies revealed reactivities of RA sera not only with RA 33, but also with additional nuclear antigens in the molecular weight regions of 36, 31, 25 and 20 kD (Fig. 3) [30]. Similar to anti-RA 33, antibodies against these antigens were found almost exclusively in RA sera and not in sera from patients with various other autoimmune diseases. For unknown reasons, these reactivities were not observed with all extracts prepared and were particularly common when frozen cells were used for extraction. Similar to RA 33, the only treatment that eliminated the reactivity with the other nuclear antigens was proteinase digestion, indicating that these antigens were proteins. When 25 selected RA sera were analyzed for their patterns of reactivity with RA 33 and the additional antigens, different sera had different reactivities, in both qualitative and quantitative terms. As shown in Table 3, in terms of frequency, antibodies to RA 33 and to the 36-kD protein were the predominant reactivities. Occassionally, however, RA sera were seen with antibodies to the 36-kD anti-

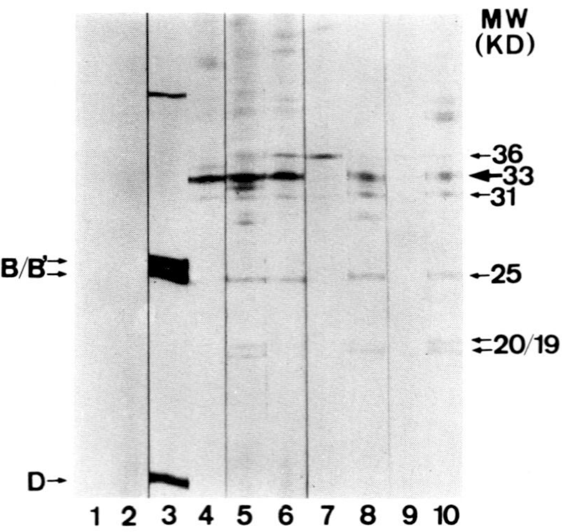

Fig. 3. Immunoblot analysis of a nuclear extract containing RA 33 and other antigens frequently reacting with RA sera. *Lane 1,* Healthy control; *lane 2,* no serum; *lane 3,* anti-Sm serum from an SLE patient; *lanes 4–10,* sera from RA patients. Reactivities directed against RA 33 were detected in sera 4–6, 8, and 10; sera 5, 6, 8, and 10 contained additional reactivities directed against antigens with estimated molecular weights of 36, 31, 25, and 20/19 kD; serum 7 reacted only with the 36-kD antigen. (see Fig. 2 for additional details of the band patterns)

Table 3. Patterns of autoantibodies to RA 33 and/or other nuclear antigens in 25 selected RA sera (determined semiquantitatively by immunoblotting)

Serum	36 kD	RA 33	31 kD	25-kD	19-/20-kD
1	−	+	−	−	−
2	−	+	−	−	−
3	−	+ +	+	+	−
4	+	−	−	−	−
5	+	−	−	−	−
6	+ +	−	−	−	−
7	+ +	+	−	−	−
8	+ +	−	+	−	−
9	+	+	−	−	−
10	+	+ +	+	−	+
11	+	+ +	+	+	−
12	+	+ +	+	+ +	−
13	+	+ + +	+	+ + +	+ + +
14	+	+ + +	+ +	+ + +	+ +
15	+	+ + +	+ + +	+ + +	+ + +
16	+ +	+ + +	+	+ +	+
17	+ +	+ + +	+	+ + +	+
18	+ +	+ + +	+ +	+ + +	+ + +
19	+ +	+ + +	+ + +	+ + +	+ +
20	+ +	+ + +	+ + +	+ +	+ + +
21	+ +	+ + +	+ + +	+ + +	+ + +
22	+ +	+ + +	+ + +	+ + +	+ + +
23	+ + +	+	+	+	−
24	+ + +	+	+	+	−
25	+ + +	+ + +	+ +	+	−

+ + +, Strong; + +, intermediate; +, weak activity
Strong anti-RA 33 reactivity is frequently associated with elevated reactivities with the other antigens; some sera contain antibodies to RA 33 (1, 2) or the 36 kD antigen (4–6), but lack reactivity with the other moieties

gen but only weak or absent reactivity to RA33 and the other antigens (sera 4–8, 23, and 24 in Table 3).

Similar to RA33, the additional antigens were shown to have no relation to previously described nuclear autoantigens or EBV-encoded structures. Furthermore, there was no cross-reaction with rheumatoid factor, as was evident by immunoblot analysis of RF-depleted serum fractions, which retained the reactivitiy with RA33 and the other moieties (Fig. 2). Although it cannot be completely excluded that RA33 and the other antigens constitute degradation products of a larger protein, we consider this unlikely in view of the differential reactivities of RA sera with the particular proteins. The apparent association of the 33-kD antigen with antigens of other molecular weights leads us to hypothesize that these proteins may constitute parts of a much larger molecular complex, similar to the Sm/RNP particles [3, 29].

In fact, most recent data obtained in our laboratory have indicated that RA33 and some of the associated proteins belong to the family of heterogeneous nuclear ribonucleoproteins (hnRNP) [31].

Conclusion

The experiments discussed reveal that screening for potentially new serologic parameters in RA has led to the detection of autoantibodies to a nuclear antigen in the molecular weight range of 33 kD, therefore termed anti-RA33. Although the frequency of anti-RA33 was lower than that of rheumatoid factor in RA, it was similar to or even higher than that of several other antibodies with disease specificity, such as anti-Sm in SLE, anti-Scl70 in PSS, or anti-Jo1 in polymyositis. Furthermore, RA33 was detected in patients with early stages of RA and may therefore be useful in serologic investigations of patients suspected of having RA.

It will be of particular importance to elucidate the nature of RA33 and possibly associated antigens in order to understand their function in cell biology as well as their potential role in the pathogenesis of rheumatoid arthritis.

References

1. Tan EM (1985) The LE-cell and antinuclear antibodies: a breakthrough in diagnosis. In: McCarthy DJ (ed) Landmark advances in rheumatology. American Rheumatism Association, Atlanta
2. Hardin JA, Rahn DR, Shen C, Lerner MR, Wolin SL, Rosa MD, Steitz J (1982) Antibodies from patients with connective tissue diseases bind specific subsets of cellular RNA protein particles. J Clin Invest 70:141–147

3. Reichlin M, Harley JB (1987) ANA subsets in SLE. In: Smolen JS, Zielinski CC (eds) Systemic lupus erythematosus – clinical and experimental aspects. Springer, Berlin Heidelberg New York

4. Douvas AS, Achten M, Tan EM (1979) Identification of a nuclear protein (Scl 70) as a unique target of human antinuclear antibodies in scleroderma. J Biol Chem 254:10514–10522

5. Mathews MB, Bernstein RM (1983) Myositis autoantibody inhibits histidyl-tRNA synthetase: a model for autoimmunity. Nature 304:177–179

6. Tan EM, Cohen AS, Fries JF et al. (1982) The 1982 revised criteria for the classification of systemic lupus erythematosus. Arthritis Rheum 25:1271–1277

7. Yoshida S, Akizuki M, Mimori T et al. (1983) The precipitating antibody to an acidic nuclear protein antigen, the Jo-1, in connective tissue diseases. Arthritis Rheum 26:604–610

8. Franco HL, Weston WL, Peebles C, Forstat SL, Phanaphak P (1981) Autoantibodies directed against sicca syndrome antigens in the neonatal lupus syndrome. Am J Acad Dermatol 4:67

9. Scott JS, Maddison PJ, Taylor PV, Esscher E, Scott O, Skinner RP (1983) Connective-tissue disease, antibodies to ribonucleoprotein, and congenital heart block. N Engl Med 309:209–212

10. Ropes MW, Bennet EA, Cobb S, Jacox R, Jessar R (1958) Revision of diagnostic criteria for rheumatoid arthritis. Bull Rheum Dis 9:175

11. Arnett FC, Elworth SM, Bloch DA et al. (1988) The American Rheumatism Association 1987 revised criteria for the classificatin of rheumatoid arthritis. Arthritis Rheum 31:315–324

12. Waaler E (1940) On the occurrence of a factor in human serum activating the specific agglutination of sheep blood corpuscles. Acta Pathol Microbiol Scand 17:172

13. Mannik M (1985) Rheumatoid factors - their discovery and possible role in pathogenesis of rheumatoid arthritis. In: McCarty DJ (ed) Landmark advances in rheumatology. American Rheumatism Association Atlanta, pp 103–110

14. Carson DA (1985) Rheumatoid factor. In: Kelley WN, Harris ED, Ruddy S, Sledge CB (eds) Textbook of rheumatology. Saunders, Philadelphia, pp 664–679

15. Dresner E, Trombly P (1958) The latex-fixation reaction in rheumatic diseases. N Engl J Med 261:981–986

16. Hassfeld W, Steiner G, Harthmuth K, Kolarz G, Scherak O, Graninger W, Thumb N, Smolen JS (1989) Demonstration of a new antinuclear antibody (anti-RA 33) that is highly specific for rheumatoid arthritis. Arthritis Rheum 32:1515–1520

17. Mimori JT, Akizuki M, Yamagata H, Inada S, Yoshida S, Homma M (1981) Characterization of a high-molecular-weight acidic nuclear protein recognized by autoantibodies in sera from patients with polymyositis-scleroderma overlap. J Clin Invest 68:611–620

18. Reichlin M, Maddison PJ, Targoff I, Bunch T, Arnett F, Sharp GC, Treatwell E Tan EM (1984) Antibodies to a nuclear/nucleolar antigen in patients with polymyositis-overlap syndromes. J Clin Immunol 4:40–44

19. Miyachi I, Fritzler MJ, Tan EM (1978) Autoantibody to a nuclear antigen in proliferating cells. J Immunol 121:228

20. Fritzler MJ, Kinsella TD, Garbutt E (1980) The CREST syndrome – a distinct serologic entity with anticentromere antibodies. Am J Med 69:520

21. Menzel J, Steffen C, Kolarz G, Kojer M, Smolen JS (1978) Demonstration of anticollagen antibodies in rheumatoid arthritis synovial fluids by ^{14}C-radioimmunoassay. Arthritis Rheum 21:243–248

22. Kataaha PD, Mortazavi SM, Russel G, Holborow EJ (1985) Anti-intermediate filament antibodies, antikeratin antibody, and antiperinuclear factor in rheumatoid arthritis and infectious mononucleosis. Ann Rheum Dis 44:446–449

23. Westgeest AAA, van Loon AM, van der Logt JTM, van de Putte LBA, Boerbooms AM (1989) Antiperinuclear factor, an RA-specific autoantiody. J Rheumatol 16:626–630

24. Hannestad K, Stoller BD (1978) Certain rheumatoid factors react with nucleosomes. Nature 275:671–673

25. Alspaugh MA, Jensen FC, Rabin H, Tan EM (1978) Lymphocytes transformed by the Epstein-Barr virus: induction of nuclear antigen reactive with antibody in rheumatoid arthritis. J Exp Med 147:1018–1027
26. Luka J, Kreofsky T, Pearson GR, Hennessy K, Kieff E (1984) Identification and characterization of a cellular protein that cross-reacts with the Epstein-Barr virus nuclear antigen. J Virol 52:833–838
27. Steinbocker O, Traeger CH, Battermann RC (1949) Therapeutic criteria in rheumatoid arthritis. JAMA 140:659–662
28. Hartmuth K, Barta A (1987) In vitro processing of the human growth hormone primary transcript. Nucleic Acids Res 15:7005–7025
29. Lerner MR, Steitz JA (1979) Antibodies to small nuclear RNAs complexed with proteins are produced by patients with systemic lupus erythematosus. Proc Natl Acad Sci USA 76:5495–5499
30. Hassfeld W, Steiner G, Smolen JS (1990) Rheumatoid arthritis – autoantibodies. N Engl J Med (letter) 323:995–996
31. Steiner G, Hartmuth K, Barta A, Hassfeld W, Smolen JS. The rheumatoid arthritis specific autoantigen RA 33 is a member of the heterogeneous ribonucleoprotein (hn RNP) family (Submitted)

Acute-Phase Response and Amyloid*

G. Husby

Department of Rheumatology, The University Hospital of Tromsø, 9000 Tromsø, Norway

The acute phase is described as a series of events that occur in response to infection or tissue injury. Inflammation, as expressed clinically by the classical tetrad of dolor, calor, rubor et tumor represents the local reaction to such insults to tissue integrity, whereas the acute-phase phenomena reflect the systemic response in this recpect [56]. The ultimate goal of the inflammatory and acute-phase responses is to restore and maintain homeostasis by destruction and elimination of causative agents, limination of the extent of injury, removal of damaged tissue constituents, and repair.

The acute-phase response is highly heterogeneous, qualitatively as well as quantitatively. This variability depends on the nature of the initiating insult, the extent, duration, and type of injury, and factors related to the host. Induction of acute-phase phenomena (Table 1) may follow a variety of bacterial, viral, parasitic, or fungal infections, traumatic lesions including surgery and childbirth, tissue necrosis including infarction, various acute and chronic inflammatory states of known or unknown etiology, and malignancies.

Being of systemic nature, the acute-phase response in its most florid form affects many biological parameters (Table 2). Fever, leukocytosis, and thrombocytis occur, together with changes in protein (increased catabolism),

Table 1. Factors involved in induction of the acute-phase response

---

Chemicals, toxic agents
Physical trauma: surgical, thermal, irradiation, blunt
Infections: bacterial, viral, parasitic
Inflammation, acute and chronic
Malignancies
Tissue necrosis, e.g., myocardial infarction
Immunization

---

* This work was supported by the Norwegian Council for Science and the Humanities, the Norwegian Women's Public Health Association, and the *Norsk Revmatikerforbund.*

Smolen, Kalden, Maini (Eds.)
Rheumatoid Arthritis
© Springer-Verlag Berlin Heidelberg 1992

Table 2. Clinical and metabolic features of the acute-phase response

---

Fever
Leukocytosis
Thrombocytosis
Metabolic alterations: Increased protein catabolism
                                   Negative nitrogen balance
                                   Increased total protein synthesis
                                   Increased gluconeogenesis
                                   Lipid changes
Hormonal changes
Altered serum concentrations of minerals and amino acids

---

carbohydrate (increased gluconeogenesis) and lipid metabolism [55, 56, 87].
Changes in the synthesis of various hormones and the serum concentrations of
amino acids and minerals can also be added to this list. Such changes result in a
variety of functional disturbances, for example of the immune, reticuloendothelial, and nervous systems.

The Acute-phase Reactants

The term "acute phase" was originally used to describe certain alterations in the
concentration of a number of plasma proteins – so-called acute phase reactants
– the first one described being C-reactive protein (CRP; reviewed by Pepys and
Baltz [87]). These alterations represent an important, and probably the best-
studied aspect of the acute-phase response. Indeed, it is possible that all plasma
proteins to some extent are subjected to anabolic or catabolic changes during
the acute phase [56].

In general, the acute-phase proteins are synthesized by the liver, which is
therefore a central organ in such situations, but some are also produced at
extrahepatic sites, for example by macrophages. The alterations in plasma
proteins are heterogeneous; some proteins increase whereas other decrease their
concentrations in the acute phase, and magnitude of these alterations and the
time patterns of increase and normalization vary greatly among the various
proteins (Table 3). The alterations of individual proteins may also be stimulus
dependent.

The plasma proteins that increase their concentration by 25% or more in the
acute phase have in general been included among these proteins [56], whereas
those that decrease, e.g., albumin, prealbumin, transferrin, have been called
"negative acute-phase reactants".

Most acute-phase proteins increase their concentration by 50% to about
fourfold (Table 3), and many of these have a known functional significance,
such as being involved in transport, enzyme inhibition, coagulation, or
complement activation [55, 87].

Table 3. Best-studied human acute-phase proteins, classified on the basis of usual magnitude of increase in plasma concentration (From Kushner and Mackiewicz [57], with kind permission of authors and publisher)

Group I: about 50%	Group II: about 2–4×increase	Group III: up to 1000×increase
Ceruplasmin Complement components C3, 4	α1 Acid glycoprotein α1 Proteinase inhibitor (α1 Anti-trypsin) α1 Anti-chymotrypsin Haptoglobin Fibrinogen	C-reactive protein (CRP) Serum amyloid A (SAA)

Two serum proteins, namely CRP and serum amyloid A (SAA), which are outstanding in their magnitude of response (Table 3), increase several hundred-fold or more, i.e., from 1 mg/l or less in the normal state up to more than 1000 mg/l in the acute phase [56, 71–73, 75]. It is an interesting paradox that the functional aspect of these two most characteristic acute-phase proteins is rather obscure. Brief descriptions of CRP and SAA follow.

C-Reactive Protein

CRP, the classical acute-phase reactant, was detected in 1930 because sera from patients were found to precipitate pneumococcal C-polysaccharide. Normal sera did not show this precipitation, but more sensitive techniques later showed that CRP is a normal serum protein present in very low concentration in normal individuals, it increases rapidly to several hundred-fold following proper stimulation. CRP is an "old" protein; it has been found in an invertebrate, the horeseshoe crab, and its structure has been well conserved in evolution. It has very special ligand binding properties, and binds strongly to phosphorylcholine [87]. As mentioned, the function of CRP is rather obscure, although it may be involved in complement fixation and phagocytosis [22]. CRP seems to be produced exclusively by hepatocytes, its increased secretion being a result of increased transcription following induction [29, 67]. Measurement of CRP is now established as a useful laboratory test to monitor the acute-phase response for both clinical and experimental purposes [87]; it is more accurate and reliable than the erythrocyte sedimentation rate in many clinical situations [57].

Structurally, CRP consists of five polypeptide subunits non-covalently associated in a diskline configuration with cyclic pentameric symmetry [87], because of this structure, CRP belongs to a group of proteins called pentraxins [87]. CRP shares 70% amino acid homology with serum AP (SAP), the precursor of amyloid P-component (AP), which is an extrafibrillar constituent of amyloid [87].

Serum Amyloid A

SAA was detected in 1972 [42, 61] because of its reactivity with antisera to amyloid A protein (AA), the chief fibril protein in reactive amyloidosis [10, 39, 43]. In addition to being associated with amyloidosis, SAA is, as mentioned, one of the two most characteristic and sensitive acute-phase reactants, the other being CRP [72, 73]. We have measured serum concentrations of SAA of up to 1280 mg/l in patients with inflammation, while the lowest value recorded by us is 0.02 mg/l; this means a multiplum of 64000. The mean concentration in normal human sera as measured by radioimmunoassay in our laboratory is 1 mg/l [69]. SAA is therefore, a clinically sensitive indicator of inflammation in diseases known to stimulate the acute-phase response [69,75, 76, 87]. In addition to monitoring activity of chronic inflammatory disorders, measurement of SAA is of significance for the early detection of infectious compications in cystic fibrosis [71] and of opportunistic infections in AIDS [48] and has prognostic value with regard to determining the amount of tissue necrosisin myocardial infarction [72, 73]. High SAA has also been shown to be associated with dissemination of cancer [91] and rejection of homografts [74].

SAA behaves by and large similar to CRP in inflammation, and because of problems regarding standardization of test systems for SAA, CRP measurements are presently advocated for use in clinical practice [69].

SAA is present on high-density lipoprotein (HDL) in the circulation as an apolipoprotein [9, 70, 97]. This and other properties of SAA, particularly its structure, regulation, and significance in AA amyloidosis, will be dealt with in more detail later in this chapter.

Induction of the Acute-phase Response

Since the acute-phase response is by definition a systemic response to local tissue injury, circulating soluble or cell-bound mediators should be required for its mediation at sites distant from the initial event. Furthermore, the signals brought about by such mediators would require receptors present on the cells to be activated. The recent developments in molecular biology and gene technology have provided a large body of new knowledge regarding the cellular and humoral mechanisms operating in the acute-phase response.

The events that lead to increased acute-phase protein concentrations following tissue injury or infection can be summarized as follows: Activation of macrophages induces monokines that, via the circulation, provide signals for hepatic acute-phase protein expression, which is thereafter turned off following removal of insulting agents and restoration of injured tissue. In long-standing situations, however, e.g., in rheumatoid arthritis, the stimulatory mechanisms are not sufficiently turned off and the "acute" phase becomes chronic.

Monokine Production of Activated Mononuclear Phagocytes

The macrophage is a multipotent cell and plays an important role in host defense against infections and neoplasia [20]. It secretes more than 50 different proteins, including the monokines. The multiple activities of the macrophage are brought about by a wide variety of stimuli that are only partly understood [20, 60]. These include various microorganisms, microbial products, inflammatory agents, antigens, lymphokines, and pharmacological agents. The best-studied monokines involved in the acute-phase response are interleukin-1 (IL-1), tumor necrosis factor (TNF), and interleukin-6 (IL-6). There are described in detail elsewhere in this book.

Induction of these three monokines and their interactions in the regulation of hepatic acute-phase protein synthesis represents a highly complicated network of mechanisms [21, 22, 57, 60, 109]. There is still much to be learnt about how these mechanisms work in vivo in different pathological situations. It appears that IL-1, TNF, and IL-6 can mutually stimulate each other; they appear capable of inducing themselves, and via their individual receptors they may act synergistically on target cells. The mechanisms for regulation of these monokines also appear to be partly overlapping and partly independent [12]. The literature is not yet consistent regarding their functional distinctions, which may be explained by the use of different species or cells for study and different experimental conditions, but the availability of complementary DNAs and recombinant messenger and receptor molecules will provide a better understanding of these complex mechanisms.

Other Mediators Involved in Acute-phase Responses

Cytokines other than these monokines are also involved in the regulation of inflammatory acute-phase reactions. These include the hematopoietic colony-stimulating factors and the interferons. It appears that inferferon-γ is an important early mediator of the acute-phase response because of its ability to stimulate macrophage expression of monokines, either directly or by priming activation by other signals, for example bacterial lipopolysaccharide (LPS) [104]. The arachidonic acid metabolites prostaglandins and leukotrienes, which can be produced by practically all cell types, interact with the cytokines in a complex and only partly understood way.

In addition, materials present in the urine of febrile patients and pregnant women, or produced by Epstein-Barr-infected B cells and human neutrophils, have been shown to inhibit IL-1 [60, 84, 93]. A distinct urinary inhibitor of TNF has also been described [94]. Such agents could be utilized to prevent unwanted effects of macrophage activation; however, as long as more specific inhibitors are lacking, the beneficial activities of these important monokines will probably also be inhibited.

More "conventional" hormones are involved in the regulation of the acute-phase response. Glucocorticosteroids appear to be essential for the acute-phase protein expression in hepatocytes [27], but they can also down-regulate monokine expression via a negative feedback mechanism: IL-1 induces ACTH production by the pituitary gland, which in turn stimulates the glucocorticoids that inhibit IL-1 expression by macrophages [56, 60].

Recently a fourth monokine, called "macrophage inflammatory protein-1", has been shown to induce fever as well as increase SAA concentrations in mice to the same extent as TNF [14].

Definition and Classification of Amyloidosis

Amyloidosis comprises a heterogeneous group of disorders caused by extracellular deposition of a characteristic proteinaceous material, the amyloid fibrils, in various organs and tissues [17, 28, 40, 41]. The pathophysiological consequences of amyloid deposition depend on its tissue and organ distribution, and the symptoms and signs are caused partly by functional disturbances due to displacement of normal tissue structures, and partly by organ enlargement [37]. The amyloid fibrils have very low solubility in physiological conditions, which is thought to be responsible for the irreversible and often progressive course of the disease, in many cases leading to death within months or years of diagnosis [37, 38]. In 1968, Pras et al. established a water extraction method for the purification of amyloid fibrils which permitted chemical and immunologic analyses of isolated amyloid fibrils and their protein subunits [40].

Gel filtration of solubilized amyloid fibrils obtained from different clinical and experimental types of amyloidosis has, in many instances, revealed an elution pattern consisting of two main protein peaks [36]. The second of these peaks represents a distinct protein subunit with a molecular weight ranging from about 4 to 30 kD in different amyloid preparations [28, 40]. Several apparently nonrelated proteins can constitute this subunit in different cases of amyloidosis. However, a common feature of these proteins appears to be β-pleated sheets, a structure which is present in all amyloid fibrils so far studied [28]. A steadily increasing number of such fibril proteins are characterized by their amino acid sequence, and in some cases complementary DNA has also been established [41]. The different amyloid proteins are often related to specific clinical forms of amyloidosis. Indeed, many types of amyloid disease (Table 4) can now be defined by structural analysis of the fibril proteins and/or the genes coding for them [8, 28, 36, 41].

Certain serum proteins are precursors for the different fibril proteins in the various systemic forms of amyloidosis (Table 4). Two important types of fibril protein related to systemic amyloidosis are the amyloid L (light-chain, AL) and amyloid A (AA) proteins. Protein AL, which consists of homogeneous

Table 4. Human systemic amyloid fibril proteins verified by amino acid sequencing[a]

Clinical type	Amyloid protein	Related protein
Idiopathic (primary) amyloidosis		
Systemic	AL(A$\varkappa$, Aλ)	IgL, (V$\varkappa$, Vλ)
Localized	AL(A$\varkappa$, Aλ)	IgL, (V$\varkappa$, Vλ)
Myeloma-associated amyloidosis	AL(A$\varkappa$, Aλ)	IgL, (V$\varkappa$, Vλ)
Reactive (secondary) amyloidosis	AA	SAA
Heredofamilial amyloidosis		
Recessive, autosomal:		
Familial Mediterranean fever (FMF)	AA or AA variant	SAA
Dominant, autosomal:		
Familial amyloid nephropathy with urticaria and deafness (Muckle-Wells syndrome)	AA[b]	SAA
Familial amyloid polyneuropathy (FAP)	Prealbumin variants Apo AI variant	Prealbumin Apo AI
Familial amyloid cardiomyopathy (FAC)	Prealbumin variant	Prealbumin
Senile amyloidosis	Prealbumin (variant)	Prealbumin
Amyloidosis associated with chronic hemodialysis	β2-Microglobulin	β2-Microglobulin

[a] The nomenclature and abbriviations are according to those proposed by Benditt et al. [11] with small modifications.
[b] Only residues 2–30 are sequenced.

(monoclonal) immunoglobulin kappa or lambda light chains or the aminoterminal fragments thereof is seen in idiopathic and myeloma-associated amyloidosis (AL amyloidosis) [28, 37]. Protein AA is associated with amyloidosis reactive to long-standing inflammation and some malignancies, familial Mediterranean fever (FMF), familial nephropathic amyloidosis with febrile urticaria – the Muckle-Wells syndrome [64, 82] – and spontaneous and experimental amyloidosis in animals [28, 41]. These forms of amyloidosis could therefore also be called AA amyloidosis, the pathogenetic aspects of which will be focused on below.

Reactive, AA amyloidosis occurs in about 5% of cases of both adult and juvenile rheumatoid arthritis, and although the prevalence has declined during the past three decades, it is still a severe complication and an important cause of early death, particularly in the juvenile cases. For more detailed descriptions of the epidemiological diagnostic, clinical, and therapeutic aspects of amyloidosis reactive to chronic arthritis, the reader is referred to Husby [38] and Dilon et al. [19].

Table 5. Human SAA and AA

					5					10					15					20
SAA[a]	Arg	Ser	Phe	Phe	Ser	Phe	Leu	Gly	Glu	Ala	Phe	Asp	Gly	Ala	Arg	Asp	Met	Trp	Arg	Ala
AA[b]																				
					25					30					35					40
SAA	Tyr	Ser	Asn	Met	Arg	Glu	Ala	Asn	Tyr	Ile	Gly	Ser	Asp	Lys	Tyr	The	His	Ala	Arg	Gly
AA																				
				45 ↓					50					55					60
SAA	Asn	Tyr	Asp	Ala	Ala	Lys	Arg	Gly	Pro	Gly	Gly	Ala/Val	Trp	Ala	Ala	Glu	Ala/Val	Ile/Leu	Ser	Asn
AA												Val[c]					Ala[c]	Ile		
			↓ 65					70					75		↓			80
SAA	Ala	Arg	Glu	Asn	Ile	Glu	Arg	Phe	Phe	Gly	His	Gly	Ala	Glu	Asn	Ser	Leu	Ala	Asp	Glu
AA																	–COOH			
		↓	↓	85					90					95					100
SAA	Ala	Ala	Asn	Glu	Trp	Gly	Arg	Ser	Gly	Lys	Asp	Pro	Asn	His	Phe	Arg	Pro	Ala	Gly	Leu
				104															
SAA	Pro	Glu	Lys	Tyr	–COOH															

[a] Sletten et al. [99]
[b] Sletten and Husby [98]
[c] Ala or $\frac{\text{Ala}}{\text{Val}}$ have been found in position 52 and Val in position 57 in other human AA proteins [61, 81]

Serum and Tissue Amyloid A Proteins

The unique protein AA was first described by Benditt and co-workers [10]. The precursor for tissue AA is SAA, as evidenced by several experiments [46, 49]: Human HDL-SAA complexes from acute-phase sera were introduced into mice during the induction of amyloidosis with LPS. Human AA was detected in the amyloid fibrils that developed in these animals. The precursor-product relationship between SAA and AA was thereby established and later confirmed by others [103].

Human SAA consists of 104 amino acid residues corresponding to a molecular weight of about 11.5 kD (Table 5) and is larger but otherwise essentially identical to protein AA in its primary structure [86, 98, 99]. Protein AA is formed by cleavage of SAA at different positions varying from 45 up to 83 in different cases, leaving the N-terminal largely intact [40]. The sequence 46–104 is apparently not critical for fibrillogenesis [45], although the most typical human AA consists of 76 amino acid residues, thus lacking the 28 C-terminal amino acids of SAA (Table 5).

The pronounced hydrophobicity of the sequence consisting of the 11 first N-terminal amino acids is the most striking feature of SAA and AA (Tables 5 and 6), while residues 25–49 of the two proteins and 76–104 of SAA have unspecified function [47, 86, 105, 106]. The sequence between residues 33 and 51 is highly conserved in the evolution, pointing to an important biological function [45], which is largely unknown, however, except for the fact that it participates in amyloidosis. Computer analyses and wet-gel-ray studies of SAA [105, 106] confirm the hydrophobicity at the N-terminal residues 1–11. These residues form an α-helix and are probably involved in lipid binding, strongly indicating that this part of the molecule is involved in the complexing of SAA with HDL [86].

Table 6. Partial N-terminal amino acid sequence of human, milk, and murine SAA and AA

					5					10			
Human SAA/AA	Arg	Ser	Phe	Ser	Phe	Leu	Gly	Glu	Ala	Phe	Asp	Gly	Ala
Mink SAA[a]		PCA	Trp				Phe				Ile/Val	Gln	
Mink AA[b]		PCA	Trp				Phe				Val	Gln	
Murine SAA[c]	Gly						Ile/Val					Gln	
Murine AA[d]	Gly						Ile					Gln	

[a] Waalen et al. [107]
[b] Syversen et al. [102]
[c] Anders et al. [2]
[d] Hoffmann et al. [33]

Table 7. Murine SAA genes and protein products [77, 79, 90]

Isotype	Gene expression	Protein product
SAA 1	Mainly liver	Nonamyloidogenic, 50% of normal and acute-phase SAA
SAA 2	Mainly liver	Amyloidogenic, 50% of normal and acute-phase SAA. Decreases in serum during amyloidogenesis
SAA 3	Liver + extrahepatic, macrophages	Protein product not discovered in serum or elsewhere. Remains intracellularly?

Chemical analyses of SAA from man, mouse [2], mink [102], and horse [100] (Table 6) have revealed the protein to be polymorphic in all of these species [45].

Studies using complementary DNA for murine and human SAA have confirmed that more than one SAA gene exists in both species. Thus Lowel et al. [65] reported the complete nucleotide sequence of two nonallelic murine SAA genes encoding two SAA isotypes (SAA 1 and SAA 2) which, together with a third SAA gene (SAA 3) and a pseudogene [112], make up the entire murine SAA gene family (Table 7).

Furthermore, two human SAA mRNAs have been identified [54, 95], and there appears to be a family of three SAA genes also in man [92], in addition, probably a pseudogene as well (P. Woo, personal communication).

Induction, Production, and Regulation of SAA

As mentioned, signals for SAA induction are monokine mediated, and it is generally accepted that the liver (i.e., the hepatocyte) is its chief producer [40], although expression of murine SAA genes had been demonstrated in various extrahepatic sites [77, 90].

The dramatic increase in hepatic production of SAA in acute-phase situations is regulated by increases in SAA mRNA, 500-fold or more in murine liver during the acute-phase response. Studies in mice [29, 66] further suggest that acute-phase SAA mRNA is regulated at the transcriptional and post-transcriptional levels. The upstream sequences of the SAA gene family were shown to have common sequences with genes for another acute-phase protein, fibrinogen, which could explain the coordinate expression of acute-phase protein genes.

Studies of human SAA regulation were previously hampered by the lack of hepatoma cell lines expressing this protein. However, a human SAA genomic clone has been successfully transfected into mouse L-cells, and regulatin of SAA synthesis was achieved using IL-1 and TNF [110]. Furthermore, cultured adult human hepatocytes were recently shown to produce SAA in response to recombinant IL-6 stimulation [13, 80], and induction of SAA by IL-1, IL-6, or TNF in human hepatoma Hep 3B [26] and PLC/PRF/5 cells [58, 89] had been observed. The increased synthesis of SAA in Hep 3B cells was accompanied by a similar increase in SAA mRNA, suggesting regulation at the pretranslational level, also in man. The mechanism by which these monokines control SAA expression is unknown, but recent analysis of the 5'-flanking region of a human SAA gene have revealed a number of putative regulatory sequences [23].

The bulk of SAA is complexed to HDL in serum [9, 70, 97]. Indeed, it has been shown [15, 70] that SAA can constitute up to 87% of the total apolipoprotiens of HDL in human acute-phase sera, while only minute amounts are present on HDL in the normal state.

Small amounts of protein AA-like molecules have also been observed among the HDL apolipoproteins in acute-phase sera [46, 47, 49], suggsting that some SAA had been converted to AA in the circulation. This is in line with the findings that enzymes present on the surface of circulating monocytes [59], as well as in serum [96], are capable of transforming SAA to AA-like fragments in vitro. Whether the existence of AA-like molecules in the circulation is of importance for amyloid formation is not clear.

When SAA increases in acute-phase serum it displaces apo AI from the HDL particle [16, 85]. The reverse process, namely the displacement of SAA from acute-phase HDL by apo AI or apo AII, has been shown to take place in vitro [49, 50]. High concentrations of these "normal" apoproteins in vivo may thus release SAA from HDL and make it available for amyloid formation. It is interesting that tissues like the liver and intestines that actually produce apo AI and apo AII are also predilection sites for AA-type amyloidosis.

Formation and Deposition of AA Amyloid

SAA is precursor for tissue AA, and availability of the precursor is obviously one prerequisite for amyloidogenesis. It is well known that those of the chronic inflammatory diseases like rheumatoid arthritis that are associated with high concentrations of acute-phase proteins including SAA also underlie reactive amyloidosis [38, 45]. However, only a minority of patients with chronic arthritis develop amyloidosis, despite chronically raised SAA [38], and there is no absolute correlation between SAA concentration and the development of amyloidosis [77]. Additional amyloid-promoting factors are therefore required.

Besides the mere presence of SAA, the structure of this precursor protein appears to be of importance. SAA is heterogeneous (Table 5), and in 1977, amino acid sequence studies of murine SAA revealed two residues, namely valine and isoleucine at position 7 (Table 6), probably representing two isotypes of this protein [2], later designated SAA 1 and SAA 2, whereas only isoleucine is present in murine AA [33]. Thus, only SAA 2 forms amyloid (Table 7), and although hepatic mRNA for SAA1 and SAA2 was expressed at the same magnitude in the acute phase, SAA2 was selectively removed from the circulatin during amyloidogenesis [79]. Furthermore, murine SAA2 appears to have a lower affinity for HDL than SAA1 in vitro [50], which could facilitate the selective release of SAA2. In addition, the expression of the "amyloid-prone" SAA2 has been shown to be defective in SJL mice that are resistant to amyloid induction [112], futher supporting the importance of this SAA isotype in amyloidogenesis.

In order to examine whether these observations in murine AA amyloidosis are relevant for other species, an experimental model for AA amyloidosis induced with LPS in the mink was established [1, 44]. The structure of AA [107] and SAA [102] in this species revealed striking analogy to the situation in the mouse, with both valine and isoleucine indicating two SAA isotypes at position 10, while only valine was present at this position in AA (Table 6). This polymorphism of mink SAA has very recently been confirmed at the DNA level: At least two SAA genes are present in this animal (Marhaug, Husby and Dowton, manuscript in preparation). Comparative studies in the horse similarly indicate amyloidogenic and nonamyloidogenic molecular species of SAA [100].

The importance of the N-terminal half of SAA in amyloidosis is further illustrated by recent experiments in the rat, an animal that does not develop amyloidosis. SAA is not found in rat acute-phase HDL [6]. A rat liver SAA mRNA codes for an amino acid sequence lacking the 50-residue N-terminal portion of the human protein [63, 78]. This N-terminal sequence therefore appears to contain the region(s) which both binds to HDL and is important for amyloid formation.

What then, is the situation in man? In contrast to mouse and mink, there are no obvious "amyloidogenic" or "nonamyloidogenic" sequences in the N-terminal half of human SAA (Tables 5 and 6) [86, 99]. However, a heterogeneity at position 58 (leucine and isoleucine in SAA [99] does not occur in any human AA protein so far sequenced (Table 5). But residue 58 of SAA clearly belongs to a part of the molecule which is apparently not critical for fibril formation. On the other hand, an AA protein associated with FMF, consisting of 76 amino acids, has threonine at residue 69 [61], whereas all AA proteins related to reactive amyloidosis have phenylalanine at this position. This substitution in FMF amyloid involving all three nucleotides, which has been confirmed by the structure of a corresponding human SAA gene [110], may be important for this inherited form of AA amyloidosis.

Interestingly, the amino acid sequence deduced from the structure of a human SAA gene recently determined [54] differed from any human AA protein so far studied, supporting the existence of "nonamyloidogenic" SAA gene products also in man.

Incomplete Degradation of SAA

SAA has a half-life of approximately 24 h in man [75]. Enzymes bound to while blood cels [59], serum proteases [7, 96], and Kupffer cells in the liver [25] degrage SAA in vitro, compatible with both hepatic and extrahepatic catabolism of SAA in vivo. The degradation is inhibited by SAA [7], supporting the observation [88] that it takes place by a specific mechanism. An intermediate fragment in the catabolism of SAA is an AA-like molecule [59, 96]. Insufficient breakdown and removal of SAA or this AA-like fragment may lead to its deposition in amyloid [59]. Supporting this is the experimental evidence of defective reticuloendothelial (i.e., Kupffer cell) function in preamyloidotic mice [25].

The question remains, however, whether limited degradation of SAA is a prerequisite for amyloid formation. Apparently intact SAA makes up the fibrils in amyloid isolated from man [52] and the duck [24] and is also present, together with different-size AA molecules, in many other amyloid preparations [45, 51]. Intriguing in this respect is the theory [103] that the enzymatic cleavage of SAA is a post fibrillar event.

Amyloid Enhancing Factor and Glycosaminoglycans

Amyloid enhancing factor (AEF) is a poorly defined material which probably consists of both protein and carbohydrate, is induced in the spleen, liver, and kidney during persistent inflammation, and is probably synthesized and secreted by reticuloendothelial cells in these organs [4, 34, 53]. AEF consistently precedes the occurrence of amyloid induced in these organs in the mouse [53] and the hamster [83]. Intravenously administered AEF has been shown to shorten the induction time of experimental amyloidosis from weeks to between 24 and 48 h, possibly by altering the catabolism of SAA, because AEF is not capable of inducing SAA [18].

Glycosaminoglycans (GAGs) have been proposed to account for the carbohydrate moiety in AEF [101]. GAGs occur in the tissues in close temporal and morphological relationship to amyloid deposition [101]. Recent experiments [68] showed, by direct chemical evidence, that GAGs identified as chondroitin sulphate, dermatan sulphate, and heparin/heparan sulphate are specifically co-purified with AA-type fibrils, supporting the suggestion [83, 101] that GAGs (or proteoglycans) constitute the amyloid fibrils together with protein or are closely associated with them in vivo. The large negative charge of GAGs indicates an involvement in precursor folding and incorporation in the fibrils [101]. This property of GAGs may explain why precursor proteins with such diverse primary structures as SAA and immunoglobulin light chains make up fibrils with identical ultrastructure in the tissues.

Protein AP – the Amyloid "P Component"

Protein AP is an α-glycoprotein which is invariably present in amyloid deposits, regardless of the chemical nature of amyloid fibrils and the clinical type of amyloidosis [32, 35, 87]. AP is not a part of the amyloid fibrils but is closely bound to them in a calcium-dependent fashion [35, 87]. AP has been shown to bind heparan sulphate and dermatan sulphate in a calcium-dependent manner, and such GAGs may be responsible for the association between AP and amyloid [30].

A normal plasma petraxin protein, SAP, is identical to protein AP in its structure and binding properties [3, 87]. Studies using radiolabeled SAP injected intravenously [5] showed that SAP is the precursor of tissue AP. Further, the radionuclide imaging could be used in the diagnosis of various types of human amyloidosis [32]. Although the serum concentration of SAP is not increased in the acute phase or in patients with amyloidosis, the synthesis of the protein may be increased 100-fold in amyloidotic patients, pointing to a specific role of SAP in amyloidogenesis [32]. Otherwise, the biological significance of AP/SAP is largely unknown, although purified human AP has been shown to inhibit proteolytic activity of elastase in vitro [62]. This may have implications for amyloidogenesis, since AP could inhibit the enzymatic breakdown of amyloid precursor protein at the site of fibril deposition. A DNA polymorphic site, 5′ to the SAP gene, was significantly associated with AA amyloidosis in juvenile rheumatoid arthritis, supporting an active role of AP in amyloidogenesis [111], although this finding was not supported by others [31].

Conclusions

In all forms of systemic amyloidosis the fibril precursor is a serum protein – in AA amyloidosis, the characteristic acute-phase apolipoprotein SAA. Amyloidosis may be caused by excess amounts of precursor protein as the result of increased production and/or decreased clearance. However, only a minor proportion of patients with inflammation develop AA amyloidosis, in spite of chronically raised SAA. On the other hand, individuals with presumably low concentrations of SAA may develop AA amyloidosis. Additional factors are obviously needed for the formation of AA amyloidosis. Genetically determined "amyloid-prone" SAA molecules are one such factor, together with diverse or altered expression of the SAA genes. Other genes may also be important, for example those coding for and regulating SAP. In addition, the strong resistance of the A/J mouse strain to amyloid induction has been shown to be accounted for by a single gene [108]. Still another factor is AEF: virtually all CBA/J mice receiving stimulus for persistent inflammation plus AEF develop amyloidosis within 2 days. This suggests that a proper combination of different amyloid-promoting factors is operating in this model [53]. GAGs may be involved in the conversion of diverse precursor proteins into fibrils with identical ultrastructure.

There is reason to believe that the relative importance of the various etiologic and pathogenetic factors operating in AA amyloidosis may differ in different cases of this disorder. The ongoing research, particularly that in the field of molecular biology of amyloidosis, which has received increasing interestin recent years, will no doubt shed new light on the mechanisms of this often lethal disorder.

Acknowledgement. The author is grateful to Ms. Marit Espejord for her skillful secretarial assistance.

References

1. Anders RF, Nordstoga K, Natvig JB, Husby G (1976) Amyloid-related serum protein SAA in endotoxin-induced amyloidosis of the mink. J Exp Med 143:678–683
2. Anders RF, Natvig JB, Sletten K, Husby G, Nordstoga K (1977) Amyloid-related serum protein SAA from three animal species: comparison with human SAA. J Immunol 118:229–234
3. Andersson JK, Mole JE (1982) Large-scale isolation and partial primary structure of human plasma amyloid P-component. Ann NY Acad Sci 389:216–234
4. Axelrad MA, Kisilevsky R (1980) Biological characterization of amyloid-enhancing factor. In: Glenner GG, Costa PP, de Freitas AF (eds) Amyloid and amyloidosis. Exerpta Medica, Amsterdam pp 527–533
5. Baltz ML, Caspi D, Evans DJ, Rowe IF, Hind CRK, Pepys MB (1986) Circulating serum amyloid P component is the precursor of amyloid P component in tissue amyloid deposits. Clin Exp Immunol 66:691–700
6. Baltz ML, Rowe IF, Capsi D, Turnell WG, Pepys MB (1987) Acute-phase high-density lipoprotein in the rat does not contain serum amyloid A protein. Biochem J 242:301–303
7. Bausserman LL, Saritelli AL, van Zuiden P, Collaher CJ, Herbert PN (1987) Degradation of serum amyloid A by isolated perfused rat liver. J Biol Chem 262:1583–1589
8. Benditt EP, Eriksen N (1971) Chemical classes of amyloid substance. Am J Pathol 65:231–252
9. Benditt EP, Eriksen N (1977) Amyloid protein SAA is associated with high-density lipoprotein from human serum. Proc Natl Acad Sci USA 74:4025–4028
10. Benditt EP, Eriksen M, Hermodsen MA, Ericsson LH (1971) The major proteins of human and monkey amyloid substance: common properties including unusual N-terminal amino acid sequences. FEBS Lett 19:169–173
11. Benditt EP, Cohen AS, Costa PP, Franklin EC, Glenner GG, Husby G, Mandema E, Natvig JB, Ossermann EF, Sohar E, Wegelius O, WEstermark P (1980) Guidelines for Nomenclature. Pp XI–XII in GG Glenner, PP Costa and AF de Freitas (Eds) Amyloid and Amyloidosis. Excerpta Medica, Amsterdam, Oxford, Princeton
12. Burchett SK, Weaver WM, Westall JA, Larsen A, Kronheim S, Wilson CB (1988) Regulation of tumor necrosis factor/cachetin and IL-1 secretion in human mononuclear phagocytes. J Immunol 140:3473–3481
13. Castel JV, Gómez-Lechón MJ, David M, Hirano T, Kishimoto T, Heinrich PC (1988) Recombinant human interleukin-6 (IL-6/BSF-2/HSF) regulates the synthesis of acute-phase proteins in human hepatocytes. FEBS Lett 232:347–350

14. Cerami A, Beutler B (1988) The role of cachectin/TNF in endotoxic shock and cachexia. Immunol Today 1:28–31
15. Clifton PM, Mackinnon AM, Barter PJ (1985) Effects of serum amyloid A protein (SAA) on composition, size, and density of high-density lipo-proteins in subjects with myocardial infarction. J Lipid Res 26:1389–1398
16. Coetzee GA, Strachan AF, van der Westhuyzen DR, Hoppe HC, Jeenan MS, de Beer FC (1986) Serum amyloid A-containing human high-density lipoproteins. J Biol Chem 261:9644–9651
17. Cohen AS (1967) Amyloidosis. N Engl J Med 277:522–530, 574–583, 628–638
18. Deal CL, Sipe JD, Tatsuta E, Skinner M, Cohen AS (1982) The effect of amyloid enhancing factor (AEF) on the acute – phase serum amyloid A (SAA) and serum amyloid P (SAP) response to silver nitrate. Ann NY Acad Sci 389:439–441
19. Dillon V, Woo P, Isenberg D (1989) Amyloidosis in the rheumatic diseases. Ann Rheum Dis 47:696–701
20. Dinarello CA (1984) Interleukin-1. Rev Infect Dis 6:51–95
21. Dinarello CA, Mier JW (1987) Lymphokines. N Engl J Med 317:940–945
22. Dowton SB, Colten HR (1988) Acute-phase reactants in inflammation and infection. Semin Hematol 25:84–90
23. Edbrooke MR, Burt DW, Cheshire JK, Woo P (1989) Identification of *cis*-acting sequences responsible for phorbol ester induction of human serum amyloid A gene expression via a nuclear factor kappa B-like transcription factor. Mol Cell Biol 9:1908–1916
24. Ericsson LH, Eriksen N, Walsh KA, Benditt EP (1987) Primary structure of duck amyloid protein A. FEBS Lett 218:11–16
25. Fuks A, Zucker-Franklin D (1985) Impaired Kupffer cell function precedes the development of secondary amyloidosis. J Exp Med 161:1013–1028
26. Ganapathi MK, Schultz D, Mackiewicz A, Samold D, Hu SI, Brabenec A, Macintyre S, Kushner I (1988) Heterogenous nature of the acute-phase response. Differential regulation of human serum amyloid A, C-reactive protein, and other acute-phase proteins by cytokines in Hep 3B cells. J Immunol 141:564–569
27. Gauldie J, Richards C, Harnish D, Landsorp P, Baumann H (1987) Interferon β2/B-cell stimulatory factor type 2 shares identity with monocyte-derived hepatocyte-stimulating factor (HSF) and regulates the major acute-phase protein response in liver cells. Proc Natl Acad Sci USA 84:7251–7255
28. Glenner GG (1980) Amyloid deposits and amyloidosis. N Engl J Med 302:1283–1292
29. Goldberger G, Bing DH, Sipe JD, Rits M, Colton HR (1987) Transcriptional regulation of genes encoding the acute-phase proteins CRP, SAA and C3. J Immunol 138:3967–3971
30. Hamazaki H (1987) CA^{2+}-mediated association of human serum amyloid P component with heparan sulfate and dermatan sulfate. J Biol Chem 262:1456–1460
31. Harats N, Kluve-Beckerman B, Skinner M, Paso M, Quinn L, Benson MD (1989) Lack of association of a restriction fragment length polymorphism for serum amyloid P gene with reactive amyloidosis. Arthritis Rheum 32:1325–1327
32. Hawkins PN, Lavender JP, Myers MJ, Pepys MB (1988) Diagnostic radionuclide imaging of amyloid: biological targeting by circulating human serum amyloid P component. Lancet 1:1413–1418
33. Hoffman JS, Ericsson LH, Eriksen N, Walsh KA, Benditt EP (1984) Murine tissue amyloid protein AA. NH2-terminal sequence identity with only one of two serum amyloid protein (ApoSAA) gene products. J Exp Med 159:641–646
34. Hol PR, Snel FWJJ, Niewold TA, Gruys E (1986) Amyloid enhancing factor (AEF) in the pathogenesis of AA-amyloidosis in the hamster. Virchows Arch [B] 52:273–281
35. Holck M, Husby G, Sletten K, Natvig JB (1979) The amyloid P component (protein AP): an integral part of the amyloid substance? Scand J Immunol 10:55–60
36. Husby G (1980) A chemical classification of amyloid correlation with different clinical types of amyloidosis. Scand J Rheumatol 9:60–64

37. Husby G (1983) Immunoglobulin-related (AL) amyloidosis. Clin Exp Rheumatol 1:353–358
38. Husby G (1985) Amyloidosis and rheumatoid arthritis. Clin Exp Rheumatol 3:173–180
39. Husby G, Natvig JB (1974) A serum component related to non-immunoglobulin amyloid protein AS. A possible precursor of the fibrils. J Clin Invest 53:1054–1061
40. Husby G, Sletten K (1986) Chemical and clinical classification of amyloidosis 1985. Scand J Immunol 23:253–265
41. Husby G, Sletten K (1986) Amyloid proteins. In: Marrink J, van Rijswijk MH (eds) Amyloidosis. Nijhoff, Dordrecht, pp 23–24
42. Husby G, Sletten K, Michaelsen TE, Natvig JB (1972) An alternative nonimmunoglobulin origin of amyloid fibrils. Nature 238:187
43. Husby G, Natvig JB, Michaelsen TE, Sletten K, Høst H (1973) Unique amyloid protein subunit common to different types of amyloid fibril. Nature 244:362–364
44. Husby G, Natvig JB, Sletten K, Nordstoga K, Anders RF (1975) An experimental model in mink for studying the relation between amyloid fibril protein AA and the related serum protein SAA. Scand J Immunol 4:811–816
45. Husby G, Husebekk A, Marhaug G, Skogen B, Sletten K (1988) Serum amyloid A (SAA): the precursor for protein AA in secondary amyloidosis. Adv Exp Med Biol 243:148–192
46. Husebekk A, Skogen B, Husby G, Marhaug G (1985) Transformation of amyloid precursor SAA to protein AA and incorporation in amyloid fibrils in vivo. Scand J Immunol 21:283–287
47. Husebekk A, Husby G, Sletten K, Marhaug G (1986) Characterization of amyloid protein AA and its serum precursor SAA in the horse. Scand J Immunol 23:703–709
48. Husebekk A, Permin H, Husby G (1986) Serum amyloid protein A (SAA) – an indicator of inflammation in AIDS and AIDS-related complex (ARC). Scand J Infect Dis 18:389–394
49. Husebekk A, Skogen B, Husby G (1987) Characterization of amyloid proteins AA and SAA as apolipoproteins of HDL. Displacement of SAA from the HDL-SAA by apo AI and apo AII. Scand J Immunol 25:375–381
50. Husebekk A, Skogen B, Husby G (1988) Replacement of SAA from the SAA-HDL complex by Apo AI and Apo AII. Relevance for amyloid formation? In: Jsobe S, Araki F, Uchino S, Kito and E Tsubura (eds) Amyloid and Amyloidosis. Plenum, New York and London, pp 223–228
51. Husebekk A, Husby G, Sletten K, Skogen B, Nordstoga K (1988) Characterization of bovine amyloid proteins SAA and AA. Scand J Immunol 27:739–743
52. Isobe T, Husby G, Sletten K (1980) Characterization of an amyloid protein AA similar to SAA. In: Glenner GG, Costa PP, de Freitas AF (eds) Amyloid and amyloidosis. Exerpta Medica, Amsterdam pp 331–336
53. Kisilevsky R (1987) From arthritis to Alzheimer's disease: current concepts on the pathogenesis of amyloidosis. Can J Physiol Pharmacol 65:1805–1815
54. Kluve-Beckerman B, Long GL, Benson MD (1986) DNA sequence evidence for polymorphic forms of human serum amyloid A (SAA). Biochem Genet 24:795–803
55. Koj A (1974) Acute-phase reactants. In: Alison AC (ed) Structure and function of plasma proteins. Plenum, New York pp 73–132
56. Kushner I (1982) The phenomenon of the acute-phase response. Ann NY Acad Sci 389:39–48
57. Kushner I, Mackiewicz A (1987) Acute-phase proteins as disease markers. Dis Markers 5:1–11
58. Kushner I, Ganapathi MK, Macintyre SS (1989) Regulation of biosynthesis and secretion of human C-reactive protein and serum amyloid A. In: Pepys MB (ed) Acute-phase proteins in the acute-phase response. Springer, Berlin Heidelberg New York, pp 69–83
59. Lavie G, Zucker-Franklin D, Franklin EC (1978) Degradation of serum amyloid A protein by surface-associated enzymes of human blood monocytes. J Exp Med 148:1020–1031

60. Le J, Vilcek J (1987) Tumor necrosis factor and interleukin-1: cytokines with multiple overlapping biological activities. Lab Invest 56:234–248
61. Levin M, Franklin EC, Frangione B, Pras M (1972) The amino acid sequence of a major non-immunoglobulin component of some amyloid fibrils. J Clin Invest 51:2773–2776
62. Li JJ, McAdam PW (1984) Human amyloid P component: an elastase inhibitor. Scand J Immunol 20:219–226
63. Liao WS, Stark GS (1986) Cloning of rat cDNAs for eight acute-phase reactants and kinetics of induction of mRBAs following acute inflammation. Adv Inflamm Res 10:220–222
64. Linke RP, Heilmann KL, Nathrath WBJ, Eulitz M (1983) Identification of amyloid A protein in a sporadic Muckle-Wells syndrome. N-terminal amino acid sequence after isolation from formalin-fixed tissue. Lab Invest 48:698–704
65. Lowell A, Potter DA, Stearman RS, Morrow JF (1986) Structure of the murine serum amyloid A gene family. J Biol Chem 261:88442–8452
66. Lowell CA, Stearman RS, Morrow JF (1986) Transcriptional regulation of serum amyloid A gene expression. J Biol Chem 261:8453–8561
67. Macintyre S, Samols D, Kushner I (1986) Regulation of C-creative protein secretion by cultured rabbit hepatocytes. Protides Biol Fluids 34:251–254
68. Magnus JH, Husby G, Kolset SO (1989) Glycosaminoglycans are present in purified AA-type amyloid fibrils associated with juvenile rheumatoid arthritis. Ann Rheum Dis 48:215–219
69. Marhaug G (1983) Three assays for the characterization and quantitation of human serum amyloid A. Scand J Immunol 18:329–338
70. Marhaug G, Sletten K, Husby G (1982) Characterization of amyloid-related serum protein SAA complexed with serum lipoproteins (apo SAA). Clin Exp Immunol 50:382–393
71. Marhaug G, Permin H, Husby G (1983) Amyloid-related serum protein (SAA) as an indicator of lung infection in cystic fibrosis. Acta Paediatr Scand 72:861–866
72. Marhaug G, Hårklau L, Olsen B, Husby G, Husebekk A, Wang H (1986) Serum amyloid A protein in acute myocardial infarction. Acta Med Scand 220:303–306
73. Marhaug G, Østensen M, Husby G, Kolmannskog S, Flaegstad T, Stokland T, Husebekk A (1986) Clinical acute-phase pattern of serum amyloid A. Protides Biol Fluids 34:375–378
74. Maury CPJ, Teppo A-M, Ahonen J, v Willebrand E (1984) Measurement of serum amyloid A protein concentrations as a test of renal allograft rejection in patients with initially non-functioning grafts. Br Med J 288:340–341
75. McAdam KPWJ, Elin RJ, Sipe JD, Wolff SM (1978) Changes in human serum amyloid-A and C-reactive protein after etiocholanolene-induced inflammation. J Clin Invest 61:390–394
76. McAdam KPWJ, Li J, Knowles J, Foss NT, Dinarello CA, Rosenwasser LJ, Selinger MJ, Kaplan MM, Goodman R (1982) The biology of SAA: identification of the inducer, in vitro synthesis, and heterogeneity demonstrated with monoclonal antibodies. Ann NY Acad Sci 389:126–136
77. Meek RL, Benditt EP (1986) Amyloid A gene family expression in different mouse tissues. J Exp Med 164:2006–2017
78. Meek RL, Benditt EP (1989) Rat tissues express serum amyloid A protein-related mRNAs. Proc Natl Acad Sci USA 86:1890–1894
79. Meek RL, Hoffmann JS, Benditt EP (1986) Amyloidogenesis. One serum amyloid A isotype is selectively removed from the circulation. J Exp Med 163:499–510
80. Moshage HJ, Roelofs HMJ, v Pelt JF, Hazenberg BPC, v Leeuwen MA, Limburg PC, Aarden LA, Yap SH (1988) The effect of interleukin-1, interleukin-6 and its interrelationship on the synthesis of serum amyloid A and C-reactive protein in primary cultures of adult human hepatocytes. Biochem Biophys Ress Commun 155:112–117
81. Møyner K, Sleten K, Husby G & Natvig JB (1980) An unusually large (83 amino acid residues) amyloid fibril protein AA from a patient with Waldenstrø's macroglobulinaemia and amyloidosis. Scand J Immunol 11:549–554

82. Muckle TJ (1979) The "Muckle-Wells" syndrome. Br J Dermatol 100:87–92
83. Niewold TA, Hol PR, van Andel ACJ, Lutz ETG, Gruys E (1987) Enhancement of amyloid induction by amyloid fibril fragments in hamster. Lab Invest 56:554–549
84. Oppenheim JJ, Kovacs EJ, Matusushima K, Durum SK (19869 There is more than one interleukin-1. Immunol Today 7:45–56
85. Park JS, Rudel LL (1985) Alteration of high-density lipoprotein subfraction distribution with induction of serum amyloid A protein (SAA) in the non-human primate. J Lipid Res 26:82–91
86. Parmelee DC, Titani K, Ericsson LH, Eriksen N, Benditt EP, Walsh KA (1982) Amino acid sequence of amyloid-related apoprotein (apoSAA) from human high-density lipoprotein. Biochemistry 21:3298–3303
87. Pepys M, Baltz ML (1983) Acute-phase proteins with special reference to C-reactive protein and related proteins (pentraxins) and serum amyloid A protein. Adv Immunol 34:141–212
88. Prelli F, Pras M, Frangione B (1987) The degradation and deposition of amyloid AA fibril is tissue specific. Biochemistry 26:8251–8256
89. Ramadori G, Van Damme J, Rieder H, Meyer zum Büschenfelde KH (1988) Interleukin-6, the third mediator of acute-phase reaction, modulates hepatic protein synthesis in human and mouse. Comparison with interleukin 1 β and tumor necrosis factor-α. Eur J Immunol 18:1259–1264
90. Rokita H, Shirahama T, Cohen AS, Meek RL, Benditt EP, Sipe J (1987) Differential expression of the amyloid SAA3 gene in liver and peritoneal macrophages of mice undergoing dissimilar inflammatory processes. J Immunol 139:3849–3853
91. Rosenthal CJ, Sullivan LM (1979) Serum amyloid A to monitor cancer dissemination. Ann Intern med 91:383–390
92. Sack GH Jr (1988) Serum amyloid (SAA) gene variations in familial Mediterranean fever. Mol Biol Med 5:61–67
93. Seckinger P, Williamson K, Balavoine J-F, Bach B, Mazzei G, Shaw A, Dayer J-M (1987) A urine inhibitor of interleukin-1 activity affects both interleukin-1 α and -1 β but not tumor necrosis factor α1. J immunol 139:1541–1545
94. Seckinger P, Isaaz S, Dayer J-M (1988) A human inhibitor of tumor necrosis factor α. J Exp Med 167:1511–1516
95. Sipe JD, Colten HR, Goldberger G, Edge MD, Tack BF, Cohen AS, Whitehead AS (1985) Human serum amyloid A (SAA): biosynthesis and postsynthetic processing of preSAA and structural variants by complementary DNA. Biochemistry 24:2931–2935
96. Skogen B, Natvig JB (1981) Degradation of amyloid proteins by different serine proteases. Scand J Immunol 14:389–396
97. Skogen B, Børresen AL, Natvig JB, Berg K, Michaelsen TE (1979) High-density lipoproteins as carrier for amyloid-related protein sAA in rabbit serum. Scand J Immunol 10:39–45
98. Sletten K, Husby G (1974) The complete amino acid sequence of non-immuno-globulin amyloid fibril protein AS in rheumatoid arhritis. Eur J Biochem 41:117–125
99. Sletten K, Marhaug G, Husby G (1983) The covalent structure of amyloid-related serum protein SAA from two patients with inflammatory disease. Hoppe-Zeyler's Physiol Chem 364:1039–1046
100. Sletten K, Husebekk A, Husby G (1989) The primary structure of equine serum amyloid A (SAA) protein. Scand J Immunol 30:117–122
101. Snow AD, Willmer J, Kisilevsky R (19879 A close structural relationship between sulfated proteoglycans and AA amyloid fibrils. Lab Invest 57:687–698
102. Syversen V, Sletten K, Marhaug G, Husby G, Lium B (1987) The amino acid sequence of serum amyloid A (SAA) in mink. Scand J Immunol 26:763–767
103. Tape C, Tan R, Nesheim M, Kisilevsky R (1988) Direct evidence for circulating apoSAA as the precursor of tissue AA amyloid deposits. Scand J Immunol 28:317–324
104. Trinchieri G, Perussia B (1985) Immune interferon: a pleiotropic lymphokine with multiple effects. Immunol Today 6:131–136

105. Turnell W, Sarra R, Glover ID, Baum JO, Caspi D, Baltz ML, Pepys MD (1986)
     Secondary structure prediction of human SAA 1. Presumptive identification of calcium
     and lipid binding sites. Mol Biol Med 3:387–407
106. Turnell W, Sarra R, Baum JO, Caspi D, Baltz ML, Pepys MB (1986) X-ray scattering and
     diffraction by wet gels of AA amyloid fibrils. Mol Biol Med 3:409–424
107. Waalen K, Sletten K, Husby G, Nordstoga K (1980) The primary structure of amyloid
     fibril protein AA in endotoxin-induced amyloidosis of the mink. Eur J Biochem
     104:407–412
108. Wohlgethan JR, Cathcart ES (1980) Amyloid resistance in A/J mice. Studies with a
     transfer model. Lab Invest 42:663–67
109. Wong GG, Clark SC (1988) Multiple actions of interleukin-6 within a cytokine network.
     Immunol Today 9:137–139
110. Woo P, Sipe J, Dinarello CA, Colten HR (1987) Structure of a human serum amyloid A
     gene and modulation of its expression in transfected L cells. J Biol Chem 262:15790–
     15795
111. Woo P, O'Brien J, Robson M, Ansell BM (1987) A genetic marker for systemic
     amyloidosis in juvenile arthritis. Lancet 2:767–769
112. Yamamoto KI, Shiroo M, Migita S (1986) Diverse gene expression for isotypes of murine
     serum amyloid A protein during acute-phase reaction. Science 232:227–229

Markers of Cartilage Destruction

F. A. Wollheim[1] and T. Saxne[2],*

[1] Professor and Chairman, Department of Rheumatology, Lund University Hospital, Lund, Sweden
[2] Department of Rheumatology and Department of Physiological Chemistry, University of Lund, Sweden

Introduction

Progressive destruction of the normal architecture of the joint is a hallmark of chronic joint diseases such as rheumatoid arthritis and osteoarthritis. Cartilage and juxta-articular bone are degraded, resulting in functional impairment and disability. However, progressive destruction does not always occur. Therefore, it is desirable to identify patients at risk for developing severe joint damage as candidates for early aggressive but also toxic drug therapy in selected cases [1]. Biochemical markers of disease activity in routine use primarily reflect inflammation, which is not necessarily linked to the destructive process [2]. Therefore, levels of inflammatory markers are usually not suitable for monitoring tissue destruction. Radiography can be used only to show late events in the process, since when changes are visible on radiograms the damage at the molecular level is already advanced. Treatment at this stage may be too late to affect the destructive process. These limiations in the currently used measures also reduce the possibility of identifying the beneficial effects of new drugs on joint destruction.

However, the increased knowledge of cartilage biochemistry gained during the past several decades has provided new tools for monitoring tissue damage in joint disease (for reviews see [3–6]. It is thus now becoming possible to quantify cartilage-specific macromolecules in body fluids their tissue specificity and release during early phases of the destructive process will facilitate the understanding of this process and should provide new means for detecting early cartilage damage.

In this review we will give a brief overview of the biochemical structure of cartilage and outline the rationale for quantifying cartilage macromolecules in

* T. S. is presently the recipient of a research grant from the German Center for Rheumatic Research in Berlin

Smolen, Kalden, Maini (Eds.)
Rheumatoid Arthritis
© Springer-Verlag Berlin Heidelberg 1992

body fluids. The markers, which have been measured in clinical studies, will be presented with relevant examples. Finally, the future potentials and limitations of this new technology will be discussed.

Structure of Cartilage

Cartilage is a specialized connective tissue, the few cells of which – the chondrocytes are dispersed in an abundant extracellular matrix. The chondrocytes synthesize all matrix components, and they are also capable of producing enzymes which participate in cartilage degradation both during normal turnover and in pathological conditions [7]. Seventy-five percent of the extracellular matrix is water. The organic material consists of three main components. Collagen, predominantly type II, constitutes about 70% of the dry weight [5], but also minor collagens (types VI, IX, X, and XI) are present in small amounts (for reviews see [8–10]. Proteoglycans, mainly of the large, aggregating type, make up about 20% of the dry weight (for reviews see [4, 5 and 11]). A heterogeneous group of other non-collageneous matrix proteins constitutes approximately 10% of the organic material (for review see [4]). The type-II collagen fibers create a network in which the

Table 1. Cartilage matrix macromolecules (for references see [4, 8–10, 33–35]

Protein	Properties
Large, aggregating proteoglycan	Provides resilience
Link protein	Stabilizes proteoglycan aggregate
PG-S1 (biglycan)	Homology with decorin and fibromodulin; no known function
PG-S2 (decorin)	Modulates collagen fibril formation
Fibromodulin (59-kD protein)	Modulates collagen fibril formation
Cartilage matrix protein (CMP, 148-kD protein)	Interacts with proteoglycans(?)
Cartilage oligomeric matrix protein (COMP)	No known function
58-kD protein	Chondrocyte attachment?
36-kD protein	Chondrocyte attachment
Anchorin	Binds to type-II collagen
Collagen II carboxylterminal propeptide (chondrocalcin)	No known function. Binds to hydroxylapatite
Type-II collagen	Fibril forming, tensile strength
Type-VI collagen	Function unknown
Type-IX collagen	Binds to type-II collagen fibrils – stabilizes fibrillar network?
Type-X collagen	Role in remodeling and bone formation?
Type-XI collagen	Binds to type-II collagen fibrils – stabilizes fibrillar network?

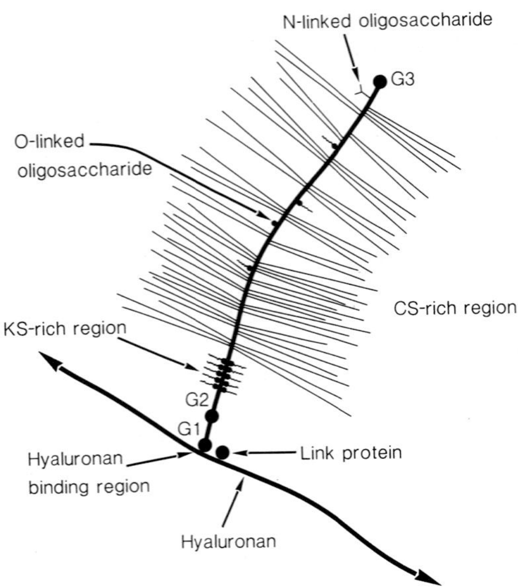

Fig. 1. Principal structure of the large, aggregating cartilage proteoglycan. The central protein core with three globular domains (*G1, G2,* and *G3*) is substituted with a large number of negatively charged chondroitin sulfate chains (*CS*), keratan sulfate chains (*KS*), and oligosaccharides. For references see [4] and [11]

other components are entrapped. Table 1 outlines the principal components of cartilage.

The large, aggregating proteoglycan has an Mr of about 3.5×10^6. Its principal structure is shown in Fig. 1. The molecule consists of a central protein core with an Mr of around 220000 [12]. Negatively charged side chains of chondroitin sulfate and keratan sulfate are covalently attached at two distinct parts of the core protein. The keratan sulfate-rich region represents approximately 10% of the core and contains most of the some 30 keratan sulfate chains [13], whereas the chondroitin sulfate-rich region contains about 100 chondroitin sulfate side chains and is situated closer to the C-terminal end of the core protein. This C-terminal globular part of the core protein shows homology with a lectin specific for galactose [14]. The N-terminal part of the core protein contains two homologous, globular domains [15]. The one situated most N-terminally binds specifically to hyaluronan (hyaluronic acid). Thus, several proteoglycans can bind to one hyaluronan molecule, creating a large aggregate. This aggregate is further stabilized by another matrix protein, the link protein, that binds both to the hyaluronan-binding domain of the proteoglycan monomer and to hyaluronan (for references see [11]). The aggregating proteoglycans are found only in cartilage, although many connective tissues contain large proteoglycans which can bind to hyaluronan [16]. The N-terminal and C-terminal globular domains appear to have structures related to those of the cartilage proteoglycans, and these proteoglycans show extensive cross-reactivity in immunoassays for the hyaluronan-binding region [17]. However, the protein backbone of the chondroitin sulfate-rich region is different.

Cartilage, like most connective tissues, contains small proteoglycans of two types. They have protein cores with an Mr of around 32000 [18–20]. PG-S1 (biglycan) contains two chondroitin sulfate or dermatan sulfate side chains, depending on the tissue origin. PG-S2 (decorin) contains only one chondroitin/dermatan sulfate side chain [17]. Fibromodulin, another matrix protein with wide distribution, has a tyrosine-rich domain characteristic of glycosaminoglycans containing tyrosine sulfate [19]. Thus, these three molecules all contain polyanionic structures in their N-terminal domain. In addition, fibromodulin also contains keratan sulfate chains attached to the molecule [19]. Fibromodulin and decorin both bind to the fibril-forming collagens with high affinity, and in vitro they inhibit collagen fibrillogenesis [21].

Cartilage matrix protein (148-kD protein) is a cartilage-specific protein, particularly enriched in tracheal cartilage [22]. Notably, it is present in neither normal adult nor arthritic articular cartilage [23, 24]. It contains three subunits with Mr of approximately 50000, linked via disulfide bridges [22, 25]. The function of the protein is not known; however, it has been shown to interact with the large, aggregating proteoglycans (Heinegård, personal communication). Cartilage oligomeric matrix protein (COMP) is also specific for cartilage and is particularly enriched in articular cartilage ([26]; D. Heinegård, personal communication). It consists of several subunits with apparent Mr 100000. The protein is anionic, seemingly due to its content of acidic carbohydrate substituents (D. Heinegård, personal communication). The function of the protein is not clear. The 58-kD protein is found in most connective tissues [27], and the 36-kD protein is prominent in both cartilage and bone [4, 28]. The functions of these proteins are not known, but they may promote chondrocyte attachment [4]. Anchorin is a protein which binds to type-II collagen and may mediate anchoring of collagen to chondrocytes [29]. Fibronectin, the classical mediator of cell attachment and binding of matrix constituents, is a minor constituent of normal adult cartilage. However, the concentration increases in osteoarthritic cartilage [30]. Chondrocalcin is an oligomeric protein present in all types of cartilage and is most prominent in articular and mineralized cartilage. Upon reduction, the protein forms subunits with apparent Mr 35000. The protein is identical with the C-terminal propeptide of procollagen II [31].

Type-II collagen is the predominating collagen of cartilage. It consists of a triple helix formed from three identical α-chains. Type-II collagen forms the fibrils responsible for the tensile properties of the tissue. It is cross-linked by covalent cross-links, e.g., the pyridinoline cross-link [8]. The fiber-forming collagens in different tissues are structurally very similar, although sufficiently different to allow specific antibodies to be raised [32]. Type-IX collagen is found only in cartilage and contains three α-chains which are structurally different from those of type-II collagen (for references see [8]). In addition this collagen contains a chondroitin sulfate side chain [33]. Type-IX collagen can bind to type-II collagen [34]. Types-X and -XI collagen are unique to cartilage, the former being found predominantly in hypertrophic cartilage (for references see [8, 9]). Type-XI collagen also binds to type-II collagen fibrils [35].

Rationale for Measuring Cartilage Components in Body Fluids

During normal turnover, and in increased amounts in disease, cartilage macromolecules are continuously degraded and new ones are formed. The regulation of this process is insufficiently known [36], but it is well established that proteoglycans are degraded early in a pathological process such as rheumatoid arthritis (for references see [5]). The subsequent events are less well known, but it is hypothesized that then the noncollagenous matrix proteins and finally the collagen fibers are degraded. This process is shown schematically in Fig. 2. Notably, there is always a close connection between anabolic and catabolic processes. Thus, degradation of matrix components always results in a repair process, attempting to build fresh matrix, which means that the result of analysis of a released marker is always influenced by both facets of the cartilage metabolism.

The degraded fragments are released into the synovial fluid and leave the joint cavity mainly by the lymphatic drainage [37], subsequently reaching the

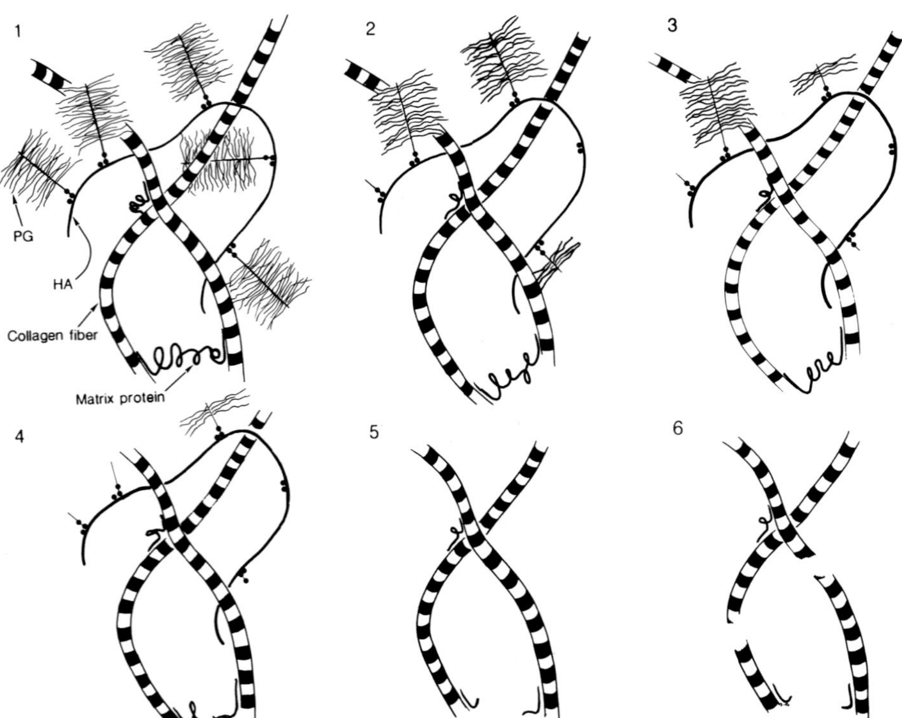

Fig. 2. Fragmentation and loss of macromolecules from cartilage during progressive matrix degeneration. *PG,* Proteoglycan, *HA,* hyaluronan. (Courtesy of Prof. D. Heinegård. Reproduced with permission from Frymoyer and Gordon [8])

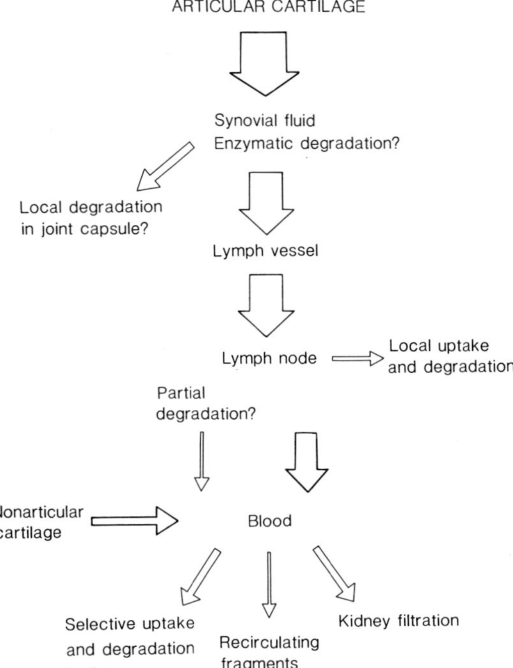

Fig. 3. Putative pathways for release and catabolism of articular cartilage macromolecules. Macromolecules are fragmented by proteases and released into the surrounding synovial fluid. The fragments are eliminated by lymphatic drainage to the blood and are then removed by liver uptake or kidney filtration. Note influx of fragments from other cartilage types

circulation. A fraction of the fragments are presumably entrapped in the lymphatic system [38]; a significant proportion is eliminated through uptake and metabolism in the liver endothelial cells [39]. Finally, smaller fragments may be eliminated through kidney filtration. It should be noted that limited information is available about the quantitative importance of each of these extra-articular metabolic pathways, making interpretation of results of serum or urinary measurements difficult [40, 41]. Serum and urinary results are also influenced by the release of cartilage antigens from extra-articular sites, such as the tracheobronchial tree and the intervertebral disks. Figure 3 outlines the metabolic pathways for released cartilage molecules. This chain of events forms the basis for the efforts to develop assays for measuring cartilage markers in synovial fluid, blood, and urine.

Macromolecules, with Potentials as Cartilage Markers

All cartilage matrix components or fragments of these are presumably released during tissue turnover and thus have the potential of being measurable cartilage markers in synovial fluid and possibly also in blood and urine.

Proteoglycans

Determinations of proteoglycan antigens in body fluids initially employed chemical methods of detecting glycosaminoglycans [42]. These polysaccharides are not tissue specific, however, which creates difficulties in determining the source of the molecules. Measured values in synovial fluid are also difficult to interpret, since the synovial tissue cells produce glycosaminoglycans [43]. Analyses of these compounds have therefore been of limited value in clinical practice. However, in recent reports results from such assays have been shown to correlate with results obtained with the more tissue-specific methods described below ([44, 45], S. Björnsson, personal communication).

The development of sensitive, specific immunochemical techniques for measuring proteoglycan epitopes in body fluids provides more reliable tools for studying the metabolic disturbance of cartilage in joint disease. The approaches applied in patient studies are shown in Table 2.

Making use of the limited tissue distribution of the glycosaminoglycan keratan sulfate, immunochemical assays for its determination using monoclonal antibodies have been developed [46–49]. Since more than 95% of the keratan sulfate in the body is present in cartilage and the intervertebral disks, the bulk of the circulating keratan sulfate originates from cartilage [5]. Several antibodies with slightly different specificities have been used. Most published results have been obtained using antibodies which recognize highly sulphated keratan sulfate chains [47, 49, 50]. One problem with this is that the extent of sulfatation may vary considerably between individuals [6]. It should also be noted that the antibodies raised by different investigators are not identical. Since cleavage of the molecule may give rise to various fragments under different conditions, different results from different investigators may occur.

Another approach is to develop assays for the detection of epitopes on the core protein of the cartilage proteoglycan. Most clinical studies have been performed with an ELISA using a polyclonal antibody preferentially recognizing the chondroitin sulfate-rich region of the core protein of the large, aggregating proteoglycan of cartilage [51, 66]; for references see [5, 52], but

Table 2. Immunochemical assays used to quantify proteoglycan fragments

Year	Reference	Test and specificity	Antiserum
1985	Saxne et al. [66]	ELISA, core protein	Polyclonal
1985	Gysen and Franchimont [53]	RIA, core protein	Polyclonal
1985	Thonar et al. [47]	ELISA, keratan sulfate	Monoclonal
1987	Witter et al. [48]	RIA, keratan sulfate on core protein	Monoclonal
1988	Ratcliffe et al. [50]	RIA, keratan sulfate	Monoclonal
1989	Carroll [45]	RIA, hyaluronan-binding region	Polyclonal

antibodies with other specificities have also been described ([53], for references see [48]).

Keratan sulfate and epitopes on the core protein can be measured in both synovial fluid and blood. One drawback concerning the serum analyses of these antigens is their rapid elimination from the circulation [40].

Noncollagenous Cartilage Matrix Proteins

Only a few studies measuring noncollagenous cartilage matrix proteins in patients have been reported [24, 52, 54–56]. It is possible that the elimination of some of these proteins from the circulation is slower than for proteoglycans, and serum analyses of some of these markers might therefore be more feasible.

Collagen

Information on the presence of collagen degradation products in body fluids in relation to cartilage metabolism in joint disease is scarce. Measurements of hydroxyproline or hydroxylysine in urine using colorimetric assays have been used to monitor collagen degradation [57, 58], but the value of these techniques is limited. These amino acids are not tissue specific and reach the blood stream or urine during normal or accelerated metabolism in most tissues. Furthermore, they are also released during collagen biosynthesis and maturation [59]. During degradation a large proportion is further metabolized, which means that only a fraction appears in the urine [58]. It should also be noted that the complement component C1q contributes to circulating levels [58].

The collagen cross-link pyridinoline is released during collagen breakdown, both in cartilage and in bone, and may be a marker for collagen degradation [8, 60, 61]. As yet this marker has been quantified only in urine, which limits its value, but promising results have been obtained [62, 63].

Recently, immunochemical and immunohistological assays for the detection of type-II collagen in synovial fluid using well-characterized monoclonal antibodies have been developed [64, 65], but only limited results from clinical studies are so far available.

Clinical Applications

Proteoglycan Antigens

The ELISA for proteoglycan core protein developed in Lund [51] has been used extensively for synovial fluid analyses. High levels were found in reactive arthritis and crystal-induced synovitis [66, 67], as well as in acute inflammation of the hip in children [68]. In rheumatoid arthritis a wide range of concentrations were observed, which stay remarkably constant in exudates obtained from individual joints at various points in time [69]. Expectedly low levels are characteristic of exudates from joints with advanced cartilage destruction [66]. Thus, proteoglycan levels in exudates must always be related to the condition of the joint cartilage. Proteoglycan levels in early rheumatoid arthritis may be useful prognostic markers [69]. Both synovial fluid and serum proteoglycan levels are higher in osteoarthritic patients with advanced disease than in those with advanced rheumatoid arthritis [70]. Intra-articular glucocorticoid injection results in reduced proteoglycan levels [71], most likely due to reduced release from the cartilage matrix.

Serum levels in adults are only 1% of synovial fluid levels and do not differ significantly from normal levels [67]. Whereas no age-dependent variation has been observed in adults, normal children have distinctly higher levels than normal adults. Serum levels are slightly lower in patients with juvenile chronic arthritis than in age-matched controls. In children below the age of 20 years an inverse relation between age and proteoglycan serum concentration was found [72].

A number of immunoassays based on monoclonal antisera to keratan sulfate have yielded results that conform with the results of the core protein assays, although differences also exist. Thus, Thonar et al. have also shown an age dependency for serum values of keratan sulfate, although the curve was more "bell shaped", with the highest concentrations at the age of 10–12 years [73]. A direct comparison of the tests has been undertaken, and they show good agreement although two of 22 sera showed discrepantly high core protein levels [74].

No correlations have been found between acute-phase reactants and proteoglycan core protein levels ([67], T. Saxne, unpublished data). More important is the absence of correlation between serum or synovial fluid core protein concentrations and concentrations of the aminoterminal collagen-III propeptide or hyaluronan ([75], P. Geborek, T. Saxne, A. Engström-Laurent, unpublished data). These markers, although not acute – phase reactants, nevertheless correlate to synovitis activity. In contrast, Poole and co-workers have found an inverse relation between serum levels of keratan sulfate and levels of orosomucoid or hyaluronan in patients with rheumatoid arthritis [76].

Carroll [45] compared an RIA for proteoglycans, using antibodies recognizing epitopes on the hyaluronan-binding region, with spectrophotometrical quantification of sulphated glucosaminoglycans in joint fluids from patients with rheumatoid arthritis, osteoarthritis, Reiter's syndrome, and gout, and found linear correlations with r-values between 0.95 and 0.65. Interestingly, the ratio of glycosaminoglycans over proteoglycans varied and was higher in rheumatoid arthritis than in osteoarthritis and gout, indicating qualitative differences in composition of synovial fluid glycosaminoglycans.

Although not tested in formal studies, neither nonsteroidal anti-inflammatory drugs nor second-line treatment had any noticeable influence on concentrations of cartilage-derived proteoglycans in synovial fluid or serum [67].

Low-dose oral prednisolone treatment (2.5–7.5 mg daily) seems to increase serum and synovial fluid concentrations of proteoglycans [67]. High-dose intramuscular glucocorticoid treatment (methylprednisolone 120 mg weekly; Panayi G and Saxne T, unpublished data) as well as high-dose oral prednisolone treatment (40–60 mg daily) [77], on the other hand, reduce circulating levels of proteoglycans.

CMP (148-kD Protein)

CMP has been studied with an RIA [23, 24]. The absolute synovial fluid concentrations are lower than serum levels, in agreement with the extra-articular origin of the protein. Concentrations were found to be elevated in rheumatoid arthritis [24], which is evidence for extra-articular cartilage involvement in this disease. CMP is also, as expected, a marker for disease activity in relapsing polychondritis [24].

COMP

COMP concentrations in synovial fluid have been studied by an ELISA in rheumatoid arthritis and found to relate to cartilage destruction as measured by the Larsen score in much the same way as proteoglycans [52]; the absolute levels were in the same order of magnitude. We have found higher concentrations of this marker in advanced osteoarthritis than in exudates from correspondingly destructive rheumatoid arthritis knees (T. Saxne, unpublished data). The levels of this marker in serum are approximately 10% of synovial fluid levels. The ratio is thus ten times higher than for proteoglycans, and this could make COMP useful as a serum marker for cartilage pathology.

Collagen-derived Components

Attempts to develop assays for collagen fragments with monoclonal antisera specific for type-II collagen epitopes have, in general, not been successful, although immunohistological evidence indicates the presence of type-II collagen-related material in synovial fluid phagocytes [65]. Promising results have been reported by Robins and co-workers [60–63], who developed HPLC assays and ELISAs for pyridinoline and deoxypyridinoline. The former was found in increased amounts in the urine from patients with rheumatoid arthritis, and the levels correlated with ESR and CRP.

Conclusions

Identification of a number of cartilage-specific matrix components in recent years has opened up a new field for exploration of putative markers of altered matrix metabolism. Clinically useful results have been obtained with regard to proteoglycan core protein, proteoglycan keratan sulfate epitopes, CMP, and COMP. No simple immunoassay for collagen-derived material has been reported, but urinary determination of excretion of hydroxy-pyridinium cross-links is available. Presently available assays of marker molecules usually do not allow distinction between increased release and reduced elimination, or between accelerated catabolism and stimulated synthesis with overflow into the joint fluid. Future work should be aimed at identifying markers that specifically represent either of these processes, e.g., the type-II collagen C-terminal propeptide, which holds promise as a marker for matrix synthesis. The combined use of markers with differing release patterns may generate information on pathophysiology and stage of disease, as has been exemplified in this review. Futhermore, as the knowledge of cartilage biochemistry increases, it may become possible to find markers which have a restricted distribution to a single tissue compartment. Release of such a marker could then be used to monitor involvement of that particular locus. Although serum samples are easily obtained, the problems of interpreting results of serum measurements of presently available markers previously discussed make such measurements less informative. We strongly urge that studies of processes in joint cartilage using the marker technique initially always be focused on synovial fluid analyses. In this compartment, the predominating factors which influence levels of cartilage-specific markers are release from cartilage and elimination from the joint cavity. Synovial fluid results may later be correlated to serum measurements in order to identify markers that reach the circulation and have adequately slow removal rates to be reliably quantified in serum.

References

1. Rasker JJ, Cosh JA (1984) The natural history of rheumatoid arthritis: a fifteen-year follow-up study. The prognostic significance of features noted in the first year. Clin Rheumatol 3:11–20
2. Harris ED Jr (1989) The clinical features of rheumatoid arthritis. In: Kelley WN, Harris ED Jr, Ruddy S, Sledge CB (eds) Textbook of rheumatology. Saunders, Philadelphia, pp 943–981
3. Heinegård D, Paulsson M (1987) Cartilage. In: Cunnigham LW (ed) Methods Enzymol 145:336–363
4. Heinegård D, Oldberg Å (1989) Structure and biology of cartilage and bone matrix noncollagenous macromolecules. FASEB J 3:2042–2051
5. Lohmander LS (1988) Proteoglycans of joint cartilage. Structure, function, turnover and role as markers of joint disease. In: Dixon JS, Bird H (eds) Bailliere's Clinical

Rheumatology. Biochemical Aspects of Rheumatic Disease. Bailliere Tindall, London, pp 37–62

6. Hascall VC, Glant TT (1987) Proteoglycan epitopes as potential markers of normal and pathologic cartilage metabolism. Arthritis Rheum 30:586–588

7. Stockwell RA (1979) Biology of cartilage cells. University Press, Cambridge

8. Eyre D, Benya P, Buchwalter J, Caterson B, Heinegård D, Oegema T, Pearce R, Pope M, Urban J (1989) Macromolecular constituents of cartilage and intervertebral disc. In: Frymoyer JW, Gordon SL (eds) New perspectives on low back pain. American Academy of Orthopedic Surgeons Symposium, Park Ridge, pp 147–207

9. Miller EJ, Gay S (1987) The collagens: an overview and update. Methods Enzymol 144:3–41

10. Mayne R, Irwin MH (1986) Collagen types in cartilage. In: Kuettner K, Schleyerbach R, Hascall V (eds) Cartilage biochemistry. Raven, New York, pp 23–35

11. Heinegård D, Sommarin Y (1987) Proteoglycans: an overview. Methods Enzymol 144:305–319

12. Doege K, Sasaki M, Horigan E, Hassel JR, Yamada Y (1988) Complete primary structure of the rat cartilage proteoglycan core protein deduced from cDNA clones. J Biol Chem 262:17757–17767

13. Antonsson P, Oldberg Å, Heinegård D (1989) The keratan sulfate-enriched region of bovine cartilage proteoglycan consists of a consecutively repeated hexapeptide motif. J Biol Chem 264:16170–16173

14. Halberg DF, Proulx G, Doege K, Yamada Y, Drickamer K (1988) A segment of the cartilage proteoglycan core protein has lectin-like activity. J Biol Chem 263:9456–9490

15. Mörgelin M, Paulsson M, Hardingham T, Heinegård D, Engel J (1988) Cartilage proteoglycans: assembly with hyaluronate and link proteins as studied by electron microscopy. Biochem J 253:175–185

16. Mörgelin M, Paulsson M, Malmström A, Heinegård D (1989) Shared and distinct structural features of interstitial proteoglycans from different bovine tissues revealed by electron microscopy. J Biol Chem 264:12080–12090

17. Heinegård D, Björne-Persson A, Cöster L, Franzen A, Gardell S, Malmström A, Sandfalk R, Vogel K (1985) The core protein of large and small interstitial proteoglycans from various connective tissues form distinct subgroups. Biochem J 230:181–194

18. Rouslahti E (1988) Structure and biology of proteoglycans. Annu Rev Cell Biol 4:229–255

19. Oldberg Å, Antonsson P, Lindblom K, Heinegård D (1989) A collagen-binding 59-kDa protein (fibromodulin) is structurally related to the small interstitial proteoglycans PG-S1 and PG-S2 (decorin). EMBO J 8:2601–2604

20. Fischer L, Termine J, Young M (1989) Deduced protein sequence of bone small proteoglycan I (biglycan) shows homology with proteoglycan II (decorin) and several nonconnective tissue proteins in a variety of species. J Biol Chem 264:4571–4576

21. Hedbom E, Heinegård D (1989) Interactions of a 59-kDa connective tissue matrix protein with collagen I and collagen II. J Biol Chem 264:6898–6905

22. Paulsson M, Heinegård D (1981) Purification and structural characterization of a cartilage matrix protein. Biochem J 197:367–375

23. Paulsson M, Heinegård D (1982) Radioimmunoassay of the 148-kilodalton cartilage protein: distribution of the protein among bovine tissues. Biochem J 207:207–213

24. Saxne T, Heinegård D (1989) Involvement of nonarticular cartilage as demonstrated by release of a cartilage-specific protein in rheumatoid arthritis. Arthritis Rheum 32:1080–1086

25. Kiss I, Deak F, Holloway Jr RG, Delius H, Mebust KA, Frimberger E, Argraves WS, Tsonis PA, Winterbottom N, Goetinck PF (1989) Structure of the gene for cartilage matrix protein, a modular protein of the extracellular matrix. J Biol Chem 264:8126–8134

26. Fife RS, Brandt KD (1984) Identification of a high-molecular-weight (>400000) protein in hyaline cartilage. Biochim Biophys Acta 802:506–514

27. Heinegård D, Larsson T, Sommarin Y, Franzen A, Paulsson M, Hedbom E (1986) Two novel matrix proteins isolated from articular cartilage show wide distribution among connective tissues. J Biol Chem 261:13866–13872

28. Larsson T (1989) Cartilage matrix biology. Studies on factors of relevance for tissue homeostasis. Thesis, University of Lund
29. Fernandez MP, Selmin O, Martin GR, Yamada Y, Pfäffle M, Deutzmann R, Mollenhauer J, von der Mark K (1988) The structure of anchorin CII, a collagen-binding protein isolated from chondrocyte membrane. J Biol Chem 263:5921–5925
30. Wurster NB, Lust G (1982) Fibronectin in osteoarthritic canine articular cartilage. Biochem Biophys Res Commun 109:1094–1101
31. Van der Rest M, Rosenberg LC, Olsen BR, Poole AR (1986) Chondrocalcin is identical with the C-propeptide of type-II procollagen. Biochem J 237:923–925
32. Timpl R (1984) Immunology of the collagens. In: Piez K, Reddi K (eds) Extracellular matrix biochemistry. Elsevier, New York, pp 159–190
33. Konomi H, Seyer JM, Ninomiya Y, Olsen BR (1986) Peptide-specific antibodies identify the $\alpha 2$ chain as the proteoglycan subunit of type-IX collagen. J Biol Chem 261:6742–6746
34. Vaughan L, Mendler M, Huber S, Bruckner P, Winterhalter KH, Irwin MI, Mayne R (1988) D-periodic distribution of collagen type IX along cartilage fibrils. J Cell Biol 106:991–997
35. Mendler M, Eich-Bender SG, Vaughan L, Winterhalter KH, Bruckner P (1989) Cartilage contains mixed fibrils of collagen types II, IX and XI. J Cell Biol 108:191–197
36. Morales TI, Hascall VC (1989) Factors involved in the regulation of proteoglycan metabolism in articular cartilage. Arthritis Rheum 32:1197–1201
37. Weinberger A, Simkin PA (1989) Plasma protein in synovial fluids of normal human joints. Semin Arthritis Rheum 19:66–76
38. Fraser JRE (1989) Hyaluronan: sources, turnover and metabolism. In: Lindh E, Thorell J (eds) Clinical impact of bone and connective tissue markers. Academic, London, pp 31–49
39. Smedsrød B (1989) Catabolism in liver sinusoids. In: Lindh E, Thorell J (eds) Clinical impact of bone and connective tissue markers. Academic, London, pp 51–73
40. Heinegård D, Saxne T (1991) Connective tissue macromolecules as markers for tissue processes in joint disease. Eur J Rheumatol Inflamm 11:91–99
41. Brandt KD (1989) A pessimistic view of serologic markers for diagnosis and management of osteoarthritis. Biochemical, immunologic and clinicopathologic barriers. J Rheumatol 16 [Suppl 18]:39–42
42. Seppälä PO, Kärkkäinen J, Lethonen A, Mäkisara P (1972) Chondroitin sulphate in the normal and rheumatoid synovial fluid. Clin Chim Acta 36:549–553
43. Marsh JM, Wiebkin OW, Gale S, Muir H, Maini RN (1979) Synthesis of sulphated proteoglycans by rheumatoid and normal tissue in culture. Ann Rheum Dis 38:166–170
44. Carroll GJ (1987) Spectrophotometric measurement of proteoglycans in osteoarthritic synovial fluid. Ann Rheum Dis 46:375–379
45. Carroll GJ (1989) Measurement of sulphated glycosaminoglycans and proteoglycan fragments in arthritic synovial fluid. Ann Rheum Dis 48:17–24
46. Caterson B, Christner JE, Baker JR (1983) Identification of a monoclonal antibody that specifically recognizes corneal and skeletal keratan sulfate: monoclonal antibodies to cartilage proteoglycan. J Biol Chem 258:8848–8854
47. Thonar EJ-MA, Lenz ME, Klintworth GK, Caterson B, Pachman LM, Glickman P, Katz R, Huff J, Kuettner KE (1985) Quantification of keratan sulfate in blood as a marker of cartilage catabolism. Arthritis Rheum 28:1367–1376
48. Witter J, Roughley PJ, Webber C, Roberts N, Keystone E, Poole AR (1987) The immunologic detection and characterization of cartilage proteoglycan degradation in synovial fluids of patients with arthritis. Arthritis Rheum 30:519–529
49. Zanetti M, Ratcliffe A, Watt FM (1985) Two subpopulations of differential chondrocytes identified with a monoclonal antibody to keratan sulfate. J Cell Biol 101:53–59
50. Ratcliffe A, Doherty M, Maini RN, Hardingham TE (1988) Icreased concentrations of proteoglycan components in the synovial fluids of patients with acute but not chronic joint disease. Ann Rheum Dis 47:826–832
51. Heinegård D, Inerot S, Wieslander J, Lindblad G (1985) A method for the quantification of cartilage proteoglycan structures liberated to the synovial fluid during developing degenerative joint disease. Scand J Clin Lab Invest 45:421–427

52. Saxne T (1989) Molecular markers for joint disease. In: Lindh E, Thorell J (eds) Clinical impact of bone and connective tissue markers. Academic, London, pp 223–228
53. Gysen P, Franchimont P (1984) Radioimmunoassay of proteoglycans. J Immunoassay 5:221–243
54. Fife RS (1988) Identification of cartilage matrix glycoprotein in synovial fluid in human osteoarthritis. Arthritis Rheum 31:553–556
55. Fife RS, Myers SL, Brandt KD, Ehrlich J, Shelbourne D (1989) Failure to detect "early" osteoarthritis of the knee by a screening test for cartilage matrix glycoprotein in serum (abstract). Arthritis Rheum 32 [Suppl 4]:107
56. Shinmei M, Naramatsu Y, Tanaka O, Inamori Y, Shimomura Y, Matsuyama S, Matsuzawa K (1989) Increased levels of chondrocalcin (type-II collagen C-propeptide) in osteoarthritic synovial fluids (abstract). Arthritis Rheum 32 [Suppl 4]:108
57. Kivirikko KI (1970) Urinary excretion of hydroxyproline in health and disease. Int Rev Connect Tissue Res 5:93–163
58. Krane SM, Kantrowitz FG, Byrne M, Pinnell SR, Singer FR (1977) Urinary excretion of hydroxylysine and its glycosides as an index of collagen degradation. J Clin Invest 59:819–827
59. Bienkowski RS, Engels CJ (1981) Measurement of intracellular collagen degradation. Anal Biochem 116:414–424
60. Robins SP (1983) Cross-linking of collagen: isolation, structural characterization and glycosylation of pyridinoline. Biochem J 215:167–173
61. Robins SP (1982) An enzyme-linked immunoassay for the collagen cross-link pyridinoline. Biochem J 207:617–620
62. Robins SP, Stewart P, Astbury C, Bird HA (1986) Measurement of the cross-linking compound, pyridinoline, in urine as an index of collagen degradation in joint disease. Ann Rheum Dis 45:969–973
63. Black C, Marabani M, Sturrock RD, Robins SP (1989) Urinary excretion of the hydroxypyridinium cross-links of collagen in patients with rheumatoid arthritis. Ann Rheum Dis 48:641–644
64. Stewart TE, Mestecky J, Moreland LW, Gay S (1989) Immunoassay for collagen type II in synovial fluid and serum of patients with erosive joint disease (abstract). Arthritis Rheum 32 [Suppl 4]:84
65. Moreland LW, Stewart T, Gay RE, Guo Qiang Huang, McGee N, Gay S (1989) Immunohistologic demonstration of type-II collagen in synovial fluid phagocytes of osteoarthritis and rheumatoid arthritis patients. Arthritis Rheum 32:1458–1464
66. Saxne T, Heinegård D, Wollheim FA, Pettersson H (1985) Difference in cartilage proteoglycan level in synovial fluid in early rheumatoid arthritis and reactive arthritis. Lancet 2:127–128
67. Saxne T, Heinegård D, Wollheim FA (1987) Cartilage proteoglycans in synovial fluid and blood in inflammatory joint disease. Relation to systemic treatment. Arthritis Rheum 30:972–979
68. Lohmander LS, Wingstrand H, Heinegård D (1988) Transient synovitis of the hip in the child: increased levels of proteoglycan fragments in joint fluid. J Orthop Res 6:420–424
69. Saxne T, Wollheim FA, Pettersson H, Heinegård D (1987) Proteoglycan concentration in synovial fluid: predictor of future cartilage destruction in rheumatoid arthritis? Br Med J 295:1447–1448
70. Saxne T, Carlsson Å (1990) Cartilage markers in synovial fluid and blood in osteoarthritis and rheumatoid arthritis. Scand J Rheum (abstr) 19:171
71. Saxne T, Heinegård D, Wollheim FA (1986) Therapeutic effects on cartilage metabolism in arthritis as measured by release of proteoglycan structures into the synovial fluid. Ann Rheum Dis 45:491–497
72. Saxne T, Castro F, Rydholm U, Svantesson H (1989) Cartilage-derived proteoglycans in body fluids of children. Inverse correlation with age. J Rheumatol 16:1341–1344
73. Thonar E J-M A, Pachman LM, Lenz ME, Hayford J, Lynch P, Kuettner KE (1988) Age-related changes in the concentration of serum keratan sulphate in children. J Clin Chem Clin Biochem 26:57–63

74. Saxne T, Hayford J, Heinegård D, Lenz ME, Thonar E, Wolheim FA, Pachman L (1989) Serum levels of the proteoglycan core protein and keratan sulfate correlate in juvenile rheumatoid arthritis (abstract). Arthritis Rheum 32 [Suppl 4]:105
75. Hörslev-Petersen K, Saxne T, Haar D, Thomsen BS, Bendtsen KD, Junker P, Lorenzen I (1988) The aminoterminal-type-III procollagen peptide and proteoglycans in serum and synovial fluid in patients with rheumatoid arthritis or reactive arthritis. Rheumatol Int 8:1–9
76. Poole AR, Witter J, Roberts N, Piccolo F, Brandt R, Paquin J, Baron M (1990) Inflammation and cartilage metabolism in rheumatoid arthritis: studies of the blood markers hyaluronic acid, orosomucoid and keratan sulfate. Arthritis Rheum 33:790–799
77. Campion G, Schnitzer T, Zeitz H, Thonar E (1989) The effect of oral administration of prednisolone and of the non-steroidal anti-inflammatory drug piroxicam on serum keratan sulfate (abstract). Arthritis Rheum 32 [Suppl 4]:105

Therapy

Progress in the Therapy of Rheumatoid Arthritis

J. R. Kalden

Institute of Clinical Immunology and Rheumatology, Department of Internal Medicine III, Friedrich Alexander-Universität Erlangen-Nürnberg, Krankenhausstr. 12, W-8520 Erlangen, FRG

Introduction

Despite intensive efforts over the past several decades to widen the therapeutic repertoire for the treatment of rheumatoid arthritis (RA), there has been little change. The current treatment facilities can be illustrated by the traditional pyramid, following the disease activity in the therapeutic regimens. On the first level are the nonsteroidal anti-inflammatory drugs (NSAIDs), which, however, have not proven to be sufficient over the long term. Thus, second-level agents, which are characterized by a delayed onset of action and which lack the analgetic properties of NSAIDs, are subsequently used, compounds such as gold, anti-malarials, D-penicillamine, or sulfasalazine, which have been specified as disease-modifying antirheumatic drugs (DMARDs). If these DMARDs do not prove to be effective, immunosuppressive agents such as methotrexate, azathioprine, or cytotoxic substances, mainly cyclophosphamide, are applied. In parallel, following the first- and second-line drugs within this classical pyramid, steroids are used intermittently or additionally – either in low doses or even as a high-dose pulse therapy [1]. Furthermore, treatment of RA has always been complemented by surgery, and if necessary by intra-articular inoculation of steroids and rehabilitive therapies.

Although the classical pyramid of drug treatment in RA might be of some help for general practitioners and rheumatologists in treating RA patients, this concept is not altogether satisfactory. While in short-term studies a positive effect on synovial inflammation has been shown, long-term observations indicate that this effect is not maintained. In addition, as recently shown by Kushner [2] fewer than 20% of patients remain on a second-line drug for 5 years, mainly due to side effects. With regard to the efficacy of a specific therapeutic regimen, some interesting studies have demonstrated that a progression or an arrest of radiographic erosions was correlated with clinical and laboratory parameters of inflammation, regardless of the medication administered [3–5]. With regard to 2-year follow-up studies, only gold, cyclophosphamide, and cortisone prevented a radiographic progression in at least 70% of the patients studied [6, 7, 8].

Smolen, Kalden, Maini (Eds.)
Rheumatoid Arthritis
© Springer-Verlag Berlin Heidelberg 1992

This lack of effective treatment regimes for RA has triggered a search for new treatment approaches. Thus cyclosporin A, a potent immunosuppressive agent, has been used in open, controlled and randomized trials. Although a significant effect was found with regard to the suppression of the inflammatory activity in three published studies, therapy had to be interrupted because of frequent and severe side effects, including nephrotoxicity [9–11]. There have also been attempts to improve the therapeutic repertoire for RA with different combinations of second-line and immunosuppressive agents. However, the combination of D-penicillamine and hydroxychloroquine produced no improvement of the clinical course of relative treatment with the single compounds over a period of 2 years [12, 13]. In contrast to these results, some positive effects were reported with the combination of gold and hydroxychloroquine [14]. With the combination of hydroxychloroquine, azathioprine, and cyclophosphomide [15] in the treatment of patients with severe nodular RA complicated by systemic vasculitis, a complete remission was observed in 51%. Another 41% were nearly in complete remission or showed partial depression of the disease activity. Of special interest in this study is the fact that in 65% of the patients treated improvement or arrest of the radiographic erosions was recorded.

Methotrexate is currently experiencing a renaissance in RA medication. There are several communications demonstrating a significant beneficial effect on the course of the disease with administration of 12–15 mg/week [16–18]. Although methotrexate was shown to be effective at least over a period of 36–53 months, in a study by Kremer and Lee [16], radiologic evidence of a disease progression was noted after 24 months of treatment, and in addition, toxic effects, especially with regard to the liver, were defined as major factors in limiting long-term treatment [19, 20]. Other trials such as that performed by Rau et al. [21] revealed no significant difference in the liver histology between biopsies of 16 patients with RA before the application of methotrexate and 40 biopsies taken during the treatment.

Besides the application of new drug compounds or a combination therapy of different immunosuppressive and immunomodulating agents, attempts have also been made to influence effectively the clinical course of RA with the pentapeptide thymopoietin (TP 5) [22–25]. In a placebo-controlled double-blind randomized study in which 21 patients received intravenous injections of Thymopentin, a significant improvement was seen after 3 weeks in the Thymopentin-treated group [25]. However, further studies are necessary to prove the efficacy of TP 5 therapy, including a dose-finding study as well as long-term treatment investigations.

There is ample evidence linking sex hormones with autoimmunity [26]. Thus changes in the clinical course of systemic and organ-related autoimmune diseases have been reported. The effect of sex hormones has been demonstrated on regulatory T cells as well as on different subsets of B cells, mainly CD5 positive, which are thought to be responsible for autoantibody production [27]. The finding that in several experimental animal models of arthropathies both estrogenic and androgenic hormones modulate the severity of arthritis [28, 29]

Table 1. New therapeutic approaches in the treatment of rheumatoid arthritis

A. Total lymphoid irradiation	D. Peptides
B. Antibodies	E. Others
a. Immunoglobulin preparations	a. Collagen II
b. Monoclonal antibodies	b. Immunotoxins
C. Cytokines and cytokine inhibitors	c. Photopheresis
a. IL-1 and IL-1 inhibitors	F. T-cell vaccination*
b. IL-2 and IL-2 inhibitors	
c. Interferon gamma	

See contribution by Breedveld et al., this volume

has lead to attempts using estrogen treatment in RA patients. However, as reported by Bijlsma et al. [30], the efficacy of estrogen treatment in RA patients was less impressive.

From this short summary on the different treatments available for RA, it is ovbious that the therapeutic repertoire has to be improved by the search for and/or development of new treatment modalities, based upon our increasing knowledge of immunopathogenic mechanisms underlying tissue-destructive mechanisms in rheumatoid arthritis.

New Approaches to the Therapy of RA

During the plast few years, various new avenues to treating RA have been explored and, in certain situations, they have already been applied clinically (Table 1). On the other hand, some of the therapeutic approaches shown in Table 1 are still rather hypothetical.

Total Lymphoid Irradiation

Total lymphoid irradiation (TLI) has been applied in patients with refractory rheumatoid arthritis in several therapeutic trials. According to a communication by Brahn et al. [31], after completion of TLI, a significant improvement was noted in several disease parameters, including number of swollen joints, duration of morning stiffness, and 50 ft. walking time. Additionally, blood lymphopenia and a decrease in T helper cells were noted. A beneficial effect of TLI in refractory arthritis was suggested. Further data were subsequently published by Strober et al. [32]. In a randomized double-blind study, 13 patients with intractable rheumatoid arthritis were subjected to full-dose total lymphoid irradiation (2000 rad), and 11 patients were assigned to receive a control low-dose total lymphoid irradiation (220 rad). Alleviation of joint disease activity was significantly greater in the high-dose group, as judged on the basis of morning stiffness, joint tenderness, and functional assessment 3 and 6 months after radiotherapy. Complications following high-dose therapy, were transient neutropenia, thrombocytopenia, pericarditis, and pleurisy. Using TLI, significant changes in immunologic parameters such as suppression of pokeweed mitogen-induced stimulation of immunoglobulin production [33], changes in T-cell subsets [34], and a marked decrease in the number and function of peripheral blood helper/inducer T lymphocytes as well as a significant decrease in the spontaneous secretion of interleukin 1 in synovial biopsy specimens were recorded [35]. Although 2000 cGy were found to be sufficient to produce measurable therapeutic benefits for 6 at least months in patients with otherwise refractory RA [36], major side effects have raised serious questions with regard to the feasibility of this treatment approach. In a study by Sherrer et al. [37], patients who had received either total lymphoid irradiation or immunosuppressive treatment for intractable RA were compared. Stability levels and motility were equal in both groups. However, there were more hospitalizations for infections in the TLI group, and the infecting organisms tended to be staphylococcus or gram-negative organisms. In our own experiments [38] in 11 patients with intractable RA, a significant improvement of the clinical symptoms was observed after 6 months of treatment; this was followed, however, by a rapid deterioration. Our study also exhibited severe side effects, including septic arthritis and an accelerated amyloidosis, and in some cases death of unknown origin. A critical summary of the use of fractionated total lymphoid irradiation was published recently by Zvaifler [39].

Total nodal lymphoid irradiation in RA has been developed from observations in patients with malign lymphomas and rheumatoid arthritis who experienced an obvious beneficial effect of irradiation therapy and from experimental animal studies [40, 41]. The effect of TLI on the disease activity of RA seems to be comparable to effects observed during thoracic duct drainge treatment used earlier, as well as to the outcome of treatment with anti-CD4 monoclonal antibodies, namely due to a depletion of T lymphocytes. Thus, as already stated, a clear-cut correlation between changes in T-cell subsets [34] and a marked decrease in the number of CD4-positive peripheral blood helper/inducer T cells was reported in patients benefiting from TLI. However, although this treatment modality is further evidence for the important role of cellular immune mechanisms in the pathogenesis of inflammatory synovitis in RA, this therapeutic regime is not yet a clinical routine, due particularly to the many toxicities which have been described as being associated with the use of TLI in the studies reported thus far. In addition, a long-term risk for the development of cardiac toxicity in cancer, as seen in Hodgkin's patients, is not yet clarified. Furthermore, the development of secondary malignancies has not yet been excluded, nore are side effects such as the observed acceleration of amyloidosis in an advanced state of RA. In summary, TLI has to be regarded as an experimental form of RA treatment. Modifications in the administration and the dose of radiotherapy – possibly diminishing adverse side effects – might prove to be of therapeutic value in at least some cases of intractable RA, however.

Antibodies

Immunoglobulins

The administration of high-dose intravenous immunoglobulins has been found to be effective in the treatment of idiopathic thrombocytopenia (ITP) [42, 43] and has also been applied successfully in the management of Kawasaki disease and certain autoimmune disoders [44]. In ITP, the response to high-dose intravenous immunoglobulins has been attributed to a transient blockade of the reticuloendothelial system, while in long-term responses, more specific immunomodulating effects have been discussed [43]. In 1982 and 1985, Sany et al. [45, 46] published data demonstrating that immunoglobulins eluted from human placenta (placenta-eluted gammaglobulin, PEGG) might beneficially affect the clinical course of RA. This therapeutic approach goes back to studies performed by Riggio et al., showing that PEGG has immunosuppressive properties [47]. In a more recent communication by Moynier et al. [48], evidence was presented that 99% of placenta-eluted gammaglobulins belong to the IgG antibody class and that treatment success was attributed to the presence of alloantibodies to class-II HLA antigens. This observation was confirmed by findings demonstrating (a) that IgG from PEGG were cytotoxic for the non-T-cell population, (b) that IgG or Fab2 fragments from PEGG were bound only to class-II HLA-bearing cells, and (c) that Fab2 fragments from PEGG were able to block complement-mediated cytotoxicity of anti-HLA-DR- and anti-DQ-w1 alloantibodies. Thus, the reason why PEGG influences the clinical course of RA seems to be the presence of high titers of class-II HLA antibodies.

In other rheumatic diseases, the use of intravenous immunoglobulins has also been reported as being successful, for example in patients suffering from dermatomyositis, polymyositis, and rheumatoid arthritis [49] and in patients with lupus erythematosus or Sjögren's syndrome [50]. With the exception of idiopathic thrombocytopenic purpura, however, control studies are necessary to determine the real efficacy of high-dose intravenous immunoglobulin therapy in patients with collagen and/or vascular disorders and to prove whether PEGG is superior to normally prepared immunoglobulin preparations.

Monoclonal Antibodies

Monoclonal antibody therapy for nonmalignant diseases was introduced in organ transplantation and this led to new immunosuppressive treatments (Fig. 1). Thus injections of the anti-CD3 monoclonal antibody OKT3, directed against mature T cells, led to a significant reversal of kidney transplant rejections [51–53]. In autoimmune situations, treatment with monoclonal antibodies against T-helper/inducer subsets were first investigated in animal models. In these studies, anti-DC4 treatment resulted in a depletion of this T-cell subset, inducing a state of immune tolerance to antigens that had been administered during the phase of treatment [54–58]. Hence, it was shown that monoclonal antibodies directed against a shared idiotype on rat T-cell receptors specific for myelin basic protein protected the animals from developing

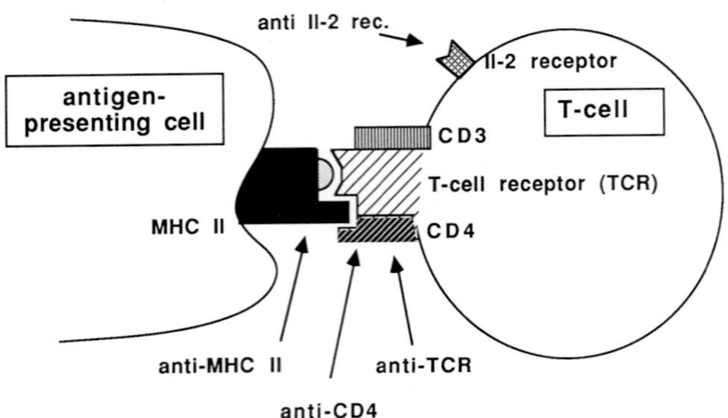

Fig. 1. Possibilities of blocking T-cell activation by monoclonal antibodies, using either anti-MHC class-II antibodies or antibodies directed against molecules of the CD4 epitope or the T-cell or IL-2 receptor on CD4-positive T cells. In addition, not showing here, there is the administration of peptides, at least in those cases where the autoantigen has been defined, competing with and thus inhibiting the autoantigen presentation by MHC class II to CD-4-positive T lymphocytes

experimental allergic encephalomyelitis [59], and that antibodies to the L3T4 epitopes were able to retard autoimmunity in NZB/NZW mice as well as in BXSB mice, which are prone to develop systemic lupus erythematosus [60]. In addition, Shizuro et al. [61] reported that in nonobese diabetic mice a spontaneous diabetes mellitus was blocked by treatment with a monoclonal antibody against the L3T4 determinants present on the cell membrane of T-helper cells. In the human situation, first reports on the use of monoclonal antibodies in the treatment of autoimmune diseases have been published by Hafler et Weiner [62] and Hafler et al. [63] involving patients suffering from multiple sclerosis. Based on these experimental and clinical findings, and on data demonstrating a beneficial therapeutic effect of thoracic duct drainage [64] as well as leukapheresis [65, 66] – and in certain respects of TLI – on the clinical course of RA, first pilot studies have been performed with monoclonal anti-CD4 antibodies in RA [67, 68].

In our own studies (Horneff et al, [6, 8a]) the treatment with an anti-CD4 monoclonal antibody was studied in ten patients with severe intractable rheumatoid arthritis. In a phase-I trial, the monoclonal antibody was infused in a dosage of 0.3 mg/kg body wt. on 7 consecutive days. Kinetic studies demonstrated a drastic depletion of CD4-positive cells down to a minimum of 25 cells/ml 1 h after infusion. A subsequent recovery of CD4-positive cells 24 h after infusion did not reach the initial values, and the full 7-day treatment resulted in an overall significant reduction of CD4-positive cells (Fig. 2). In addition, there was an inverse CD4/CD8 ratio that persisted 3–4 weeks in general. Lymphocyte transformation assays demonstrated significantly reduced reactivity in six of the ten patients. Four individuals exhibited an unexpected T-cell responsiveness to mitogens and common antigens. Parallel laboratory studies showed a reduction of the ESR, C-reactive protein,

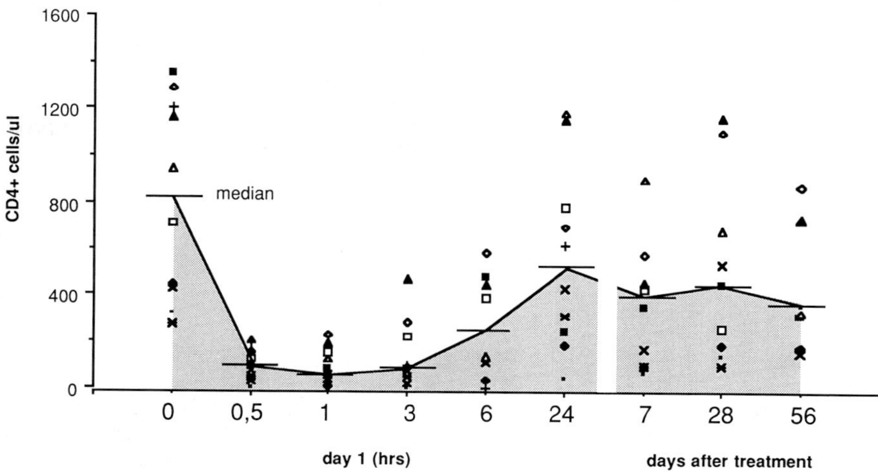

Fig. 2. Kinetics of CD4-positive cells of ten patients treated with 0.3 mg/kg body wt. of an anti-CD4 monoclonal antibody for 30 min. Each *symbol* denotes one individual patient. *Bars* demonstrate the medium value. Except for the time point of 24 h after the first infusion, all CD4-positive cell counts were significantly decreased compared with the value prior to treatment. (from [68a]; Published with permission of the authors)

rheumatoid factor, and total immunoglobulin values in seven of the nine patients who completed the treatment regimen.

Clinical improvements consisted of a significant reduction of the Richie index, increased strength, and a reduced number of swollen joints. Adverse effects were skin urticaria in two patients, leading to a withdrawal of therapy for one individual, and chills with fever suggestive of a lymphokine release syndrome in another two patients. Only low levels of human anti-mouse immunoglobulin antibodies developed, not exceeding 0.5 mg/l. In four patients it was possible to repeat the treatment cycle with better efficacy. Similar although not identical data have been published by Herzog et al. and Walker et al. [69, 70]. First therapeutic trials have also been conducted using monoclonal antibodies to the interleukin-2 receptor [7], and prolonged improvement in refractory rheumatoid arthritis was observed after brief antithymocyte globulin therapy [72].

With regard to the efficacy of anti-CD4 monoclonal antibody therapy, a significant reduction of synovitis was particularly remarkable in our own study as well as in that published by Herzog et al. [69]. To summarize our data treatment with a monoclonal anti-CD4 antibody led to a significant and immediate depletion of CD4-positive cells in all individuals investigated. Furthermore, this therapy resulted in a marked immunomodulation, as documented by a reduction of lymphocyte proliferation, and, finally, anti-CD4 treatment was followed by significant changes in laboratory and clinical parameters, without any major side effects. However, further studies and double-blind, randomized trials are necessary to evaluate the efficacy of anti-

CD4 treatment in RA patients as well as in other clinical situations such as systemic vasculitis [73]. Moreover, possible side effects have to be evaluated, such as the induction of human anti-mouse antibodies as well as anti-idiotypic antibody formation. From the present studies, however, it seems feasible that RA patients who are refractory to conventional treatment regimes might benefit from the administration of a monoclonal anti-CD4 antibody. Studies are now in progress to determine whether anti-CD4 antibody-induced partial remission can be maintained by subsequent immunosuppressive medication with long acting anti-inflammatory drugs such as gold, D-penicillamine or methrotrexate.

One problem of treatment with monoclonal antibodies, i.e., immunogenicity, might possibly be avoided, although not completely, with chimeric antibodies, using humanized monoclonal antibody preparations [74]. However, even humanized monoclonal antibodies do not preclude the possibility of inducing anti-idiotypic antibodies which might interfere with immunomodulating mechanisms in RA. Furthermore, the choice of the anti-CD4 monoclonal antibody appears to be of critical importance; even though directed against the same cell surface molecule, various known anti-CD4 antibodies have different immunomodulating effects, as shown in primate studies [75–77]. In these experiments, some antibodies led only to a coating of CD4-positive cells, while others induced a strong modulation with subsequent clearance of CD4-positive cells from the peripheral blood. Apparently, many of the immunomodulatory effects depend on the proximity of the epitope recognized to the HIB binding region [78, 79].

Besides the described administration of monoclonal antibodies to MHC class-II antigens, T-cell receptor molecules, or CD4 and IL-2 epitopes of T-cell helper cells, new monoclonal antibodies directed against molecules of the integrin family such as LFA-1, LFA-3 [80], or lymphocyte homing receptors [81], being part of the integrin family, which might be involved in ongoing inflammatory tissue reaction in RA might prove to be effective therapeutic tools.

With increasing knowledge about the linkage of autoimmune diseases and especially class–II molecules, it is reasonable to expect that more specific monoclonals against certain domains on the MHC class-II molecules will prevent autoimmunity [82]. In the same context, a therapy with monoclonal antibodies to different V-regions of the T-cell receptor might become clinically important; this has already been demonstrated in experimental allergic encephalitis, where an anti-V-beta-VIII-antibody reversed paralytic disease in immunized animals [83, 84]. Thus, as we gain more information on the immunogenic side of a given autoantigen as well as increase our knowledge with regard to the MHC molecules that bind immunogenic "auto"-peptides, and with a better understanding of the T-cell receptor immunogenetics, including the identification of sequences which recognize antigen-MHC complexes, highly specific approaches for immunotherapy in autoimmune diseases including RA will become feasible.

Cytokines and Cytokine Inhibitors

Cytokines have been implicated as important mediators of inflammation in joint-destructive mechanisms in RA. This is based on many in vitro and in vivo clinical and experimental studies [85–90]. The clear-cut evidence for the involvement of cytokines in synovitis and cartilage destruction-perpetuating mechanisms in RA, as well as in other rheumatic disease entities, has led to intensive research into the possible clinical application of cytokines in natural or recombinant form – especially interferon gamma – on the one hand and into inhibitors – both natural and synthetic – of different cytokines on the other.

Interleukin 1 and IL-1 Inhibitors

An increasing amount of evidence has been published suggesting that IL-1 plays a central role in pathogenic mechanisms in RA, as summarized by Arend and Dayer [86]. Recent studies focusing on the identification of IL-1 inhibitors indicate that natural inhibitors of IL-1 exist that potentially modulate local effects of IL-1 in the rheumatoid joint. Levels of activity of IL-1 inhibitors include the reduction of IL-1 synthesis, the binding and blocking of the IL-1 receptor, and interference on a post-receptor level [90–92]. However, it is worth mentioning that many of the so-called IL-1 inhibitors have not yet been purified; thus, their mechanisms of action have still to be defined. Besides a well-characterized 22-kD IL-1 inhibitor as obtained from human monocytes cultured on adherent IgG [91], a 25-kD IL-1 inhibitor has been demonstrated in synovial fluid from RA patients; it is thought to be due partly to TGF beta activities [93]. Furthermore, cells in the synovial fluid have been reported to produce IL-1 inhibitory substances in vitro [94, 95], and, as in adult RA, inhibitory activity has also been found in the sera and urine of patients with juvenile RA, in whom maximum levels were correlated with the presence of fever [96]. The relevance, however, of the 25-kD IL-1 inhibitor found in rheumatoid synovial fluid remains to be established. Increased levels of IL-1 on the one hand and the presence of IL-1 inhibitor activity in the rheumatoid joint on the other might indicate that there is a specific balance between the agonist and antagonist, which might be disturbed in the process of perpetuating active synovitis. This could be due either to a decreased production of antagonist proteins or to an excessive production of the agonist IL-1. The therapeutic application of cytokine inhibitors is clearly hypothetical, and further studies are necessary to determine whether in RA patients as well as in patients suffering from other rheumatic diseases the application of IL-1 inhibitors is of clinical value.

Similar data have been obtained with TNF alpha, which also seems to be involved in ongoing tissue-destructive mechanisms in the joints of RA patients. TNF alph has been shown to be synthesized by synovial tissue [97], and, at least in vitro, a stimulated resorption and inhibition of synthesis of proteoglycan in cartilage has been observed [98]. Dayer et al. [99] published evidence that TNF stimulates collagenase and prostaglandin E_2 production by human synovial cells and fibroblasts. Similar to IL-1, local effects of TNF alpha in the synovium and synovial fluid of RA patients might be antagonized by inhibitory proteins. Thus a specific inhibitor of TNF alpha has been described in the urine of febrile patients [100] as well as in supernatants of cell cultures from synovial fluid cells of RA patients [95]. Regarding the possible therapeutic use of IL-1 and TNF-alpha inhibitors, a report by Henderson and Pittiphir [101] is of interest, presenting in vivo evidence of a synergistic interaction between IL-1 and TNF alpha with regard to their arthritogenic activities.

Interleukin 1 and IL-2 Inhibitors

There is a defective interleukin-2 production in synovial T cells in RA patients [102, 103], which could be due in part to an inhibitor of IL-2 synthesis found in the synovial fluid of RA patients [104, 105]. Although elevated soluble interleukin-2 receptor levels were reported in both sera and synovial fluid of patients with rheumatoid arthritis [106], supporting the hypothesis that in vivo T-cell activation plays an important role in RA, it seems doubtful that a monoclonal antibody directed against the IL-2 receptor could be of any therapeutic benefit.

Interferon gamma

Interferon gamma is a cytokine with multiple effects on cells of the immune system. Interferon gamma has been demonstrated in the synovial fluid of RA patients, although not unequivocally [107], and has been traced by immunohistochemical studies in synovial tissue [108]. Besides its effects on cells of the immune system, interferon gamma has further activities including an influence on the growth and differentiation of normal and neoplastic cells, as well as on the production of other cytokines such as IL-1, colony-stimulating factors, and interleukin-6 [109].

Case reports demonstrating that patients with various malignancies and RA who were treated with interferon gamma and who showed a positive effect of the interferon gamma treatment on the course of RA initiated phase-I trials to examine interferon gamma as a new therapeutic principle. Besides these incidental observations, data have been reported to demonstrate that a dose-dependent inhibition of prostaglandin release was induced by interferon gamma as well as a modulation of the hyperoxygenase and cyclooxygenase production in a mouse system; furthermore, an inhibition – again dose dependent – of the interleukin-4-induced B-cell proliferation in parallel with an inhibition of immunoglobulin secretion was reported. A downregulation of class-II antigen expression of B cells, dose dependent on interferon, was also shown when the effect of recombinant human interferon on rheumatoid arthritis B lymphocytes activated by the Epstein-Barr virus was studied. Lotz et al. [110] demonstrated that interferon gamma was significantly more potent than interferon alpha and interferon beta; in reducing IgM rheumatoid factor production this was parallelled by a diminished spontaneous activation of RA B cells.

With regard to the use of interferon gamma for RA patients, therapeutic trials with recombinant human interferon gamma have recently been reported. In one study [111] including 91 patients, statistically significant improvement in clinical disease among the interferon gamma-treated patients was observed, while in a second study which included 26 patients, those who had received interferon gamma showed some clinical improvement; however, it was not significant as compared with the placebo-treated controls [112]. In a third trial [113], 105 RA patients were enrolled in a 12-week randomized, prospective, double-blind, placebo-controlled study. Similar to the data reported by Veys et al. [112], although the improvement was more obvious in interferon gamma-treated patients than in the placebo group, the difference was not statistically significant. In an open therapeutic trial with interferon gamma in 110 patients, Sprekeler et al. [114] demonstrated that in 46 patients who were followed over a 12-month period, a correlation was observed between the improvement of clinical parameters such as pain and morning siffness and the improvement of laboratory parameters such as ESR, anemia, leukocytosis, or thrombocytosis. Interferon gamma was well tolerated, and no severe side-effects were seen. In contrast to the report by Sprekeler et al., it must be mentioned that other authors published evidence that treatment with interferon gamma might lead to the onset of autoimmune diseases [115] and to the induction of antinuclear antibodies [116]. Recently, Machold and Smolen [117] also described an interferon gamma-induced exacerbation of systemic lupus erythematosus. With regard to possible side effects of interferon gamma treatment, Mauritz et al. [118] observed that interferon gamma triggers the onset of collagen arthritis in mice, which implies that it possibly enhances local inflammatory processes in the joints. In this context, Burmester et al. [119] reported that the exposure of chondrocytes to recombinant human interferon gamma induced the expression of class–II antigens, enabling these cells – at least in in vitro studies – to present antigen in an autologous tetanus toxide system.

Thus, after critically reviewing data currently available on the effect of interferon gamma treatment in RA, it seems fair to state that interferon gamma does not provide a major contribution to the existing therapeutic principles in RA, and that side effects caused by the immunomodulatory activity of interferon gamma must be expected in the patients treated, especially over longer periods.

Other cytokines also involved in the ongoing inflammatory joint reactivity in RA patients are IL-6 and various hematopoietic growth factors [86]. However, whether the inhibition of IL-6 by monoclonal antibodies or specific IL-6 inhibitors might be effective in treating RA patients is still hypothetical and lacks experimental and clinical evidence.

Pepitides

The peptide-presenting function of the major histocompatibility complex is essential for inducing an antigen-specific T-cell response and also determines

MHC-restricted immune reactivity [120]. Knowledge of this mechanism of antigen presentation has made it possible to design molecules that effectively compete with self-antigens binding to molecules of the MHC. Thus in experimental allergic encephalomyelitis (EAE) certain mice strains, for example, peptide 1–9 of the myelin-basic protein binds to class-II MHC molecules and triggers encephalogenic T cells. Peptide analogues of P1–9 were synthetically constructed and were shown to compete for binding of the encephalogenic fragment to MHC. Some of these analogues which are not encephalogenic were found to have a high avidity for MHC and thus to block the development of experimental allergic encephalomyelitis [121–123].

In similar experimental approaches, Arnon et al. [124] demonstrated that EAE could be suppressed by the copolymer of the myelin-basic protein having the amino acid sequence alanine, glutaminic acid, lysine, and thyrosine, which was called COP-1. Using this synthetic basic random copylomer, Teitelbaum et al. [125] were able to describe a specific inhibition of the T-cell response to the myelin-basic protein by COP-1. Preliminary data from experimental studies in human beings demonstrated that COP-1 might be effective in the treatment of multiple sclerosis, and that inhibition of T-cell proliferation for acetylcholine receptor epitopes related to myasthenia gravis could be induced not only by antibodies to the T-cell receptor but also by the addition of competitive synthetic polymers to the system [126]. This approach by Brocke et al. shows that a nonimmunogenic analogue of acetylcholine receptor peptides could block T-cell recognition, which might indicate a new form of treatment, not only for myasthenia gravis, but also for other autoimmune diseases where the autoantigen has been defined. With regard to rheumatoid arthritis, Yang et al. [127–129] reported recently that in mycobacterium-induced adjuvant arthritis in Lewis rats, immunization with a synthetic nonapeptide protected the rats completely against the development of adjuvant arthritis. The nonapeptide used for treating the animals had the amino-acid sequence 180–188 of the 65-kD heat-shock protein of *Mycobacterium bovis*.

Although peptide-defined autoantigens might prove in future to be useful in the treatment of different autoimmune diseases, including rheumatic disease entities, so far no clinical trials have been conducted, with the exception of ongoing therapeutic trials of the COP-1 peptide in patients with multiple sclerosis. Further investigations will be necessary, not only to define the possible autoantigen or antigens in RA, but also to look for protective and possible autoimmunity-accelerating peptides before even phase-I therapeutic trials can be started in RA patients.

Others

Collagen II
Although the nature of RA-inducing autoantigen, if it exists, is not yet clearly defined, experimental animal studies have shown that one of the potential autoantigens is collagen II, which effectively induces experimental arthritis

upon immunization. With regard to new treatment avenues, van Vollenhoven et al. [130] demonstrated that tolerance could be induced by pretreating mice intravenously with up to 500 mg of chick collagen II and starting the treatment 1 week prior to immunization with bovine collagen II in CFA. The modulation of cellular and humoral immune responses to collagen type I and collagen type II has also been shown by Butler et al. [131], using a similar experimental animal set-up. Studies are currently in progress to show if not only intravenous but also oral administration of collagen II can prevent experimental collagen-II-induced arthritis, and first trials have been initiated to see if the oral administration of collagen II can influence the clinical course of human RA.

Immunotoxins

Immunotoxins, i.e., conjugates of enzymatically active toxins with antibodies against different cell-surface structures, have repeatedly been used for cell destruction in vitro and more recently in the treatment of cancer patients [132]. Although this type of immunotherapy is of some importance not only for cancer patients but also for patients suffering from autoimmune disease, the precise antibody target has to be identified; it has also been demonstrated that the combination of immunotoxin and monoclonal antibodies is superior to monoclonal antibodies alone.

Photopheresis

Finally, an approach to the treatment of rheumatic diseases that should be stressed is photopheresis. Photopheresis has been used in the treatment of cutaneous T-cell lymphomas [133, 134], and, more recently, Wilfert et al. [135] have applied this new treatment principle to five patients with long-standing seronegative arthritis resistant to conventional therapy who were also suffering from psoriasis. Although, as the authors noted, there was a marked in vitro effect on treated lymphocytes with a reduction of viability, proliferation, and mitogen response, there was only a slight-to-moderate clinical improvement in four of the five patients treated. The improvement was seen with regard to strength of grip, swelling, pain, morning stiffness, and the necessary dosage of nonsteroidal and antirheumatic drugs and radiographic changes. In this context, it is of interest that in progressive systemic sclerosis as well [136] interferon gamma, photopheresis, and the mast cell stabilizer ketotifen seem to be promising new treatment modalities, although the mechanism of photopheresis on the ongoing immune-mediated pathogenic mechanisms is still unclear.

Qutlook

Although no major breakthrough has been recorded with regard to the treatment of rheumatoid arthritis within the plast few years, new, exciting possibilities are now emerging that may considerably improve the repertoire of treatment possibilities for this disease entity. More knowledge about the immunogenetics of molecules involved in the peptide presentation to T cells and about the immunogenetics of the T-cell receptor will facilitate new developments in immunotherapy. A substantial improvement of the available therapy for RA patients as well as for autoimmune diseases in general can also be expected from a better understanding of the physiological and pathophysiological role of cytokines and cytokine inhibitors. However, the past teaches that a rapid breakthrough in the treatment of RA should not be expected.

References

1. Sebaldt R-J (1988) Pulse steroid therapy and the search for improved drug therapy of rheumatoid arthritis. J Rheumatol 15:200–201
2. Kushner I (1989) Does aggressive therapy of rheumatoid arthritis affect outcome? J Rheumatol 16:1–4
3. Amos RS, Constable TJ, Crookson RA et al. (1977) Rheumatoid arthritis: relation of serum C-reactive protein and erythrocyte sedimentation rates to radiographic changes. Br Med J 1:195–197
4. Dawes PT, Fowler PD, Clarke S et al. (1986) Rheumatoid arthritis: treatment which controls the C-reactive protein and erythrocyte sedimentation rate reduces radiologic progression. Br J Rheumatol 24:44–49
5. Young A, Brook AS, Corbett M (1980) The clinical assessment of joint inflammatory activity in rheumatoid arthritis related to radiologic progression. Rheumatol Rehabil 19:14–19
6. Joint Committee of the Medical Research Council and Nuffield Foundation (1959) A comparison of prednisolone and aspirin or other analgesics in the treatment of rheumatoid arthritis. Ann Rheum Dis 18:173–188
7. McCarty DJ, Carrera GF (1982) Intractable rheumatoid arthritis. Treatment with combined cyclophosphamide, azathioprine, and hydroxychloroquine. JAMA 248:1718–1723
8. Sigler JW, Bluhm GB, Duncan H et al. (1974) Gold salts in the treatment of rheumatoid arthritis. A double-blind study. An Intern Med 80:21–26
9. Forre O, Bjerkhoel F, Salvesen CF et al. (1987) An open, controlled, randomized comparison of cyclosporin and azathioprine in the treatment of rheumatoid arthritis: a preliminary report. Arthritis Rheum 30:88–92
10. Dougados M, Amor B (1987) Cyclosporin A in rheumatoid arthritis: preliminary clinical results of an open trial. Arthritis Rheum 30:83–87
11. Weinblatt ME, Coblyn JS, Fraser PA et al. (1987) Cyclosporin A treatment of refractory rheumatoid arthritis. Arthritis Rheum 32:671–676
12. Martin M, Dixon J, Hickling P, Bird H et al. (1982) A combination of D-penicillamine and hydroxychloroquine for the treatment of rheumatoid arthritis (abstract). Ann Rheum dis 41:208
13. Bunch TW, O'Duffy JD, Tompkins RB, O'Fallon WM (1984) Controlled trial of hydroxychloroquine and penicillamine singly and in combination in treatment of rheumatoid arthritis. Arthritis Rheum 27:267–276
14. Singleto PT, Cervantes AG (1982) Chrysotherapy and concomiant use of antimalarial drugs therapy in rheumatoid arthritis (abstract). Arthritis Rheum 25 [Suppl]:115

15. Guka M, Carrera F, McCarty DJ (1986) Treatment of intractable rheumatoid arthritis with combined cyclophosphamide, azathioprine and hydroxychloroquine. JAMA 255:2351–2359
16. Kremer JM, Lee JK (1988) A long-term prospective study of the use of methotrexate in rheumatoid arthritis. Arthritis Rheum 41:577–584
17. Furst DE, Kremer JM (1988) Methrotrexate in rheumatoid arthritis. Arthritis Rheum 31:305–309
18. Weinblatt ME, Trentham DE, Fraser PA et al. (1988) Long-term prospective trial of low-dose methrotrexate in rheumatoid arthritis. Arthritis Rheum 31:167–175
19. Alarcon GS, Tracy IC, Blackburn WD jr (1989) Methotrexate in rheumatoid arthritis. Toxic effects as the major factor in limiting long-term treatment. Arthritis Rheum 32:671–676
20. Kremer JM, Lee RG, Tolman KG (1989) Liver histology in rheumatoid arthritis patients receiving long-term methotrexate therapy. A prospective study with baseline and sequential biopsy samples. Arthritis Rheum 32:121–127
21. Rau R, Karger T, Herborn G, Frenzel H (1989) Liver biopsy findings in patients with rheumatoid arthritis undergoing long-term treatment with methotrexate. J Rheumatol 16:489–493
22. Franchimont P, Bolla K (1985) Rationale for Thymopentin as therapeutic agent in rheumatoid arthritis. Surv Immunol Res 4 [Suppl 1]:70–75
23. Veys EM, Huskisson EC, Rosenthal M et al. (1981) Clinical response to therapy with thymopoietin pentapeptide (TP-5) in rheumatoid arthritis. Ann Rheum Dis 41:441–443
24. Veys EM, Mielants H, Verbruggen G et al. (1984) Thymopoietin pentapeptide (Thymopentin, TP-5) in the treatment of rheumatoid arthritis. A compilation of several short- and long-term clinical studies. J Rheumatol 11:462
25. Malaise MG, Franchimont P, Bach-Andersen R, et al. (1985) Treatment of active rheumatoid arthritis with slow intravenous injections of Thymopentin. A double-blind placebo-controlled randomised study. Lancet ii:4–6
26. Ansar AS, Penhale WJ, Talal N (1985) Sex hormones, immune and autoimmune responses: mechanisms of sex hormone action. Am J Pathol 121:531–559
27. Ansar AS, Dauphinee MJ, Talal N (1986) Prenatal effects of sex hormones on autoantibody-producing B cells bearing Ly-1 antigen (abstract). Arthritis Rheum [Suppl] 29:34
28. Allen JB, Blatter D, Caladra GB, Wilder RL (1983) Sex hormonal effects on the severity of streptococcal cell wall-induced polyarthritis in the rat. Arthritis Rheum 26:560–563
29. Berczi I, Nagy E, Asa SL, Kovacs K (1984) The influence of pituitary hormones on adjuvant arthritis. Arthritis Rheum 27:682–688
30. Bijlsma JWJ, Huber-Bruning O, Thijssen JHH (1987) Effect of oestrogen treatment on clinical and laboratory manifestations of rheumatoid arthritis. Ann Rheum Dis 46:777–779
31. Brahn E, Helfgott SM, Belli JA et al. (1984) Total lymphoid irradiation therapy in refractory rheumatoid arthritis. Fifteen- to forty-month follow-up. Arthritis Rheum 27:481–488
32. Strober S, Tonay A, Fiedl E et al. (1985) Efficacy of total lymphoid irradiation in intractable rheumatoid arthritis. A double-blind, randomized trial. Ann Intern Med 102:441–449
33. Kotzin BL, Strober S, Kansas GS et al. (1984) Suppression of pokeweed mitogen-stimulated immunoglobulin production in patients with rheumatoid arthritis after treatment with total lymphoid irradiation. J Immunol 2:1049–1055
34. Kotzin BL, Kansas GS, Engleman EG et al. (1983) Changes in T-cell subsets in patients with rheumatoid arthritis treated with total lymphoid irradiation. Clin Immunol Immunopathol 27:250–260
35. Gaston JSH, Strober S, Solovera JJ et al. (1988) Dissection of the mechanisms of immune injury in rheumatoid arthritis, using total lymphoid irradiation. Arthritis Rheum 321:21–30

36. Trentham DE, Belli JA, Bloomer WD et al. (1987) 2000-Centigray total lymphoid irradiation for refractory rheumatoid arthritis. Arthritis Rheum 30:980–987
37. Sherrer Y, Block D, Storber S, Fries J (1987) Comparative toxicity of total lymphoid irradiation and immunosuppressive drug-treated patients with intractable rheumatoid arthritis. J Rheumatol 14:46–51
38. Nüsslein HG, Herbst M, Manger BJ et al. (1985) Total lymphoid irradiation in patients with refractory rheumatoid arthritis. Arthritis Rheum 23:1205
39. Zvaifler N (1987) Fractionated total lymphoid irradiation: a promising new treatment for rheumatoid arthritis? Yes, no, maybe. Arthritis Rheum 30:109–114
40. Helfgott SMK (1989) Total lymphoid radiation. In: Trentham DE (ed) Rheumatic disease clinics of North America. New directions in antirheumatic therapy. Saunders, Philadelphia, p 577
41. Helfgott SM (1989) Total lymphoid irradiation. Rheum Dis Clin North Am 15:577
42. Imbach P, d'Apuzzo V, Hirt A, Rossi E, Vest M, Barandun S, Baumgartner C, Morell A, Schöni M, Wagner HP (1981) High-dose intravenous gammaglobulin for idiopathic thrombocytopenic purpura in childhood. Lancet 1:1228–1231
43. Newland AC, Treleaven JG (1983) High-dose intravenous IgG in adults with autoimmune thrombocytopenia. Lancet 1:84-87
44. Stiehm ER, Ashida E, Kwang SK, Winston DJ, Haas A, Gale RP (1987) Intravenous immunoglobulins as therapeutic agents. Ann Intern Med 107:367–382
45. Samy J, Clot J, Bonneau M, Andary M (1982) Immunomodulating effect of human placenta-eluted gamma globulins in rheumatoid arthritis. Arthritis Rheum 25:17–24
46. Combe B, Cosso B, Clot J, Bonneau M, Sany J (1985) Human placenta-eluted gamma globulins in rheumatoid arthritis. Am J Med 78:920–928
47. Riggio RR, Hopkins LE, Parrillo JE, Stenzel KH, Rubin AL (1975) Placental globulin: a new immunosuppressive agent? Transplant Proc 7:465–468
48. Moynier M, Cosso B, Brochier J, Clot J (1987) Identification of class-II HLA alloantibodies in placenta-eluted gamma globulins used for treating rheumatoid arthritis. Arthritis Rheum 30:375–381
49. Gelfand EW (1989) the use of intravenous immune globulin in collagen vascullar disorders: a potentially new modality of therapy. I Allergy Clin Immunol 84:613–616
50. Ballow M, Parke A (1989) The use of intravenous immune globulin in collagen vascular disorders. J Allergy Clin Immunol 84:608–612
51. Ortho Multicenter Transplant Study Group (1985) A randomized clinical trial of OKT3 monoclonal antibody for acute rejection of cadaveric renal transplants. N Engl J Med 313:337–342
52. Kerr PG, Atkins RC (1989) The effects of OKT3 therapy on infiltrating lymphocytes in rejecting renal allografts. Transplantation 48:33–36
53. Herbert J, Roser B (1988) Strategies of monoclonal antibody therapy that induce permanent toleance of organ transplants. Transplantation 46 [Suppl 2]:128S–134S
54. Benjamin RJ, Qin SX, Wise MP, Cobbold SP, Waldmann H (1988) Mechanism of monoclonal antibody-facilitated tolerance induction: a possible role for the DC4 (L3T4) and CD11a (LFA1) molecules in self-non-self-discrimination. Eur J Immunol 18:1079–1088
55. Cobbold SOP, Jayasuriya A, Nash A, Prospero TD, Waldmann H (1984). Therapy with monoclonal antibodies by elimination of T-cell subsets in vivo. Nature 312:548–551
56. Goronzy J, Weyand CM, Fathman CB (1986) Long-term humoral unresponsiveness in vivo induced by treatment with monoclonal antibody against L3T4. J Exp Med 164:911–925
57 Seaman WE, Wofsy D (1988) Selective manipulation of the immune response in vivo by monoclonal antibodies. Annu Rev Med 39:231–241
58. Wofsy D (1988) Treatment of autoimmune diseases with monoclonal antibodies. In: Waldmann H (ed) Monoclonal antibody therapy. Karger, Basel, pp 106–120 (Progress in allergy, vol 45)

59. Owhashi M, Heber-Katz E (1988) Protection from experimental allergic encephalomyelitis conferred by a monoclonal antibody directed against a shared idiotype on rat T cell receptors specific for myelin basic protein. J Exp Med 168:2153–2164

60. Seaman WE, Wofsy D (1987) In vivo effects of monoclonal antibody to L3T4. In: Immune regulation by characterized polypeptides. Liss, New York, pp 219–227

61. Shizuro JA, Taylor-Edwards C, Banks BA, Gregory AK, Fathman CG (1988) Immunotherapy of the nonobese diabetic mouse: treatment with an antibody to T-helper lymphocytes. Science 240:659–662

62. Hafler DA, Weiner HL (1988) Immunosuppression with monoclonal antibodies in multiple sclerosis. Neurology 38 [Suppl 2]:42–47

63. Hafler DA, Ritz J, Schlossman SF, Weiner HL (1988) Anti-CD4 and anti-CD2 monoclonal antibody infusions in subjects with multiple sclerosis. J Immunol 141:131–138.

64. Paulus HE, Machleder HI, Levine S, Yu DTY, MacDonald NS (1977) Lymphocyte involvement in rheumatoid arthritis: studies during thoracic duct drainage. Arthritis Rheum 20:1249–1262

65. Karsh J, Klippel JH, Plotz PH, Decker JL, Wright DG, Flye MW (1981) Lymphapheresis in rheumatoid arthritis. Arthritis Rheum 24:867–873

66. Wilder RL, Decker JL (1983) T-inducer lymphocytes, leukapheresis and the pathogenesis of rheumatoid arthritis. Clin Exp Rheumatol 1:89–91

67. Horneff G, Burmester GR, Strobel G, Gramatzki M, Kalden JR, Emmrich F (1989) Therapie der chronischen Polyarthritis mit einem monoklonalen Antikörper gegen das CD4-Antigen auf T-Helferzellen (abstract). Aktuel Rheumatol 14:232

68. Herzog CH, Walker CH, Pichler W, Aeschlimann A, Wassmer P, Stockinger H, Knapp W, Rieber P, Müller W (1987) Monoclonal anti-CD4 in arthritis. Lancet 2:1461–1462

68a. Horneff G, Burmester GR, Emmrich F, Kaldun JR (1991) Treatment of rheumatoid arthritis which anti-CD4 monoclonal antibody. Arthritis Rheum (in press)

69. Herzog C, Walker C, Müller W, Riethmüller G, Muller W, Pichler WJ (1989). Anti-CD4 antibody treatment of patients with rheumatoid arthritis. I. Effect on clinical course and circulating T cells. J Autoimmun 2:627–642

70. Walker C, Herzog C, Rieber P et al. (1989) Anti-CD4 antibody treatment of patients with rheumatoid arthritis. II. Effect of in vivo treatment on in vitro proliferative response of CD4 cells. J Autoimmun 2:263–269

71. Kyle V, Coughlan RJ, Tighe H, Waldmann H, Hazleman BL (1989) Beneficial effect of monoclonal antibody to interleukin-2 receptor on activated T cells in rheumatoid arthritis. Ann Rheum Dis 48:428–428

72. Shmerling RH, Trentham DE (1989) Prolonged improvement in refractory rheumatoid arthritis after antithymocyte globulin therapy of brief duration. Arthritis Rheum 32:1495–1496

73. Mathieson PW, Cobbold SP, Hale G, Clark MR, Oliveira DBG, Lockwood CM, Waldmann H (1990) Monoclonal antibody therapy in systemic vasculitis. N Engl J Med 323/4:250–254

74. Brüggemann M, Winter G, Waldmann H, Neuberger MS (1989) The immunogenicity of chimeric antibodies. J Exp Med 170:2153–2157

75. Jonker M, Nooij FMJ, Steinhof G (1987) Effects of CD4 and CD8 specific monoclonal antibodies in vitro and in vivo on T cells and their relation to the allograft response in rhesus monkeys. Transplan Proc 5:4308–4314

76. Jonker M, DenBrok JH (1987) Idiotype switching of CD4-specific monoclonal antibodies can prolong the therapeutic effectiveness in spite of host anti-mouse IgG antibodies. Eur J Immunol 17:1547–1553

77. Rose LM, Alvord EC, Hruby S, Jackevicius S, Petersen R, Warner N, Clark EA (1987) In vivo administration of anti-CD4 monoclonal antibody prolongs survival in long-tailed macaques with experimental encephalomyelitis. Clin Immunol Immunopathol 54:405–423

78. Pierson RN, Winn HJ, Russel PS, Auchincloss H (1989) CD4+ lymphocytes play a dominant role in murine xenograft rejection. Transplant Proc 21:518

79. Biddison WE, Rao PE, Talle MA, Goldstein G, Shaw S (1982) Possible involvement of the OKT4 molecule in T cell recognition of class-II HLA antigens. J Exp med 156:1065–1076
80. Hogg N (1989) The leukocyte integrins. Immunol Today 10:111–114
81. Coombe DR, Rider CC (1989) Lymphocyte homing receptors cloned – a role for anionic polysaccharides in lymphocate adhesion. Immunol Today 10:298–291
82. Steinmann L, Mantegazza R (1990) Prospects for specific immunotherapy in myasthenia gravis. FASEB J 4:2726–2731
83. Acha-Orbea H, Mitchell DJ, Timmermann L, Wraith DC, Tausch GS, Waldor MK, Zamvil SS, McDevitt HO, Steinman L (1988) Limited heterogeneity of T cell receptors from lymphocyte-mediating autoimmune encephalomyelitis allows specific immune intervention. Cell 54:263–273
84. Urban JL, Kumar V, Knoo DH, Gomez C, Horvath SJ, Clayton J, Ando DG, Sercarz EE, Hood L (1985) Restricted use of T cell receptor V genes in murine autoimmune encephalomyelitis raises possibilities for antibody therapy. Cell 54:577–592
85. Dayer JM, Demczuk S (1984) Cytokines and other mediators in rheumatoid arthritis. Springer Semin Immunopathol 7:387–413
86. Arend WP, Dayer JM (1990) Cytokines and cytokine inhibitors or antagonists in rheumatoid arthritis. Arthritis Rheum 33(3):305
87. Bendtzen K (1988) Interleukin 1, interleukin 6, and tumor necrosis factor in infection, inflammation and immunity. Immunol Lett 19:83–92
88. Alvardo-Gracia JM, Zwaifler NJ, Firestein GS (1989) Cytokines in chronic inflammatory arthritis. IV. Granulocyte/macrophage colony-stimulating factor-mediatd induction of class-II MHC antigen on human monocytes: a possible role in rheumatoid arthritis. J Exp Med 170:865–875
89. Yocum DE, Esparza L, Dubry S, Benjamin JB, Volz R, Schuder P (1989) Characteristics of tumor necrosis factor production in rheumatoid arthritis. Cell Immunol 122:131–145
90. Dayer JM, Seckingr P (1989) Natural inhibitors and antagonists of interleukin 1. In: Bomford RHR (ed) Inflammation and diseases. Amsterdam, Elsevier
91. Arend WP, Joslin FG, Thompson RC, Hannum CH (1989) An interleukin-1 inhibitor from human monocytes: production and characterization of biological properties. J Immunol 143:1851–1858
92. Larrick JW (1989) Native interleukin-1 inhibitors. Immunol Today 10:61–66
93. Lotz M, Carson DA (1989) Transforming factor β and cellular immune responses in synovial fluids (abstract). Arthritis Rheum 32 [Suppl 4]:S42
94. Lotz M, Tsoukas CD, Robinson CA, Dinarello CA, Carson DA, Vaughan JH (1986) Basis for defective responses of rheumatoid arthritis synovial fluid lymphocytes to anti-CD3 (T3) antibodies. J Clin Invest 78:713–721
95. Roux-Lombard P, Modou C, Dayer JM (1988) Inhibitors of IL-1 and TNF alpha activities in synovial fluids and cultured synovial fluid cell supernatants (abstract). Calcif Tissue Int 42:S(A47)
96. Prieur AM, Kaufmann M-T, Griscelli C, Dayer J-M (1987) Specific interleukin-1 inhibitor in serum and urine of children with systemic juvenile chronic arthritis. Lancet 2:1240–1242
97. Yocum DE, Esparza L, Dubry S, Benjamin JB, Volz R, Scuderi P (1989) Characteristics of tumor necrosis factor production in rheumatoid arthritis. Cell Immunol 122:131–145
98. Sklatvala J (1986) Tumor necrosis factor alpha stimulates resorption and inhibits synthesis of proteoglycan in cartilage. Nature 322:547–549
99. Dayer JM, Beutler B, Cerami A (1985) Cachectin/tumor necrosis factor stimulates collagenase and prostaglandin E_2 production by human synovial cells and dermal fibroblasts. J Exp Med162:2163–2168
100. Seckinger P, Isaaz S, Dayer J-M (1989) Purification and biologic characterization of a specific tumor necrosis factor alpha inhibitor. J Biol Chem 264:11966–11973
101. Henderson B, Pettipher ER (1989) Arthritogenic actions of recombinant IL-1 and tumor necrosis factor alpha in the rabbit: evidence for synergistic interactions between cytokines in vivo. Clin Exp Immunol 75:306–310

102. Firestein GS, Xu W-D, Townsend K, Broide D, Alvaro-Garcia J, Glasebrook A, Zvaifler NJ (1988) Cytokines in chronic inflammatory arthritis. I. Failure to detect T cell lymphokines (interleukin 2 and interleukin 3) and presence of macrophage colony-stimulating factor (CSF-1) and a novel mast cell growth factor in rheumatoid synovitis. J Exp Med 168:1573–1586

103. Kitas GD, Salmon M, Farr M, Gaston JSH, Bacon PA (1988) Deficient interleukin 2 production in rheumatoid arthritis: association with active disease and systemic complications. Clin Exp Immunol 73:242–249

104. Kashiwado T, Miossec P, Oppenheimer-Marks N, Ziff M (1987) Inhibitor of interleukin-2 synthesis and response in rheumatoid synovial fluid. Arthritis Rheum 30:1339–1347

105. Smith MD, Haynes DR, Roberts-Thomson PJ (1989) Interleukin 2 and interleukin-2 inhibitors in human serum and synovial fluid. I. Characterization of the inhibitor and its mechanism of action. J Rheumatol 16:149–157

106. Keystone EC, Snow KM, Bombardier C, Chasng C-H, Nelson DL, Rubin LA (1988) Elevated soluble interleukin-2 receptor levels in the sera and synovial fluids of patients with rheumatoid arthritis. Arthritis Rheum 31:96–97

107. Degré M, Mellbye OJ, Clarke-Jenssen O (1983) Immune interferon in serum and synovial fluid in rheumatoid arthritis and related disorders. Ann Rheum Dis 42:672–676

108. Husby G, Williams RC (1985) Immunohistochemical studies of interleukin-2 and alpha-interferon in rheumatoid arthritis. Arthritis Rheum 28:174–181

109. Gowen M, MacDonald BR, Russell GG (1988) Actions of recombinant human alpha-interferon and tumor necrosis factor alpha on the proliferation and osteoblastic characteristics of human trabecular bone cells in vitro. Arthritis Rheum 31:1500–1507

110. Lotz M, Tsoukas CD, Curd JG, Carson DA, Vaughan JH (1987) Effects of recombinant human interferons on rheumatoid arthritis B lymphocytes activated by Epstein-Barr virus. J Rheumatol 14:42–45

111. Lemmel EM, Brackertz D, Franke M, Gaus W, Hartl PW, Machalke K et al. (1988) Results of a multicenter placebo-controlled double-blind randomized phase-III clinical study of treatment of rheumatoid arthritis recombinant interferon-gamma. Rheumatol Int 8:87–93

112. Veys E, Mielants H, Verbruggen G, Grtosclaude JP, Merner M, Galazka A, Schindler J (1986) Interferon gamma in rheumatoid arthritis: a double-blind study comparing human recombinant interferon gamma with placebo. J Rheumatol 15:570–574

113. Cannon GW, Pincus SH, Emkey RD, Denes A et al. (1989) Double-blind trial of recombinant alpha-interferon versus placebo in the treatment of rheumatoid arthritis. Arthritis Rheum 32:9964–973

114. Sprekller R, Lemmel EM, Obert H-J (1990) Correlation of clinical and serological findings in patients with rheumatoid arthritis treated for one year with interferon-gamma. Z Rheumatol 49:1–7

115. Burman P, Karlsson FA, Öberg K, Alm G (1985) Autoimmune thyroid disease in interferon-treated patients. Lancet 2:100–101

116. Seitz M, Fanke M, Kirchner H (1988) Induction of antinuclear antibodies in patients with rheumatoid arthritis receiving treatment with human recombinant interferon gamma. Ann Rheum Dis 47:642–644

117. Machold KP, Smolen JS (1990) Interferon-gamma-induced exacerbation of systemic lupus erythematosus. J Rheumatol 17:831–832

118. Mauritz NJ, Holmdahl R, Johnsson R, van der Meide PH, Scheynius A, Klareskog L (1988) Treatment with gamma-interferon triggers the onset of collagen arthritis in mice. Arthritis Rheum 31:1297–1304

119. Burmester GR, Jahn B, Hain N, Kalden JR (1989) T-cell clones and T-cell regulation in relation to synovial inflammation. Springer Semin Immunopathology 11:259–272

120. Nagy ZA, Lehmann PV, Falcioni F, Muller S, Adorini L (1932) Why peptides? Their possible role in the evolution of MHC-restricted T cell recognition. Immunol Today 10:132–137

121. Wraith DC, Smilek DE, Mitchell DJ, Steinman L, McDevitt HO (1989) Antigen recognition in autoimmune encephalomyelitis and the potential for peptide-mediated immunotherapy. Cell 59:247–255
122. Sakai K, Mitchell DJ, Hodgkinson SJ, Zamvil SS, Rothbard JB, Steinman L (1989) Prevention of experimental encephalomyelitis with peptides blocking T-cell MHC interaction. Proc Natl Acad Sci USA 86:9470–9474
123. Urban J, Horwath S, Hood L (1989) Autoimmune T cells: immune recognition of normal and variant peptide epitopes and peptide-based therapy. Cell 59:257–271
124. Arnon R, Teitelbaum D, Sela M (1989) Suppression of experimental allergic encephalomyelitis by COP – relevance to multiple sclerosis. Isr J Med Sci 25:686–689
125. Teitelbaum D, Aharoni R, Aron R, Sela M (1988) Specific inhibition of the T cell response to myelin basic protein by the synthetic copolymer Cop 1. Proc Natl Acad Sci USA 85:9724–9728
126. Brocke S, Dayan M, Steinman L, Rothbard J, Mozes E (1990) Inhibition of T cell proliferation specific for AChR epitopes related to myasthenia gravis with antibody to T cell receptor or with competitive synthetic polymers. Int Immunol (in press)
127. Yang X-D, Gasser J, Feige U (1990) Prevention of adjuvant arthritis in rats by a nonapeptide from the 65-kD mycobacterial heat-shock protein. Clin Exp Immunol 81:189–194
128. Yang X-D, Gasser J, Riniker B, Feige U (1989) Treatment of rats with adjuvant arthritis with a synthetic peptide. Abstracts 7th international congress of immunology. Fischer, Stuttgart, p 878
129. Yang X-D, Gasser J, Riniker B, Feige U (1990) Treatment of adjuvant arthritis in rats: vaccination potential of a synthetic nonapeptide from the 65-kDa heat-shock protein of mycobacteria. J Autoimmunol 3:11
130. van Vollenhoven RF, Nagler-Anderson C, Soriano A, Siskind GW, Thorbecke GJ (1988) Tolerance induction by a poorly arthritogenic collagen II can prevent collagen-induced arthritis. Cell Immunol 115:146–155
131. Butler L, Simmons B, Zimmerman J, Deriso P, Phadke K, Hom J (1988) Regulation of cellular and humoral immune responses to collagen type I or collagen type II. Immunology 63:611–617
132. Olsnes S, Sandvig K, Petersen OW, van Deurs B (1989) Immunotoxins – entry into cells and mechanisms of action. Immunol Today 10:291–295
133. Worobec-Vitror SM (1989) Cutaneous T cell lymphoma. N Engl J Med 86:395–400
134. Wieselthier JS, Koh HK (1990) Sezary syndrome: diagnosis, prognosis, and critical review of treatment options. Transfusion 30:288
135. Wilfert H, Honigsmann H, Steiner G, Smolen J, Wolff K (1990) Treatment of psoriatic arthritis by extracorporeal photochemotherapy. Br J Dermatol 122:225–232
136. Torres MA, Furst DE (1990) Treatment of generalized systemic sclerosis. Rheum Dis Clin North Am 16:217–241

T-Cell Vaccination – A Prospect

F. C. Breedveld and R. R. P. de Vries[1]

From the Departments of Rheumatology and Immunohematology[1],
University Hospital, Leiden, The Netherlands

Introduction

T lymphocytes play an important role in the pathogenesis of a number of chronic diseases that have an autoimmune component, including rheumatoid arthritis (RA). This statement is based on the facts that the majority of inflammatory cells in the rheumatoid synovium are T cells [1, 2], that possible triggering antigens have been identified [3–5], that aberrant HLA class-II expression may be involved in the presentation of these antigens [6–8], and that T cells in the lesions may preferentially use certain T cell receptor genes [9, 10]. Novel strategies for immunotherapy of autoimmune diseases specifically directed against T cells have been developed in animal models; these are so promising that human clinical trials based on them have been started or are being considered. These strategies have in common that the intervention is targeted at the antigen presentation to or recognition by disease-inducing helper T cells. Immunologically, they may be divided into passive and active interventions. Passive interventions include the administration of antibodies at the T cell and the antigen-presenting MHC molecule or peptides that block the antigen-binding sites of MHC molecules. Basically, two strategies for active intervention have been explored: tolerance induction with the triggering or target antigen and down-regulation of the disease-inducing autoreactive T cells. Both from an immunological and from a logistic point of view active intervention is the most appropriate method for dealing with human autoimmune disease. Because in these diseases the triggering or target antigen is thus far unknown, we are focusing on exploring ways to actively down-regulate disease-inducing T cells. One of the least toxic and potentially most effective approaches to specific immunological intervention in the disease process appears to be one which has been termed "T-cell vaccination". T-cell vaccination may be defined as the administration of specifically autoimmune T cells, avirulent or attenuated, to prevent or to heal autoimmune disease. T cell vaccination has been shown to induce suppression mediated by T cells, but in this case the suppressor cells are anti-clono-typic or anti-idiotypic rather than

Smolen, Kalden, Maini (Eds.)
Rheumatoid Arthritis
© Springer-Verlag Berlin Heidelberg 1992

antigen specific. The aims of this article are to review the current status of T-cell vaccination in animal models and to describe the protocols used for T-cell vaccination in man.

Background

The isolation and in vitro growth of T lymphocytes that induce autoimmune diseases in rats and mice led to the understanding that autoimmune T-cell clones play a dominant role in disease models, including experimental autoimmune encephalomyelitis (EAE) [11, 12], experimental autoimmune thyroiditis (EAT) [13], adjuvant arthritis (AA) [14, 15] and collagen arthritis (CA) [16]. When lymph-node cells of rodents that were immunized with a disease-inducing antigen were cultured with that antigen, the T cells with antigen receptors that recognize the antigen proliferated. T-cell clones obtained in this way bore the CD4 surface marker and some were able to transfer the disease to untreated animals after intravenous inoculation. Relevant to the present communication is the observation that animals the recovered from the disease were found to have acquired resistance against further attempts to induce this disease [17, 18]. Furthermore, it was shown that disease-resistant rats continued to harbor potentially virulent T cells and yet remained healthy [13, 19]. The fact that the animals are asymptomatic carriers of potentially virulent autoimmune lymphocytes argues for the existence of some natural adjustment of the immune system. An ideal mode of therapy would be one that achieved such a control over a patient's virulent autoimmune T cells. If resistance to autoimmunity could be induced by contact with disease-inducing T cells, might such a resistance (in analogy with microbial vaccines) also be induced with attenuated T cells? The laboratory of Irun Cohen has initiated steps in the direction of this goal by employing lines and clones of autoimmune T lymphocytes to vaccinate animals against particular autoimmune diseases.

The first vaccination were done in EAE with T lymphocytes directed against myelin basic protein that had been rendered avirulent by irradiation [11, 12]. Rats receiving a single inoculation of T cells acquired after 1 week a marked resistance to EAE induced later by active immunization to myelin basic protein in complete Freund's adjuvant. Later studies showed that lymphocytes against thyroglobulin, *Mycobacterium tuberculosis,* and collagen type II vaccinate respectively against EAT, and CA [13, 16]. Besides the induction of resistance, T cell vaccination may also be applied as a form of therapy: a high percentage of rats suffering from these experimentally induced autoimmune diseases that received pretreated T lymphocyte raised from other rats underwent permanent remission of their autoimmune disease [20, 21].

Pretreatment of Lymphocytes Before Vaccination

Experimental evidence suggests that surface molecules of the T-lymphocyte vaccine induce resistance to disease by activating anti-T-cell immunity [22–24]. Therefore, several strategies were explored that augment the immunogenicity of cells. Ten thousand activated anti-myelin basic protein T cells vaccinate with greater effectiveness than 50 million inactivated T cells of the same clone. This suggests that the signal for vaccination must include an element induced by activation of the T cell [25]. Research on tumor cells had shown that pressure treatment was effective in enhancing the immunogenicity of tumor-associated through rearrangement of their membrane proteins [26]. In analogy with this observation, it was demonstrated that the capacity of activated T cells to vaccinate is markedly enhanced by treating the T cells with hydrostatic pressure or chemical cross-linkers such as formaldehyde or glutaraldehyde. Examination of the cell surface using a fluorescent antibody assay indeed indicated that pretreatment produced permanent aggregation of lymphocyte surface MHC-I and Thy-1 and -2 antigens [26]. Once the cells had been pretreated, isolated membranes from these cells were also able to vaccinate effectively. This suggests that the signals required for induction of protective immunity appear to be composed of the antigen receptor, factors related to the state of activation of the T cells, and aggregation of certain cell membrane molecules.

Mechanisms of Vaccination

Pressure-treated or fixed T lymphocytes are nonresponsive or dead, and it is not likely that they participate actively in the process of resistance. Vaccination is therefore probably accomplished by the response of the recipient to the rearranged membrane antigens of the inoculated T lymphocytes. Experiments designed to test the specificity of T-cell vaccination showed that vaccination induced specific suppression of one particular disease. Rats vaccinated with myelin basic protein-reactive T cells gained protection against EAE but not against AA; conversely, T cells reactive to arthritogenic antigens protected rats against AA but not against EAE [22, 23]. These experiments implicate an anti-clonotypic mechanism in disease resistance conferred to rats by-T cell vaccination. Lohse et al. have recently shown that T cells induced by vaccinating rats with activated syngeneic T-cell clones lacking receptors for myelin basic protein might also be potent suppressors of EAE [27]. These T cells, which have been termed "anti-ergotypic", are induced by other activated, syngeneic T cells and are not idiotype specific. The anti-ergotypic disease protection seemed to be transient compared with the anti-clonotyic response. These observations are compatible with the idea that resistance to autoimmunity induced by T-cell vaccination involves anti-idiotypic immunity, but such immunity should not be termed "anti-idiotypic" until it is proven that the marker recognized by T cells is indeed the antigen receptor of the target T cell. Other studies showed that vaccinated rats developed T cells that proliferated with the autoimmune T cells used for vaccination. The responding T cells were able to distinguish between T-cell clones with different specificity, which suggests that vaccinated rhodents possess anti-clonotypic T cells [24]. The role of T cells in the maintenance of resistance was further demonstrated by experiments that transferred resistance to a particular autoimmune disease from vaccinated rats to immunologically naive syngeneic rats by injection of T cells directed against the vaccine [28]. Vaccination with anti-myelin basic protein T cells generated anti-vaccine T cells in the regional lymph-node. Transfer of T cells isolated from the regional lymph-nodes to naive rats transferred resistance to EAE [21].

The identity of anti-clonotypic or anti-ergotypic T cells generated by T-cell vaccination, the signals that activate them, and the mechanisms of resistance induction remain to be determined. After vaccination, anti-clonotypic T cells of both the CD4 and CD8 phenotype can be isolated. The laboratory of Wekerle has shown that CD8 anti-clonotypic T cells can protect rats against EAE [29]. The anti-clonotypic T cells are cytotoxic in vitro, and destruction of idiotypic T cells may be a factor in resistance to the disease. However, virulent autoimmune T cells are able to persist in disease-resistant rats, which suggests that the immune system employs mechanisms that suppress but do not kill autoreactive T cells.

To further investigate how T-cell vaccination interacts with the immune system to affect the natural course of events, the regulatory mechanisms set in motion by the autoimmune disease itself were analyzed. Nathan Karin (Weizmann Institute) showed in AA that as early as 2 days after immunization with *Mycobacterium tuberculosis* the rats demonstrated antigen-specific suppressor cells in the spleen [30]. Another response detected before the appearance of arthritis was a specific T cell proliferative reaction to a mycobacterium-reactive T-cell line available in the laboratory. This anti-clonotypic response was detectable before T-cell responses to *M. tuberculosis* could be measured. These experiments provided a baseline for analyzing the effect of T-cell vaccination on the immunology of AA. Rats were vaccinated with pretreated mycobacterium-reactive T cells, and 1 month later they and nonvaccinated control rats were immunized with *M. tuberculosis* to induce AA. Two effects were observed: First, the vaccinated rats showed an earlier but much abbreviated response to mycobacterial antigens compared with the nonvaccinated rats who developed AA. The second effect of T-cell vaccination was that both antigen-specific and -nonspecific suppressor cells were undetectable. T-cell vaccination thus accelerated the kinetics of the antimycobacterial response and abolished conventional cells while activating anti-idiotypic T cells and inhibiting arthritis. The findings that the mycobacterial antigen induces a T-cell response to an anti-mycobacterial T cell and that vaccination with an anti-mycobacterial T cell accelerates the anti-idiotypic T cell response indicate the existence of a functional network relating mycobacterial antigens with anti-antimycobacterial antigens at the T-cell level. These observations may explain why T-cell vaccination is effective; it may both use and strengthen the idiotypic network that nature may have provided herself to prevent or control autoimmune diseases.

Experience in Patients

Irun Cohen took the initiative and organized an international workshop on T-cell vaccination for the treatment of autoimmune diseases. The workshop was convened to review the use of autoimmune T cells as vaccines to prevent and treat autoimmune diseases of laboratory animals and to assess the prospects for application of similar strategies to treat human autoimmune diseases. Stimulated by the promising results in experimental animals, Howard Weiner and David Hafler of Harvard Mecial School started a phase-I trial of T-cell vaccination in multiple sclerosis (MS) [31]. The effectiveness of T-cell vaccination in the various animal models was felt to justify embarking on this approach in incurable conditions such MS. Since current therapies involve nonspecific immunosuppression with potentially toxic regimens, nontoxic immunospecific therapies need to be explored. Because the T-cell vaccination in MS did not seem to produce unwanted side effects, other centers decided it was time to start a phase-I trial in RA patients. RA seemed to be an appropriate disease for this treatment modality because T cells are thought to play an important role in the pathogenesis, and T cells are easily obtainable from the site of inflammation. Furthermore, clinical studies that selectively suppress T-cell function, such as thoracic duct drainage [32], lymphapheresis [33], total lymph-node irradiation [34], or anti-T-cell antibody administration [35, 36], have ameliorated disease activity.

A major obstacle to the use of T-cell vaccination for treatment of human diseases is the need for antigen-specific T cells to prepare efficient vaccines. In many clinical autoimmune diseases in which cell-mediated immunity is implicated, the target self-antigen is unknown, and this rules out the possibility of specifically activating patient T cells to prepare a vaccine. An attempt to solve the problem was made by Felix Mor (Weizmann Institute), whose goal was to activate antigen-specific T cells without using specific antigen [37]. It was reasoned that T cells actively involved in an autoimmune disease might be in a state of differentiation that would distinguish them from naive, resting T cells. His strategy was to study animal models such as EAE or AA in which the specific antigen (BP or mycobacterial antigen) was known, and to test whether cells specific for the antigen could be isolated from diseased rats using nonspecific stimulators. (The particular antigen was used to monitor to what degree the specific T cells had been selected nonspecifically). They failed to obtain anti-BP or anti-mycobacterial T cells using IL-2 as a nonspecific stimulus. However, activation with concanavalin A for 48 h, followed by a period of rest for 5 days in medium containing IL-2, appeared to activate and expand antigen-specific T-cell clones. Frequencies of antigen-specific cells increased from 1:1000 to 1:25 following nonspecific activation with Con A.

Accordingly, concanavalin A was exploited to prepare a therapeutic vaccine from rats suffering from established adjuvant arthritis in order to model vaccine preparation based on the clinical situation [37]. Lymph-node cells from rats with adjuvant arthritis were activated with concanavalin A, cross-linked with glutaraldehyde, and administered to other, equally sick rats. Within 1 week of treatment, the rats went into permanent remission. Irradiated cells did not vaccinate. Thus, it was not necessary to isolate purified lines of autoimmune T lymphocytes, and vaccination was achieved with cells taken directly from the subject.

In MS patients the T-cell vaccine was prepared from the patients' own cerebrospinal fluid, where there is a mild pleocytosis consisting of greater than 90% T cells. T-cell clones were grown using a single cell methodology with autologous serum, feeder cells, PHA, and IL-2. Cells from several separate clones with the CD4 phenotype were combined and stimulated with PHA prior to vaccination. After stimulation and pretreatment of the cells with formaldehyde, the patients were inoculated with 50×10^6 autologous T cells subcutaneously and received similar booster inoculations at monthly intervals.

In RA patients the T-cell vaccine was prepared from the patients' synovial fluid or synovial tissue. Here, the first choice of T cells for preparaton of the vaccine were clones with specific antigen reactivity. Since T-cell reactivity to mycobacterial antigens was significantly more prominent in synovial fluid than in peripheral blood T cells of RA patients, T-cell clones were grown using an acetone precipitate of *M. tuberculosis* as antigen stimulation [4]. In the absence of mycobacterial reactivity of synovial T cells, clones were prepared using autologous serum and feeder cells, IL-2, and anti-CD3 monoclonal antibodies, and cross-linking was performed with formaldehyde. The vaccination procedure and the immunologic monitoring are essentially similar in the protocols for MS and RA patients. The first results were presented in the "Workshop on T-cell vaccination" held in April 1990 in Amsterdam, during the first meeting of the EEG-sponsored Concerted Action on "Immunopathogenesis and Immunotherapy of Chronic Arthritis." The data obtained in the two trials were similar. Clinically, the most important conclusion was that the procedure did not seem to be toxic. The number of patients studied and the duration of follow-up were too limited for any conclusions to be drawn about the therapeutic effect. Immunologically, T-cell vaccination induced an specific suppression of T-cell proliferation. Within 3 days after vaccination there was a marked decrease in PHA-induced proliferation of circulating T cells which lasted for more than 2 months. The ability of circulating T cells to proliferate to the T-cell clones inoculated into the patients was also investigated. In most patients an increase of peripheral blood T-cell proliferation against autologous clones was observed, but it was not directly evident that this reaction was clonotype specific. There were no pronounced changes in CD4, CD8, or CD2 T cells in peripheral blood following vaccination.

The mechanism of the decreased nonspecific proliferation and the biological significance of the T-T interactions remain to be determined, and many other questions have to be answered. T-cell vaccination is not at all an easy procedure, and we are therefore fortunate that all pioneer centers work in close collaboration and contact. Reagents will be exchanged and different protocols for expanding T cells will be used and compared. Some groups will continue to use clones for vaccine preparation, whereas others have started to use T-cell lines. However, a great deal of experimental work is still necessary, and natural T-cell networks must be studied in relation to disease activity in order to delineate the significance of T-cell vaccination in human diseases. Because the T-cell receptor is the most probable target for this type of therapy, it may be possible in the near future to use T-cell receptor peptides instead of T cells as immunotherapy and for the prevention of human autoimmune diseases [38, 39].

Acknowledgement. The authors thank Prof. Dr. I. R. Cohen for reviewing the manuscript.

References

1. Van Boxel JA, Paget SA (1975) Predominantly T-cell infiltrate in rheumatoid synovial membranes. N Engl J Med 293:517–520
2. Klareskog L, Forsum U, Scheynius A, Kablitz D, Wigzell H (1982) Evidence in support of a self-perpetuating HLA-DR-dependent delayed-type cell reaction in rheumatoid arthritis. Proc Natl Acad Sci USA 79:3632–3636
3. Holoshitz J, Drucker I, Yaretzky A, van Eden W, Klajman A, Lapidot Z, Frenkel A, Cohen IR (1986) T lymphocytes of rheumatoid arthritis patients show augmented reactivity to a fraction of mycobacteria cross-reactive with cartilage. Lancet 2:305–309
4. Res PC, Breedveld FC, van Embden JDA, Schaar CG, van Eden W, Cohen IR, de Vries RRP (1988) Synovial fluid T-cell reactivity against 65-kD heat shock protein of mycobacteria in early chronic arthritis. Lancet 2:478–480
5. Londei M, Savill CM, Verhoef A, Brennan F, Leeck ZA, Duance V, Maini RU, Feldman M (1989) Persistence of collagen type II-specific T-cell clones in the synovial membrane of a patient with rheumatoid arthritis. Proc Natl Acad Sci USA 86:636–640
6. Bottazzo GF, Pujol-Borrell P, Hanafusa T, Feldmann M (1983) Role of aberrant HLA-DR expression and antigen presentation in induction of endocrine autoimmunity. Lancet 2:1115–1118
7. Burmester GR, Jahn B, Gramatzki M, Zacher J, Kalden JR (1984) Activate T-cells in vivo and in vitro: divergence in expression of Tacand Ia antigens in the nonblastoid small T-cells of inflammation and normal T-cells activated in vitro. J Immunol 133:1230–1234
8. Teyton L, Lotteau V, Turmel P, Arenzana-Seisdedos F, Virelizier JL, Pujol JP, Loyau G, Piatier-Tonneau D, Auffray C, Charron DJ (1987) HLA-DR, DQ and DP antigen expression in rheumatoid synovial cells: a biochemical and quantitative study. J Immunol 138:1730–1738
9. Savill CM, Delves PJ, Kioussis D, Walker P, Lydyard PM, Colaco B, Shipley M, Roit IM (1987) A minority of patients with rheumatoid arthritis shown a dominant rearrangement of T-cell receptor β chain genes in synovial lymphocytes. Scand J Immunol 25:629–235
10. Stamenkovic I, Stegagno M, Wright KA, Krane SM, Amento EP, Colvin RB, Duquesnoy RJ, Kurnick JT (1988) Clonal dominance among T-lymphocyte infiltrates in arthritis. Proc Natl Acad Sci USA 85:1179–1183
11. Ben-Nun A, Wekerle H, Cohen IR (1981) The rapid isolation of clonable antigen-specific T lymphocyte lines capable of mediating autoimmune encephalomyelitis. Eur J Immunol 11:195–199

12. Ben-Nun A, Cohen IR (1983) Experimental autoimmune encephalomyelitis (EAE) medicated by T cell lines: Process of selection of lines and characterization of the cells. J Immunol 129:303–308
13. Maron R, Zerubavel R, Friedman A, Cohen IR (1983) T lymphocyte line specific for thyroglobulin produces or vaccinates against autoimmune thyroiditis in mice. J Immunol 131:2316–2322
14. Holoshitz J, Naparstek Y, Ben-Nun A, Cohen IR (1983) Lines of T lymphocytes induce or vaccinate against autoimmune arthritis. Science 219:56–58
15. Holoshitz J, Matitiau A, Cohen IR (1984) Arthritis induced in rats by cloned T lymphocytes responsive to mycobacteria, but not to collagen type II. J Clin Invest 73:211–215
16. Kakimoto K, Katsuki M, Hirofuji T, Iwata H, Koga T (1988) Isolation of a T cell line capable of protecting mice against collagen-induced arthritis. J Immunol 140:78–83
17. Cohen IR (1988) The self, the world and autoimmunity. Sci Am 258:34–43
18. Svet-Moldavsk GJ, Svet-Moldavskaya IA, Raffkina LI (1959) Various types of acquired resistance to exprimental allergic encephalomyelitis. Nature 184:1552–1559
19. Ben-Nun A, Cohen IR (1982) Spontaneous remission and acquired resistance to autoimmune encephalomyelitis (EAE) are associated with suppression of T cell reactivity: suppressed EAE effector T cells recovered as T-cell lines. J Immunol 128:1450–1457
20. Lider O, Karin N, Shinitriky M, Cohen IR (1984) Therapeutic vaccination against adjuvant arthritis using autoimmune T cells treated with hydrostatic pressure. Proc Natl Acad Sci USA 84:4577–4580
21. Cohen IR, Holoshitz J, van Eden W, Frenkel A (1985) T lymphocyte clones illuminate pathogenesis and effect therapy of experimental arthritis. Arthritis Rheum 28:841–845
22. Lider O, Reshef T, Beraud E, Ben-Nun A (1988) Anti-idiotypic network induced by T cell vaccination against experimental allergic encephalomyelitis. Science 239:181–183
23. Lider O, Beraud E, Reshef T, Friedman A, Cohen IR (1989) Vaccination against experimental autoimmune encephalomyelitis using a subencephalitogenic dose of autoimmune effector T cells. 2. Induction of a protective anti-idiotypic response. J Autoimmun 2:87–99
24. Holoshitz J, Frenkel A, Ben-Nun A, Cohen IR (1983) Autoimmune EAE mediated or prevented in T lymphocyte lines as directed against diverse antigenic determinants of myelin basic protein. Vaccination is determinant specific. J Immunol 131:2810–2813
25. Naparstek Y, Ben-Nun A, Holoshitz J, Reshef T, Frenkel A, Rosenberg M, Cohen IR (1983) T lymphocyte lines producing or vaccinating against autoimmune encephalomyelitis. Eur J Immunol 13:418–423
26. Lider O, Shinitzky M, Cohen IR (1986) Vaccination against experimental autoimmune disease using T lymphocytes treated with hydrostatic pressure. Am NY Acad Sci 475:267–273
27. Lohse AW, Mor F, Karin N, Cohen IR (1989) Control of experimental autoimmune encephalomyelitis by T cells responding to activated T cells. Science 244:820–822
28. Holoshitz J, Matitiau A, Cohen IR (1985) Role of thymus in induction and transfer of vaccination against adjuvant arthritis with a T lymphocyte line in rats. J Clin Invest 75:472–477
29. Sun D, Qin Y, Chluba J, Epplen JT, Wekerle H (1988) Supression of experimentally induced autoimmune encephalomyelitis by cytolytic T-T cell interactions. Nature 332:843–845
30. Cohen IR (1990) T cell vaccination and suppression in autoimmune disease. Prog Immunol 7:867–873
31. Cohen IR, Weiner HL (1988) T cell vaccination. Immunol Today 9:332–334
32. Paulus HE, Mackleder HI, Levine S, Yu DTY, Macdonald NS (1977) Lymphocyte involvement in rheumatoid arthritis studies during thoracic duct drainage. Arthritis Rheum 20:1249–1262
33. Karsh J, Klippel SH, Plotz PH, Decker JL, Wright DR, Flye MW (1981) Lymphapheresis in rheumatoid arthritis: a randomized trial. Arthritis Rheum 24:867–873

34. Brahn E, Helfgott SM, Belli JA, Anderson RJ, Reinherz EL, Schlossmann SF, Austen KF, Trentham DE (1984) Total lymphoid irradiation therapy of refractory rheumatoid arthritis: fifteen- to forty-month follow-up. Arthritis Rheum 27:481–488
35. Shmerling RH, Trentham DE (1989) Effect of anti-thymocyte globulin on refractory rheumatoid arthritis. Arthritis Rheum 32:[Suppl] R7
36. Herzog C, Walker C, Muller W, Rieber P, Reiter C, Riethmuller G, Wassmer P, Stockinger H, Madic O, Pichler WJ (1989) Anti-CD4 antibody treatment of patients with rheumatoid arthritis. I. Effect on clinical course and circulating T cells. J Autoimmun 2:627–642
37. Mor F, Lohse AW, Karin N, Cohen IR (1990) Clinical modeling of T cell vaccination against autoimmune disease in rats: selection of antigen-specific T cells using a mitogen. J Clin Invest 85:1594–1637
38. Acha Orbea H, Mitchell DJ, Timmermann L, Wraith DC, Tausch GS, Walder MK, Zamvil SS, McDevitt HO, Steinman L (1988) Limited heterogeneity of T cell receptors from lymphocytes mediating autoimmune encephalomyelitis allows specific immune intervention. Cell 54:263–273
39. Vandenbark AA, Hashim G, Offner H (1989) Immunization with a synthetic T-cell receptor V-region peptide protects against experimental autoimmune encephalomyelitis. Nature 341:541–544

Printing: Druckerei Kutschbach, Berlin
Binding: Buchbinderei Lüderitz & Bauer, Berlin